AF750185

UPDATE ON AMYOTROPHIC LATERAL SCLEROSIS

Edited by **Humberto Foyaca Sibat**
and **Lourdes de Fatima Ibañez Valdés**

Update on Amyotrophic Lateral Sclerosis
http://dx.doi.org/10.5772/61682
Edited by Humberto Foyaca Sibat and Lourdes de Fatima Ibañez Valdés

Contributors
Sebastiano Cavallaro, Giovanna Morello, Francesca Luisa Conforti, Antonio Gianmaria Spampinato, Maria Teresa Gonzalez Garza, Luca Diamanti, Elisabetta Zucchi, Orietta Pansarasa, Mauro Ceroni, Cristina Cereda, Boguslaw Machalinski, Anna Sobuś, Bernard Schneider, Nathalie Bernard-Marissal, Cylia Rochat, Yves Lecarpentier, Alexandre Vallée, Utpal Bhadra, Joel Eyer, Philippe Codron, Julien Cassereau, Franck Letournel, Toshiyuki Araki, Seiichi Nagano, Philip Van Damme, Bart Swinnen, Koen Van Laere, Oxana Galzitskaya, Alexander Chervyakov, Ilya Bakulin, Natalia Suponeva, Maria Zakharova, Michael Piradov, Humberto Foyaca Sibat

Published by InTech
Janeza Trdine 9, 51000 Rijeka, Croatia

© The Editor(s) and the Author(s) 2016
The moral rights of the editor(s) and the author(s) have been asserted.
All rights to the book as a whole are reserved by InTech. The book as a whole (compilation) cannot be reproduced, distributed or used for commercial or non-commercial purposes without InTech's written permission. Enquiries concerning the use of the book should be directed to InTech's rights and permissions department (permissions@intechopen.com).
Violations are liable to prosecution under the governing Copyright Law.

Individual chapters of this publication are distributed under the terms of the Creative Commons Attribution 3.0 Unported License which permits commercial use, distribution and reproduction of the individual chapters, provided the original author(s) and source publication are appropriately acknowledged. More details and guidelines concerning content reuse and adaptation can be found at http://www.intechopen.com/copyright-policy.html.

Notice
Statements and opinions expressed in the chapters are these of the individual contributors and not necessarily those of the editors or publisher. No responsibility is accepted for the accuracy of information contained in the published chapters. The publisher assumes no responsibility for any damage or injury to persons or property arising out of the use of any materials, instructions, methods or ideas contained in the book.

Publishing Process Manager Romina Rovan
Technical Editor SPi Global
Cover InTech Design team

First published September, 2016
Printed in Croatia

Additional hard copies can be obtained from orders@intechopen.com

Update on Amyotrophic Lateral Sclerosis, Edited by Humberto Foyaca Sibat and Lourdes de Fatima Ibañez Valdés
p. cm.
Print ISBN 978-953-51-2600-3
Online ISBN 978-953-51-2601-0

We are IntechOpen, the world's leading publisher of Open Access books

Built by scientists, for scientists

3,700+
Open access books available

116,000+
International authors and editors

119M+
Downloads

151
Countries delivered to

Our authors are among the
Top 1%
most cited scientists

12.2%
Contributors from top 500 universities

CLARIVATE ANALYTICS BOOK CITATION INDEX INDEXED

WEB OF SCIENCE™

Selection of our books indexed in the Book Citation Index
in Web of Science™ Core Collection (BKCI)

Interested in publishing with us?
Contact book.department@intechopen.com

Numbers displayed above are based on latest data collected.
For more information visit www.intechopen.com

For EU product safety concerns:
IN TECH d.o.o., Prolaz Marije Krucifikse Kozulić 3, 51000 Rijeka, Croatia,
info@intechopen.com or visit our website at intechopen.com.

Meet the editors

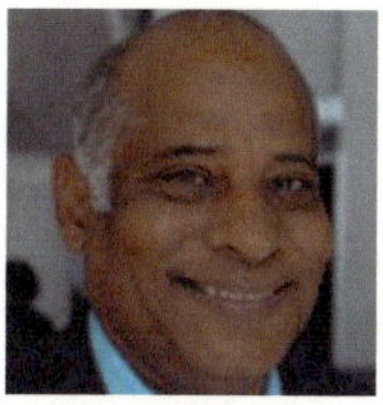

Professor Humberto Foyaca Sibat was born on May 03, 1948 in Havana City, Republic of Cuba. He graduated as a Medical Doctor in Havana University in 1971. He became specialist in neurology in 1975 and higher level specialist in 1984. Currently Dr. Foyaca has been an Associate Professor at Faculty of Health Sciences of Walter Sisulu University for more than 14 years, he is also Master in Sciences and Associate Investigator of Cuban Academy of Sciences and head of department of neurology at the Nelson Mandela Central Hospital in Mthatha since 1997. Dr. Foyaca is a member of 15 Medical Societies from all over the world; he presented more than 360 papers in different scientific events, published more than 70 manuscripts in peer-review journals and edited 3 books before this one. Since 1992 he is the Chief-Editor of The Internet Journal of Neurology, currently the largest electronic journal of neurology worldwide. He received and delivered many short training courses and organized many National and International conferences.

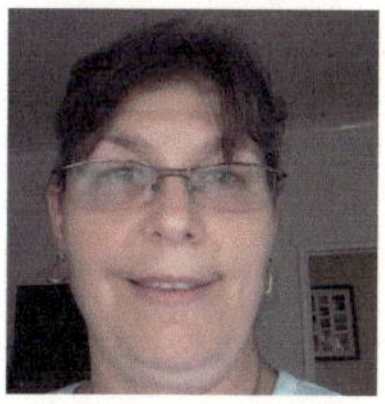

Dr. Lurdes de Fatima Ibañez Valdés, born on October 13, 1963, in Havana City, Cuba, graduated as a Medical Doctor from Havana University in 1998. She is a specialist in family medicine, holds an MSc degree, and is an aggregated scientist researcher working for the Department of Neurology at the Nelson Mandela Central Hospital in Mthatha, Eastern Cape Province, South Africa, where she is head of Epilepsy, NCC, and Neurodegenerative Clinic; she has presented more than 60 papers in National and International Medical Conferences and published 6 chapters in text books and more than 40 articles in peer-reviewed journals. She is a member of 10 medical societies worldwide.

Contents

Preface

Amyotrophic Lateral Sclerosis (ALS) causes a progressive loss of structure and function of neurons in the cerebral cortex, brainstem and the spinal cord. Usually the loss of specific functions precedes the death of affected neurons, and the related clinical features depend on localization and the degree of neurodegeneration. ALS is also related to mitochondrial dysfunctions, increased oxidative stress and atypical protein assemblies and continues being a serious health problem leading to death in a few years' time in most of the cases. Before death, patients suffer from weakness or paralysis, muscle atrophy, fasciculation, dysphagia, dysarthria, and other complications.

The introductory chapter presents, summarised, information about the progress made in ALS and published by InTech.

The information will be grouped by topics and countries in two graphics.

The number of publications written about ALS increased remarkably over the past four years. With new information consistently being presented regarding this disease, it is our hope that the information in this book is a representation of novel research to benefit the readership community and our patients. In this book, readers will find a compilation of state-of-the-art reviews about pathogenesis, aetiology, therapeutic, investigations, the molecular basis of disease progression and clinical manifestations, and the genetics familial ALS, as well as novel diagnostic criteria in the field of imagenology.

Update on Amyotrophic Lateral Sclerosis is comprised of 13 chapters from some of the world's top central nervous system researchers and neurologists to provide a timely review of the most recent developments in ALS, covering historic aspects, experimental animal models, genetics, pathogenesis, clinical aspects and imagenology among others. Contributors from Belgium, France, Japan, India, Italy, Mexico, Russia, South Africa, and Switzerland have collaborated enthusiastically and efficiently, dedicating their time to create this reader-friendly yet comprehensive work which includes many explanatory figures, tables and photos to enhance legibility and make the book clinically useful.

It is important to highlight that a lot of effort has been made to ensure the relevance of this book. After the initial review process, all chapters were peer reviewed at least two more times before final acceptance for publication. This was done in effort to ensure that the most novel information was provided to readers and researchers. We all attempted to bring in valuable updated information for all issues/topics mentioned in this book.

First of all, we would like to thanks InTech Open Access Publisher that unconditionally supported us in editing this book. Our families who supported us during this process. My Mom, Dad and my first daughter Zayra Susana, from heaven, who continue to inspire me.

My daughters Lorna Maria (32 years old) and Fatima Susana Adolfina (7 years old) who encouraged me all the time to continue moving forward with persistence. My son Thabo Humberto Jorge (8 years old) who pushed me to play physics games with him which helped me to relax and to find new ideas. My whole family contributed to this project in one way or another and they deserve our deep gratitude. I also want to thank the families, relatives, and friends of all contributors for their support. Special thanks to Walter Sisulu University (WSU), named in honour of an icon of the South Africa liberation struggle and close comrade of Nelson Mandela, the late Walter Max Ulyate Sisulu. Many thanks to Dr. EN Cishe: Acting Director Research Development of WSU, Dr. WW Chita: Dean of the Faculty of Health Sciences (WSU), Prof. A Awotedu: Head of Department of General Medicine and Therapeutic, Dr. M Mdledle: Acting Governor General Director: Clinical Governance of Nelson Mandela Central Hospital and Mrs. NP Makwedeni: Chief Executive Officer of Nelson Mandela Central Hospital for the best understanding and support. At the end, I extend my deepest sense of appreciation for the support received by Dr. Roberto Morales Ojeda: Minister of Public Health of Cuba and Dr. Jorge Delgado Bustillo: Deputy Head of the National Unit for International Cooperation in Health.

Prof. H Foyaca Sibat. MD, PhD, MSc,
First and Second Degree Specialist in Neurology
Full Scientist Research
Head of Department of Neurology
Nelson Mandela Central Hospital, Faculty of Health Sciences, WSU
Mthatha, South Africa

Dr. Lurdes de Fatima Ibañez Valdés. MD, MSc, Family Physician
Aggregate Scientist Research
Department of Neurology, Nelson Mandela Central
Hospital. Walter Sisulu University. Mthatha, South Africa.

Chapter 1

Introductory Chapter: Introduction to Update in Amyotrophic Lateral Sclerosis and Review of this Condition in Sportsmen

Humberto Foyaca-Sibat and
Lourdes de Fátima Ibañez-Valdés

Additional information is available at the end of the chapter

http://dx.doi.org/ 10.5772/64608

1. Introduction

Amyotrophic lateral sclerosis (ALS) is a progressive and almost invariably fatal neurodegenerative disease that affects motor neurons cell in the cerebral hemispheres, brainstem, and the spinal cord. The disease begins focally in the central nervous system and then spreads relentlessly. This disorder of the upper and lower motor neurons (also known as Motor Neuron Disease) can be confirmed by electromyography and is characterised by a progressive muscle weakness, spastic hypertonia, hyperreflexia, muscle wasting, dysphagia, disarthria and fasciculations in most of the patients. Less than 10% of the patients have a hereditary pattern. Mostly, ALS does not affect sphincters, sexual functions, or eyes movements. There are two well-recognised varieties: sporadic (SALS) and familial (FALS).

1.1. Recent updated information

To update knowledge about ALS, it is important to bring new information which are as follows: the FALS accounts for 5% of all ALS; an underlying mutation has been identified in approximately a third of these cases [1] and it is important to perform a screening of four principal genes (SOD1, TARDBP, FUS, C9ORF) because they cover more than 50% of FALS [2]. A recent meta-analysis of population-based studies also confirmed that 5% of ALS cases are FALS and the remaining 95% are SALS with no reported family history [3]. Both share common pathogenic mechanisms and the disease has an incidence of 2.7 cases per 100,000 people in Europe [4] and at the present moment straightforward and classical cure for ALS are not available.

INTECH
open science | open minds

© 2016 The Author(s). Licensee InTech. This chapter is distributed under the terms of the Creative Commons Attribution License (http://creativecommons.org/licenses/by/3.0), which permits unrestricted use, distribution, and reproduction in any medium, provided the original work is properly cited.

We cannot ignore the history and therefore should be mentioned that ALS is recognised back in 1850 by a British neurophysiologist Augustus Waller for the appearance of shrivelled nerve fibres and identified as a specific disease. Later, this pathological process was named and described as ALS by a French neurologist Jean-Martin Charcot. He was also a professor of anatomical pathology and is known as 'the founder of modern neurology', his name has been associated with at least 15 medical eponyms, such as: Charcot-Marie-Tooth disease, Charcot's artery (lenticulostriate artery), Charcot's joint (diabetic arthropathy), Charcot-Wilbrand syndrome (visual agnosia and loss of ability to revisualise images), Charcot-Bouchard aneurysms (tiny aneurysms of the penetrating branches of middle cerebral artery in hypertensives) and Charcot disease (better known as amyotrophic lateral sclerosis or motor neurone disease), among others. His work greatly influenced the developing fields of neurology and psychology; modern psychiatry owes much to the work of Charcot and his direct followers. He was the 'foremost neurologist of late nineteenth-century France' [5].

However, ALS was not well known until 1939 when a famous American baseball first baseman player Lou Gehrig brought national and international attention to his disease. After Lou Gehrig died, a big number of sportsman have been diagnosed with ALS or Lou Gehrig's disease, and based on their experiences a lot of knowledge about the disease have been accumulated. Most patients are diagnosed with ALS between the ages of 40-70, but the disease can also develop in younger people. The average age for an ALS diagnosis is 56. Approximately 30,000 Americans have the disease at any given time and most of them will die within 3-5 years from the beginning of the disease, although we will mention some people that are still alive. It affects people throughout the world without any racial, ethnic or socioeconomic boundaries but males are more prone to ALS. Fifty percent of affected patients live at least 3 or more years after diagnosis; 20% live 5 years or more; and up to 10% will survive more than 10 years [6]. More information is available online: http://www.hopkinsmedicine.org/neurology_neurosurgery/centers_clinics/als/conditions/als_ amyotrophic_lateral_sclerosis.html.

In our series of patients, complaints about visual disturbances, ophthalmoplegia, auditory disorders, vestibular dysfunction, olfactory problems, sensory loss or disorder of the autonomic nervous system related to ALS were not identified, although in late stages of the disease patients may develop a supranuclear gaze palsy or oculomotor palsy [7, 8], as anecdotic cases.

However, cognitive impairment can be seen in nearly a third of the patients with ALS in a pattern consistent with frontotemporal lobar dementia as has been proved [9]. These findings were also reported by many other authors [10–20]. Executive function, behaviour and speech are the most likely areas to be involved. Screening helpful in detecting abnormalities includes verbal or categorical fluency, behavioural inventories filled out by the caregiver and evaluation for the presence of depression and pseudo-bulbar signs [21]. Patients with ALS may have difficulty interpreting the emotions associated with facial expressions, even when they are otherwise cognitively normal; this may impact their relationships with their caregiver and possibly influence medical decision making [22]. In our opinion, this manifestation may occur even without confirmed lesion at the insular lobe and without insular lobe epilepsy. However, we have patients presenting ALS without cognitive disorder and very high intelligence coefficient level.

Unfortunately, due to reasons beyond our control no abstracts related to the therapy of ALS (which is not a single disease) is received. Therefore, we will mention some important aspects related to the therapy of ALS.

At the beginning of this year (29 January 2016), the following information is released: 'Results in a new mouse model of ALS indicate that delivering copper to the central nervous system can be therapeutic, according to a study published in the journal Neurobiology of Disease', and we all became very enthusiastic until Dr. Bruijn (Ph.D., M.B.A., Chief Scientist for The ALS Association) said: 'But in the meantime, it is critical to remember that oral copper supplements do not reach the central nervous system and thus cannot provide any benefit and can be quite toxic' (http://www.alsa.org/news/archive/new-copper-therapy.html), just to remind everyone that all results from animals cannot be applied to our patients. However, last year we were informed about Progress in Drug Development Reviewed at The ALS Association Drug Company Working Group Meeting (5 May 2015), where news about a new drug, a new delivery method, a new trial and a new approach to working with the Food and Drug Administration (FDA) were the highlights of the ALS Association's annual Drug Company Working Group meeting, held in April in Washington, D.C., in conjunction with the American Academy of Neurology (AAN) Meeting. From this meeting, we can summarise: (1) Induced pluripotent stem cells have been used as a drug discovery tool, leading to an upcoming clinical trial that will test a drug shown to be effective in cells derived from people with ALS. (2) Retigabine (AED) help to normalise the over-excitability of ALS cells in cell culture, and this treatment improves the survival of these cells. (3) The system to deliver glial-derived neurotrophic factor (GDNF) in ALS, based on experiments showing that GDNF can promote survival of motor neurons, is being developed. (4) A biologically based system that encapsulates protein-based growth factors or DNA-based antisense molecules can cross the blood-brain barrier, allowing peripheral administration for a drug that acts in the brain, is being developed. (5) Tirasemtiv increases muscle output at mid-levels of exertion, temporarily restoring some lost strength for everyday activities such as picking up an object, but did not meet its major objective of showing a change in the ALS Functional Rating Scale score at the end of treatment, although it improves the slow vital capacity (modified from: http://www.alsa.org/news/archive/progress-in-drug-development.html). Other results were: (6) Mexiletine is a cardiac medication that reduces hyperexcitability of motor neurons, which may help protect them from toxic excitation and it was safe to use in ALS (modified from: http://www.alsa.org/news/archive/new-clinical-pilot-studies.html). (7) One research showed that motor neurons can be protected from disease-related toxicity by human up-frameshift protein 1 (hUPF1). Promoting hUPF1 might be therapeutic and therapies for SOD1-related ALS might require different strategies and that clinical trials may have the greatest chance of success if they target people with similar forms of ALS (modified from: http://www.alsa.org/news/archive/new-therapy-rna-processing.html). All these results were preceded by the following results (2012-2015): (1) The immune system continues to grow as a target of interest in therapy design. (2) Several groups have made progress on finding biomarkers that can track disease. (3) The entire ALS community was disappointed in the negative results from the dexpramipexole trial. (4) 'Antisense' therapy against the mutation reduces the amount of aggregated RNA and may be therapeutic, according to experiments in cell culture. Antisense against the SOD1 gene has been shown to be safe in people with ALS progression. (5) The journal *The Lancet* indicates that high caloric intake is safe and tolerable in people with ALS with a feeding tube. This research sets the stage for a larger trial testing whether high caloric intake can slow progression of the disease (modified from http://www.alsa.org/news/archive/research-shows-high-calorie.html). (6) Brain storm cell therapeutics said the U.S. Food and Drug Administration has approved the start of a mid-stage clinical trial of its adult stem cell treatment for people with ALS, which have shown that it was well tolerated and safe (modified from: http://www.alsa.org/news/archive/fda-approves-brainstorm-trial.html). (7) Tocilizumab interacts with microglia to convert them from the Microglia1 to Microglia2 state. In a recent small, open-label trial in eight people with ALS, there was some evidence that the drug may be able to reduce neuroinflammation (modified from: http://www.alsa. org/news/archive/2014-drug-company-working-group.html). (8) The trial with ceftriaxone was stopped in early 2012 because data analysis indicated that it was not effective at changing the rate of progression of ALS (http://www.alsa.org/news/archive/ceftriaxone-statement.html). (9) Unexpectedly, a drug (Nuedexta) that is approved for the treatment of labile emotionality that occurs in association with ALS and other neurological disorders has been observed to improve bulbar function, primarily speech and swallowing, in a number of neurological disorders, including ALS (http://www.alsa.org/news/archive/news-from-the-international.html).

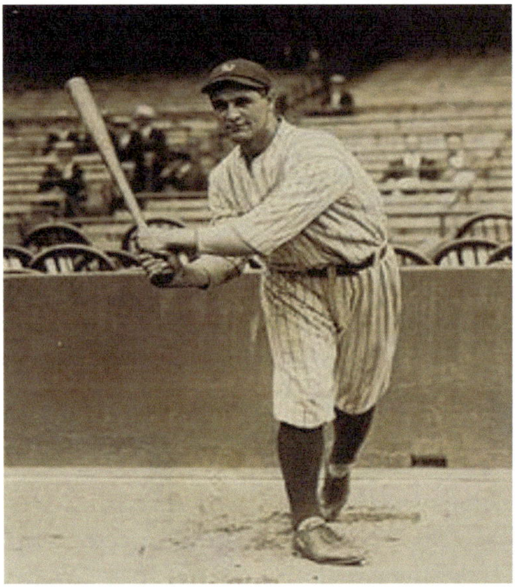

Figure 1. Henry Louis 'Lou' or 'Buster' Gehrig (Born Heinrich Ludwig Gehrig; 19 June 1903-2 June 1941) was an American baseball first baseman who played 17 seasons in Major League Baseball for the New York Yankees, from 1923 to 1939. https://en.wikipedia.org/wiki/Lou_Gehrig.

ALS is better known since 1939, when a famous American baseball first baseman player Lou Gehrig (see **Figure 1**) brought national and international attention to his disease; since then, in America this neurodegenerative disorder is better known as a Lou Gehrig's disease.

Since Gehrig died, a big number of sportsmen have been diagnosed with ALS or Lou Gehrig's disease. At this point, we like to highlight that Lou Gehrig was a very famous baseball player, but two other baseball players from the same New York Yankees team such as his friend and teammate Babe Ruth (1895-1948) who set numerous baseball records (famous for his big hitting) and won many titles with the New York Yankees, and Joe DiMaggio (1914-1999) who won the title World Series Champion nine times with the New York Yankees, were even more famous than him and they did not suffer from ALS.

2. Some sportsmen presenting amyotrophic lateral sclerosis

In 2005, Al-Chalabi and Leigh studying this topic concluded that: 'there is no evidence that football players elsewhere in the world have an increased risk of developing ALS' [23]. Other authors said that the only really consistent epidemiological risk factors for ALS are increasing age, male sex and a family history of ALS [24–28] and we agree on that. Even in Guam, where a restricted population with high risk of developing ALS has been under intense scrutiny for over 50 years, controversy persists and no environmental (or genetic) causes have been identified beyond doubt [23, 29–31]. On the other hand, cigarette smoking may also be a risk factor [27, 28, 32] but other information should be taken into consideration. For example, it is known that complex pathophysiological processes, including mitochondrial dysfunction, aggregation of misfolded protein, oxidative stress, excitotoxicity, inflammation and apoptosis, can involve both motor neurons and surrounding glial cells [33], and therefore is accepted that the aetiology of ALS likely involves a complex interaction between Multiple risk factors. Although no confirmation about the direct effect of stress or exercises on pathophysiology of ALS has been made, we cannot ignore the frequency of ALS in people practicing sport apart from the affirmation from some author saying that CNS injury is linked to an increased incidence of motor neuron degeneration [34], given the recognised association between neurodegenerative disease and activities that involve a higher risk for CNS trauma, including participation in professional full-contact sports and military service [35–39].

Most researchers investigating head injury and ALS did their studies in predisposed rats to ALS, including those with a more severe injury due to a stab-wound trauma (SOD1 rat spinal cord), and in all the studies done, those traumatic lesions did not accelerate motor neuron degeneration [40, 41], but these research protocols cannot apply to the real scenarios afforded by athletes that underwent more and repetitive instances of all kind of stress and repetitive CNS trauma leading to more chance of developing diffused axonal injury. Other authors supported this hypothesis as well [42–46] and we considerate that those results cannot be transferred to human beings.

Let us highlight one more time that a single injury is not able to hasten disease pathology, but there is enough evidence suggesting that brain injuries can be linked with ALS [47] and about the risk of developing ALS in football players [48, 49]. In our series of patients, we found that professional boxing and rugby players are the most common to be associated with ALS, but we have to mention that our job is done in a semi-rural setting where other sport modalities are not practiced. We support the hypotheses that cortical dysfunction caused by any kind of injury should be taken into consideration as part of the pathophysiology of ALS [50–52], until proven otherwise.

To practice sports or do strong exercises obviously do not cause a degenerative disorder, but if the above-mentioned activities are accompanied by prolonged and severe stress situation in a genetically predisposed person, then nobody can predict what is going to happen.

To provide better idea about this hypothesis, we decided to review some biographic aspects of these kinds of patients.

Because it is mainly an introductory chapter and due to limitations of space we had to remove some relevant aspects regarding ALS/sportsmen and a lot of illustrative material from the original chapter and to bring more attention to others topics.

2.1. Comments about some sportsmen presenting ALS

Lou Henri Gehrig is one of the most famous people affected by ALS. He was born in the Yorkville section of club and earned the nickname Columbia Lou from adoring fans. Gehrig signed his first contract with the New York Yankees Team in April 1923. Over the next 15 years he led the team to win six World Series titles. Available at the URL: http://www.biography.com/people/lou-gehrig-9308266.

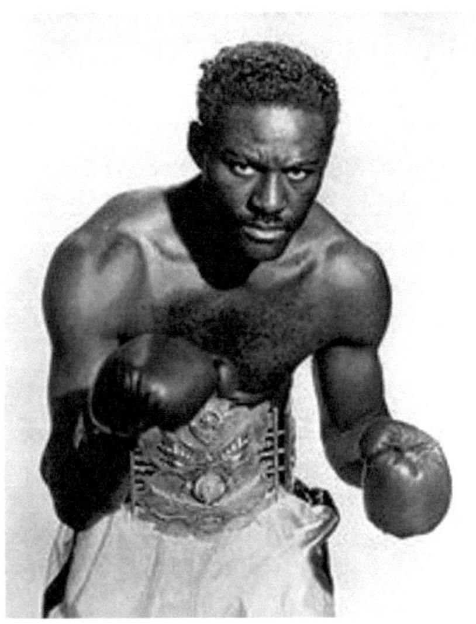

Figure 2. Ezzard Mack Charles (7 July 1921-28 May 1975) was an American professional boxer and former World Heavyweight Champion. https://en.wikipedia.org/wiki/Ezzard_Charles.

In May 1939, he noticed that his performance has been decreasing gradually due to progressive weakness all over the body and then he decided to pull himself out of the lineup of players looking for better results of his team. At that time a diagnosis of ALS was done and he died 2 years later. Lou Gehrig, also known as 'the iron man of the baseball', played in more consecutive games than any other baseball player worldwide and his record remained unbroken until 1995 (modified from: http://www.alstexas.org/understanding-als/).

Scarmeas et al. [46] published a manuscript, concluding that subjects with ALS were more likely to be slim or had once been serious athletes. Apart from Lou Gehrig, they mentioned many famous people in U.S. history who have had ALS such as: **Ezzard Charles** (see **Figure 2**) who was a quite famous heavyweight boxing champion. Charles was diagnosed with ALS. The disease affected Charles legs and eventually left him completely disabled. Charles died on 28 May 1975 in Chicago.

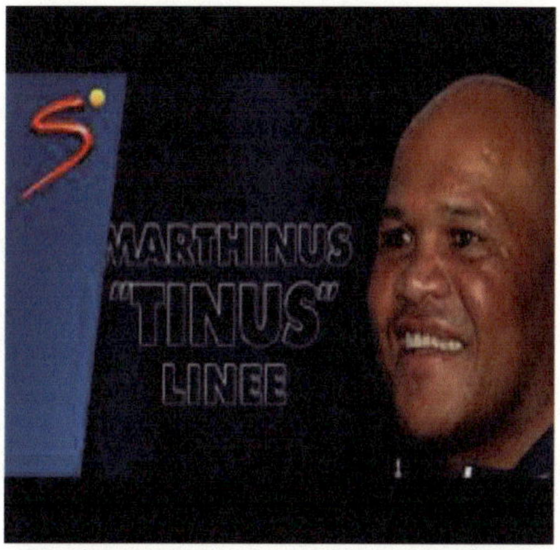

Figure 3. Marthinus 'Tinus' Linee (23 August 1969-3 November 2014) was a South African rugby player. https://en.wikipedia.org/wiki/Tinus_Linee.

Another famous baseball player affected by ALS was '**Catfish**' Hunter. From 1965 to 1979, he was a pitcher for the Kansas City Athletics, Oakland Athletics and New York Yankees. He was diagnosed with ALS in his early 50s and died of the disease about a year later. **Paul Kevin Turner** was an American professional fullback. He played eight seasons in the National Football League for the New England Patriots and Philadelphia Eagles. After Turner learned he had ALS in 2010, he created the Kevin Turner Foundation to raise awareness about sports-related brain trauma and to support research and treatment initiatives. He was involved in research that links chronic traumatic encephalopathy to ALS, and agreed to donate his brain and spinal cord when he died. On 24 March 2016, Turner died as a result of ALS at home in Vestavia Hills, Alabama. **Stephen Michael 'Steve' Gleason** (born 19 March 1977) is a former professional football player, a safety with the New Orleans Saints of the National Football League. In 2011, he revealed that he was battling ALS. **André Gerhardus Venter** (born 14 November 1970 in Vereeniging, South Africa) who was a former South African rugby union footballer and earned 66 caps playing for the South Africa national team during the mid-to-late 1990s and early 2000s. He represented South Africa during the 1999 Rugby World Cup where they finished third. Unfortunately, he was another victim of ALS. **Joost van der Westhuizen** (born 20 February 1971) was a member of the victorious South African rugby team at the 1995 World Cup. He was inducted into the International Rugby

Hall of Fame in 2007. Near the end of 2008, Van der Westhuizen first noticed weakness in his right arm. A few months later, he was play-fighting in a swimming pool with a friend who was also his personal doctor, and discovered further weakness in the arm, a diagnosis of ALS was confirmed in 2011. Modified from: http://www.eurosport.com/rugby/van-der-westhuizen-sees-a-link_sto4476535/story.shtml. **Jarrod Cunningham** (7 September 1968-22 July 2007) was a New Zealand rugby union fullback, who died from ALS. After tests at Charing Cross Hospital, Cunningham was diagnosed with ALS in June 2002. He immediately retired from professional rugby, and started the Jarrod Cunningham SALSA Foundation in March 2003 with the aim of providing hope, education and inspiration for fellow sufferers of ALS. He returned home to New Zealand in December 2004 and died at his home on 22 July 2007. **Herbert Krug** (21 June 1937-1 November 2010) was a German equestrian who won a gold medal in team dressage at the 1984 Summer Olympics in Los Angeles. He was born in Mainz and died in Hochheim am Main due to ALS. **Krzysztof Nowak** (27 September 1975-26 May 2005) was a Polish football player, best known for his stint with the VfL Wolfsburg team. He was forced to retire from the sport in early 2002 after he learned he had ALS. **Donald George "Don" Revie** was an England international footballer. In the spring of 1986, Revie moved to Kinross, Scotland where he intended to retire, but he was diagnosed with motor neurone disease in May 1987. Revie publicly announced his illness in August of that year, and made his final public appearance on 11 May 1988 at Elland Road in a wheelchair. He died in Murrayfield Hospital in Edinburgh on 26 May 1989, aged 61. Marthinus 'Tinus' Linee (see **Figure 3**) played rugby predominantly at the centre. In April 2013, Linee was diagnosed with motor neurone disease. His deteriorating health resulted in him having financial difficulties in an attempt to cover his medical costs. Linee died on 3 November 2014, aged 45 in his family home in Paarl, South Africa.

John Mudgeway was born in Masterton, he attended school in New Zealand, was an active rower and was in the school's rugby union first XV. He was diagnosed with motor neurone disease in 2002. **Ryan Walker** was born on 5 October 1978 in Pietermaritzburg (South Africa) and grew up on a beef and dairy farm in Mooi River. He was admitted in hospital for 5 days and had extensive blood tests, nerve tests, MRI and lumbar punctures. All the results came back clear. Ryan then went for his follow-up appointment with his attending doctor 4 weeks later who told him that he had ALS, and that there was no treatment available and that the prognosis was 2-5 years. More biographic information about all mentioned athletes is available at the URL: https://en.wikipedia.org.

Due to the large number of rugby players affected by ALS in South Africa, many people have questioned whether there is a link between rugby-linked head injuries and motor neuron disease in light of cases including those of Joost van der Westhuizen, Tinus Linee, John Mudgeway, Ryan Walker and Jarrod Cunningham, all professional South African rugby players who suffered from the disease [49, 53]. Due to the increasing report of sportsmen presenting ALS, of all the putative risk factors, head injury has emerged as a strong cause for initiating the neurodegenerative processes in ALS patients [38, 39].

At the present moment, there are more available facilities for confirmation of ALS, the disease is better known and the remarkable progress reached by the media and Internet has made their contribution to inform everyone about all sportsmen presenting ALS. Perhaps this is one of the reasons why we note an increase in the number of reported patients. Obviously, we also have more capacities to inform about new cases to the medical literature worldwide and this facility increase the number of reported patients.

We would like to highlight that thousands of slim athletes never developed ALS. Therefore, why a tiny few of them do develop ALS is still unknown. There is certainly no justification to avoid athletics in attempts to avoid ALS. Moreover, nothing in some authors' data can be construed as evidence that patients with ALS should not exercise [54].

3. What about other famous sportsmen?

Looking for clinical features of ALS in other sportsmen, we reviewed the biography of 100 famous sporting personalities, including Pele, Muhammad Ali, Diego Armando Maradona and Manny Pacquiao, among others (more information is available at the URL: http://www.biographyonline.net/sport/100-sporting-personalities.html), and it was a great sense of delight to find nobody was affected by ALS. Nevertheless, we also included other famous sporting personalities such as Lance Armstrong, Paula Radcliffe, Jose Mourinho, Henry Cooper, Stirling Moss, Wayne Rooney, Bill Shankly and Alex Ferguson (more information is available at the URL: http://www.biographyonline.net/sport/100-sporting-personalities.html) and we also found that nobody presented clinical manifestations of ALS.

According to the results from the study made by Turner et al., it seems that more cases than expected of ALS are associated with a prior diagnosis of asthma, celiac disease, younger-onset diabetes (younger than 30 years), multiple sclerosis, myasthenia gravis, myxedema, polymyositis, Sjögren syndrome, systemic lupus erythematosus and ulcerative colitis were confirmed, concluding that ALS raise the possibility of shared genetic or environmental risk factors [55]. These findings encouraged us to look into more groups of famous peoples to continue looking for the co-existence of ALS and other diseases. Then, we finally decided to review the biography of top 100 famous people, looking for the presence of ALS. That list of peoples was chosen mainly from the nineteenth, twentieth or twenty-first century and included famous actors, politicians, entrepreneurs, writers, artists and humanitarians (http://www.enkivillage.com/most-famous-person-in-the-world.html). From this final review, we found that only two top famous people presented ALS: Mao Tse-tung and Stephen William Hawking.

From that observation, one single question came to our mind: What is different in those particular patients?

Mao was a Chairman of China. Some authors reported that out of the billions of people in China, Mao was the only person to ever have ALS, up to that time and also the authors asked: What did he do that none of the other Chinese did? In some authors' opinion Mao had a Western diet, meaning that he did not eat rice and vegetables; instead, he ate lots of meat and they considered that this type of diet (similar to Lou Gehrig's diet) may be part of the mechanism for ALS. More information is available at the URL: http://la.indymedia.org/news/

2014/08/265540.php, http://www.scientificamerican.com/article/seeds-of-dementia-what-alzhiemers-lou-gehrigs-parkinsons-have-in-common/. Despite this coincidence, we agree that this type of diet could be a contributing factor for ALS in a predisposed patient but without doubt, it is not the direct cause of the disease.

Stephen William Hawking also has some differences compared with the rest of the patients: Why has Hawking lived for more than 50 years with ALS when so many people die 1-5 years after diagnosis? Why he remains stable? We really do not know. Of course, Hawking has a variable of SALS; probably we got a late presentation of juvenile-onset disorder, which may progress very slowly. None has survived with ALS for so long as he did, providing a big hope for patients presenting ALS. Some authors think that it is a small percentage of people for whom that actually happens [56], and we do agree.

We concluded that no famous female presenting ALS has been reported ever. Apart from Mao Tse-tung and Stephen William Hawking, no other top famous people affected by ALS have been reported and both have some differences compared with the rest of the patients. In our opinion, the prognosis of ALS is bad, especially when there are bulbar and respiratory complications but not all patients have a progressive and invariably rapid fatal outcome, as has been found.

4. More update on ALS

More than 40 chapters about ALS have been published only by INTECH since 2012, which reflect how important this problem is and how far we are from its solution. To get a graphic information about the topics published by INTECH and the countries participating, please see **Figures 4** and **5**.

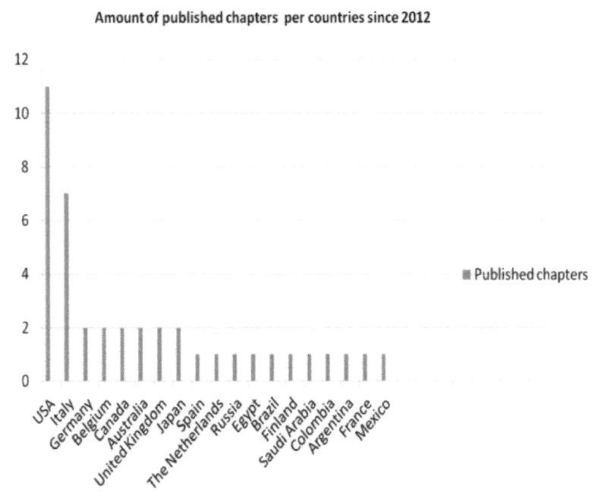

Figure 4. A graphic information about the number of topics published by INTECH since 2012 up to date.

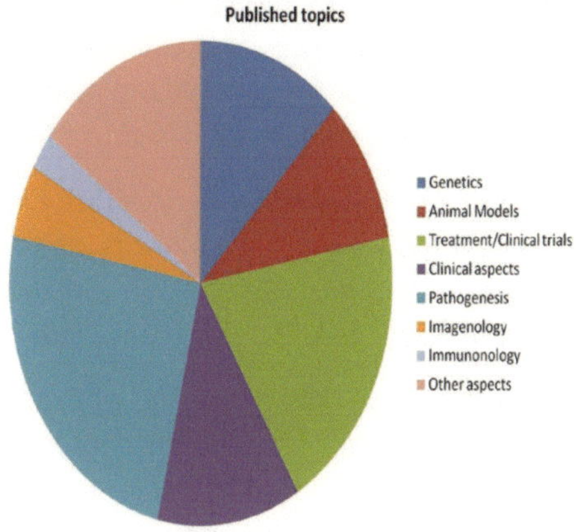

Figure 5. The number of chapters published by INTECH and participant countries since 2012 up to date.

Thanks to these publications, today we know more about genetics, immunology, pathophysiology of ALS and its pathology, and about inclusion bodies (ubiquitylated inclusions, binding protein 43, fused in sarcoma protein, bunina bodies and hyaline conglomerate inclusions). Because of these publications, the role of oxidative stress and the excitoxicity (glutamate, glutamate receptor), mitochondrial dysfunction, mitochondrial morphology, electron transport chain, calcium homeostasis, axonal transport abnormalities, glial activation, growth factors abnormalities, RNA metabolism disorders, non-cell autonomous mechanisms and apoptosis in ALS are better known. Unfortunately, most of the results were found in familial ALS (FALS) only, which represent 5% of the patients.

Nevertheless, we enjoy some advances that are reached recently: Today we know that some abnormal protein aggregates are seen in brain and spinal cord samples from patients with sporadic ALS, which suggests that protein misfolding and aggregation contribute to the pathogenesis of ALS, although a causative role remains controversial [57–59].

Increased oxidative stress promotes demyelination in brains of OXYS rats with genetically accelerated aging, which was ameliorated by feeding of affected animals [60]. In other words, increased oxidative stress associated with specific metabolic phenotypes, which promote reverse electron transport due to reduction of the membrane pool of ubiquinone by succinate or fatty acids, is a prerequisite for cases of sporadic ALS which is preferentially acquired by individuals with the mitochondrial metabolic phenotype that promotes very high levels of ROS production [61]. These authors also highlighted the importance to consider determination of metabolic phenotypes together with the disease mechanisms when working with patients or animal models of the ALS.

Recent progress has been reviewed on aggregation mechanisms of ALS pathogenic proteins, SOD1, TDP-43 and FUS/TLS, which are involved in DNA/RNA metabolism. We still have to clearly establish whether aggregation or loss of the wild-type functions of either of these two proteins is the underlying cause of the disease phenotype [62].

Mutations in Cu/Zn superoxide dismutase (SOD1) gene are linked to the motor neuron death in familial amyotrophic lateral sclerosis (FALS) and mutations in another gene, optineurin, have been linked to fALS cases, and hyaline inclusions in the anterior horn cells of spinal cord were immunoreactive for OPTN in patients with OPTN mutation (E478G) [63].

Given that the skein-like inclusions in the spinal anterior horn cells are characteristic of ALS, proteomic analysis of those inclusions will help to identify as-yet-unknown proteins pathogenic for ALS. In addition, the component analysis of skein-like inclusions will help to describe the common mechanism of sporadic and familial ALS cases [64].

In relation with the treatment for ALS, the only approved pharmacological treatment for ALS is riluzole, which extends survival by about 2 months [65]. Efforts in basic and clinical research brought some light in the understanding of pathophysiological aspects of MND. With dozens of failed neuropharmacological trials in ALS, the current concept of the design of clinical trials in ALS patients must be re-evaluated, as well as the pre-clinical models [66].

However, the development of a vaccine or immunoglobulin to remove misfolded protein in ALS is a novel therapeutic strategy because of the evidence for the existence of secretor pathways for superoxide dismutase (SOD1) mutant linked to ALS [67].

Based on recent publications and its important contributions, many aspects of respiratory care for patients with ALS, such as non-invasive ventilation and assisted cough, have brought more hope for their well-being [68–72]. And new ideas about prevention of aspiration and pneumonia and adequate management of bronchial secretions apart from an adequate management of sialorrhea, dysphagia and insufficient cough for reduction of pneumonia risk in patients with ALS [73].

Breathing pacemakers, which can delay the need for mechanical ventilation by approximately 2 years, should be offered to all patients with spinal cord injury, central alveolar hypoventilation syndrome and even in patients with ALS [74].

At present, gene and stem cell therapies are holding the hope for an efficient treatment in ALS.

Definitively, the neuroprotective role of fragment C has shed light on the understanding of the disease's neurodegeneration processes and the study of this promising property of TTC can be extended to other neurodegenerative diseases, such as Parkinson's disease, Alzheimer's disease and spinal muscular atrophy [75]. In summary, a successful neuroprotective treatment could transform neurodegenerative diseases from a relentless progressive and disabling disease to a problem that can be managed with only a modest effect on quality of life [76].

Considering other treatment modalities, we should highlight that stem cell therapy design should be aimed at neuroprotection rather than motor neuron replacement. Motor neuron replacement is technically difficult to achieve. Also, in theory it will not bring much improvement to the patients because the evidence shows that glial cells are the actual determinant of ALS disease progression. Secondly, combining stem cell transplantation and growth factor delivery provides the best result in slowing disease progression and prolonging survival, as the two greatly complement each other. Finally, some authors are now convinced that injections of stem cells in multiple sites are needed to alleviate symptoms of ALS. There should be at least one injection that focuses on protecting cell bodies of motor neurons and another that aims to maintain neuromuscular connections [77].

The SOD1 activity in the mitochondrial inter-membrane space is a relevant therapeutic target for ALS and other neurodegenerative diseases involving mitochondrial pathogenesis has been confirmed [78].

Collectively, almost all recent studies demonstrate that multiple factors including protein stability, dynamics and biophysical characteristics are likely to play a role in modulating SOD1 aggregation, and the familial ALS phenotypic characteristics are not likely to be fully explained by the aggregation behaviour of any one form of SOD1 [79].

Mitochondrial and bioenergetics defects have been claimed to play vital role in ALS pathogenesis. Altered respiratory chain enzyme activities and CNS energy hypometabolism in spinal cord and motor cortex are the hallmark of ALS [80], mitochondrial respiratory chain damage is a relevant event in ALS pathogenesis, although it is still unknown if mitochondrial abnormalities are the cause of the disease process or if they are consequence of neuronal degeneration. However, it is clear from the evidence reviewed here that mitochondria definitely play a central role in determining the fate of motor neurons and in their degeneration process [81].

Inflammation has been shown to play a critical role in the pathogenesis of ALS. Markers of inflammation, including microglial stimulating factors and pro-inflammatory cytokines, such as TNF alpha and FasL are increased in ALS [82].

The combined evidence emerging from all molecular genetic studies in chromosome 9p21-linked families and in chromosome 9p21-associated ALS/FTLD populations, suggests that it is the most important genetic factor contributing to the disease in the centre of the disease spectrum linking ALS and FTLD [83].

The role of genetics in ALS is calling for more attention among clinician gradually. Because, now almost all agree that different genes are involved in ALS disease and about the importance of a good clinical characterisation for choosing the genetic approach. Impressive progress in the understanding of the genetics of ALS has been made over the past several years with the identification of several causal genes. However, most of the genetic variability underlying ALS remains to be identified. The use of deep-sequencing techniques and functional research will be needed to further broaden our understanding of ALS pathogenesis [84].

Expansions have been identified not only in ALS-FTD pedigrees, but also in familial FTD, familial ALS and sporadic ALS. Estimated frequencies vary from 23.5 to 46.4% for familial ALS and 4.1 to 21% for sporadic ALS. The expansion, which is non-coding, is therefore the most common genetic cause of ALS identified to date [85].

The role of glial cells deserves additional comments. The identification of glial cells as an active contributor to the disease process is important. Specifically, astrocytes and microglia have been recognised as glial cell types which undeniably influence survival in rodent models of ALS. New genes have been recently linked with ALS including TDP43 and FUS, suggesting a possible role for RNA metabolism in disease pathogenesis and special efforts are underway to test therapies aimed at modifying the glial cell population in hopes of slowing ALS disease progression and extending patient survival [86]. Astrocytes clearly contribute to ALS decrease progression in both neuroinflammation and excitotoxicity [87].

Astrocytes regulate K+ buffering, glutamate clearance, brain antioxidant defence, close metabolic coupling with neurons and modulation of neuronal excitability and are involved in both exacerbations of damage and neuroprotective mechanisms. They support neurons in many ways, all of which are essential for repair and regeneration. Disturbances in astrocytic functions are implicated in neurodegenerative diseases pathogenesis; therefore, modulation of astrocytes functioning may prove to be an efficient therapeutic strategy in many chronic CNS disorders [88].

As a clinician, we dedicate more attention to those topics useful for the management of our patients and without doubt neuroimaging is one the most helpful ones particularly when genetics, immunological and others are not close to the reality of the patients. In the past, CT scan and MRI were our basic investigations supported by clinical neurophysiological tests if the clinical assessment offered some doubt. Fortunately, today we have more facilities in the field of neuroimaging and using magnetic resonance spectroscopy, positron emission tomography (PET) and functional MRI the future confirmations will be more confident.

In this book, we introduce a new experience using PET in ALS apart from the previous studies done with CT scan and MRI. In our opinion, the combination of proton magnetic resonance spectroscopy (1H-MRS) with diffusion/diffusion tensor imaging, voxel-based morphometry MRI and perfusion-weighted imaging will bring more clarification to some imagenological issues not well known as yet, and has the potential to fill the gap between pathogenesis and clinical outcome of neurodegenerative diseases and other authors also agree [89].

In conclusion, in this book we update some of the knowledge recently published by our Editorial House and introduce novel aspects on this matter and it will be a pleasure for our readership community.

Acknowledgements

Many thanks to Lic. Lorna María, Thabo Humberto Jorge and Fátima Susana Adolfina for their unconditional support.

Author details

Humberto Foyaca-Sibat* and Lourdes de Fátima Ibañez-Valdés

*Address all correspondence to: humbertofoyacasibat@gmail.com

Department of Neurology, Nelson Mandela Central Hospital, Faculty of Health Sciences, Walter Sisulu University, Mthatha, South Africa

References

[1] Kiernan MC, Vucic S, Cheah BC, Turner MR, Eisen A, et al. Amyotrophic lateral sclerosis. Lancet 2011;377:942–955.

[2] Diamanti L, Gagliardi S, Cereda C, Ceroni C. Genetics of ALS and Correlations Between Genotype and Phenotype in ALS — A Focus on Italian Population. Available at the URL: http://dx.doi.org/10.5772/56547.

[3] Byrne S, Walsh C, Lynch C, Bede P, Elamin M, et al. Rate of familial amyotrophic lateral sclerosis: a systematic review and meta-analysis. J Neurol Neurosurg Psychiatry 2011;82:623–627.

[4] Logroscino G, Traynor BJ, Hardiman O, Chio A, Mitchell D, Swingler RJ, Millul A, Benn E, Beghi E. Incidence of amyotrophic lateral sclerosis in Europe. J Neurol Neurosurg Psychiatry 2010;81(4):385–390.

[5] Kumar DR, Aslinia F, Yale SH, Mazza JL. Jean-Martin Charcot: The Father of Neurology. Clin Med Res. 2011 Mar; 9(1): 46-49.

[6] Bruijn LI, Miller TM, Cleveland DW. Unraveling the mechanisms involved in motor neuron degeneration in ALS. Annu Rev Neurosci 2004;27:723–749.

[7] Kobayashi M, Ikeda K, Kinoshita M, Iwasaki Y. Amyotrophic lateral sclerosis with supranuclear ophthalmoplegia and rigidity. Neurol Res 1999;21:661–664.

[8] Okuda B, Yamamoto T, Yamasaki M, Maya K, Imai T. Motor neuron disease with slow eye movements and vertical gaze palsy. Acta Neurologica Scandinavica 1992;85:71–76.

[9] Rippon GA, Scarmeas N, Gordon PH, Murphy PL, Albert SM, Mitsumoto H, Marder K, Rowland LP, Stern Y. An observational study of cognitive impairment in amyotrophic lateral sclerosis. Arch Neurol 2006;63(3):345–652. doi:10.1001/archneur.63.3.345.

[10] Mitsuyama Y. Presenile dementia with motor neuron disease. Dementia 1993;4(3–4): 137–142.

[11] Neary D, Snowden JS, Mann DMA, Northern B, Goulding PJ, Macdermott N. Frontal lobe dementia and motor neuron disease. J Neurol Neurosur Psych 1990;53(1):23–32.

[12] Peavy GM, Herzog AG, Rubin NP, Mesulam NM. Neuropsychological aspects of dementia of motor neuron disease: a report of two cases. Neurology 1992;42(5):1004–1008.

[13] Cavalleri F, De Renzi E. Amyotrophic lateral sclerosis with dementia. Act Neurol Scan 1994;89(50):391–394.

[14] Hudson AJ, Martzke J, Caselli RJ. Aphasic dementia and motor neuron disease. Ann Neurol 1993;34:417–418.

[15] Capitani E, Della Sala S, Marchetti C. Is there a cognitive impairment in MND? A survey with longitudinal data. Schw Arch Neurol Psych 1994:145(1):11–13.

[16] Caselli RJ, Windebank AJ, Petersen RC, et al. Rapidly progressive aphasic dementia and motor neuron disease. Ann Neurol 1993:33(2):200–207.

[17] David AS. Neuropsychological measures in patients with amyotrophic lateral sclerosis. Act Neurol Scan 1987;75(4):284.

[18] Iwasaki Y, Kinoshita M, Ikeda K, Takamiya K, Shiojima T. Neuropsychological dysfunctions in amyotrophic lateral sclerosis: relation to motor disabilities. Intl J Neurosc 1990;54(3–4):191–195.

[19] Kew J, Leigh N. Dementia with motor neurone disease. Baillieres Clin Neurol 1992;1(3): 611–626.

[20] Kew JJM, Goldstein LH, Leigh PN, et al. The relationship between abnormalities of cognitive function and cerebral activation in amyotrophic lateral sclerosis: a neuropsychological and positron emission tomography study. Brain 1993;116(6):1399–1423.

[21] Achi EY, Rudnicki SA. ALS and frontotemporal dysfunction: a review. Neurol Res Intl 2012;12:9. Article ID 806306. http://dx.doi.org/10.1155/2012/806306.

[22] Zimmerman EK, Eslinger PJ, Simmons Z, Barrett AM. Emotional perception deficits in amyotrophic lateral sclerosis. Cognitive Beh Neurol 2007;20(2):79–82.

[23] Al-Chalabi A, Leigh PN. Trouble on the pitch: are professional football players at increased risk of developing amyotrophic lateral sclerosis? Brain. 2005 Mar;128(Pt 3): 451–453.

[24] Kurtzke JF. Risk factors in amyotrophic lateral sclerosis. Adv Neurol 1991;56:245–270

[25] Mitchell JD. Amyotrophic lateral sclerosis: toxins and environment. Amyotroph Lateral Scler Other Motor Neuron Disord 2000;1:235–250.

[26] Worms PM. The epidemiology of motor neuron diseases: a review of recent studies. J Neurol Sci 2001;191:3–9.

[27] Armon C. An evidence-based medicine approach to the evaluation of the role of exogenous risk factors in sporadic amyotrophic lateral sclerosis. Neuroepidemiology 2003;22:217–228.

[28] Nelson LM, McGuire V, Longstreth WT Jr, Matkin C. Population-based case-control study of amyotrophic lateral sclerosis in western Washington State. 1. Cigarette smoking and alcohol consumption. Am J Epidemiol 2000;151:156–163.

[29] Plato CC, Garuto RM, Galasko D, Craig U-K, Plato M, Gamst A, et al. Amyotrophic lateral sclerosis and parkinsonism-dementia complex of Guam: changing incidence rates during the past 60 years. Am J Epidemiol 2003;157:149–157.

[30] Banack SA, Cox PA. Biomagnification of cycad neurotoxins in flying foxes. Implications for ALS-PDC in Guam. Neurology 2003;61:387–389.

[31] Waring SC, Esteban-Santillan C, Reed DM, Craig UK, Labarthe DR, Petersen RC, et al. Incidence of amyotrophic lateral sclerosis and of the parkinsonism-dementia complex of Guam, 1950–1989. Neuroepidemiology 2004;23:192–200.

[32] Weisskopf MG, McCullough ML, Calle EE, Thun MJ, Cudkowicz M, Ascherio A. Prospective study of cigarette smoking and amyotrophic lateral sclerosis. Am J Epidemiol 2004;160:26–33.

[33] Gordon PH. Amyotrophic lateral sclerosis: an update for 2013 clinical features, pathophysiology, management and therapeutic trials. Aging Dis 2013 Oct;4(5):295–310. Published online 2013 Oct 1. doi: 10.14336/AD.2013.0400295.

[34] Lehman EJ, Hein MJ, Baron SL, Gersic CM. Neurodegenerative causes of death among retired National Football League players. Neurology 2012;79(333):1970–1974.

[35] Veldink JH, Kalmijn S, Groeneveld GJ, Titulaer MJ, Wokke JH, Van den Berg LH. Physical activity and the association with sporadic ALS. Neurology 2005;64(415):241–245.

[36] Chio A, Calvo A, Dossena M, Ghiglione P, Mutani R, Mora G. ALS in Italian professional soccer players: the risk is still present and could be soccerspecific. Amyotroph Lateral Scler 2009;10(296):205–209.

[37] Barnes DE, Kaup A, Kirby KA, Byers AL, Diaz-Arrastia R, Yaffe K. Traumatic brain injury and risk of dementia in older veterans. Neurology 2014;83(287):312–319.

[38] Mielke MM, Savicar R, Wiste HJ, Weigand SD, Vemuri P, Knopman DS, Lowe VJ, Roberts RO, Machulda MM, Geda YE, Petersen RC, Jack CR Jr. Head trauma and in vivo measures of amyloid and neurodegeneration in a population-based study. Neurology 2014;82:70–76.

[39] Savicar R. Head trauma and neurodegeneration in veterans: an additional piece of the puzzle. Neurology 2014;83:298–299.

[40] Suzuki M, Klein S, Wetzel EA, Meyer M, Mchugh J, Tork C, Hayes A, Svendsen CN. Acute glial activation by stab injuries does not lead to overt 402 damage or motor neuron degeneration in the G93A mutant SOD1 rat model of amyotrophic lateral sclerosis. Exp Neurol 2010;221:346–352.

[41] Thomsen GM, Vit JP, Lamb A, Gowing G, Shelest O, Alkaslasi M, Ley EJ, Svendsen CN. Acute Traumatic Brain Injury Does Not Exacerbate Amyotrophic Lateral Sclerosis in the SOD1 (G93A) Rat Model (1,2,3). eNeuro. 2015 Jul 3;2(3). doi: 10.1523/ENEURO.0059-14.2015.

[42] Choo AM, Liu JZ, Dvorak M, Tetzlaffm, Oxland TR. Modeling spinal cord contusion, dislocation, and distraction: characterisation of vertebral clamps, injury severities, and node of Ranvier deformations. J Neurosci Methods 209;181(300):6–17.

[43] Jin Y, Bouyer J, Haas C, Fischer I. Behavioral and anatomical consequences of repetitive mild thoracic spinal cord contusion injury in the rat. Exp Neurol 2014;257:573–579.

[44] Mierzwa AJ, Sullivan GM, Beer LA, Ahn S, Armstrong RC. Comparison of cortical and white matter traumatic brain injury models reveals differential effects in the subventricular zone and divergent Sonic hedgehog signaling pathways in neuroblasts and oligodendrocyte progenitors. ASN Neuro. 2014 Sep 23;6(5). doi: 10.1177/1759091414551782. Print 2014.

[45] Angoa-Perez M, Kane MJ, Briggs DI, Herrera-Mundo N, Viano DC, Kuhn D. Animal models of sports-related head injury: bridging the gap between pre-clinical research and clinical reality. J Neurochem 2014;129:916–931.

[46] Mannix R, Meehan WP, Mandeville J, Grant PE, Gray T, Berglass J, Zhang J, et al. Clinical correlates in an experimental model of repetitive mild brain injury. Ann Neurol 2013;74:65–75.

[47] Prins ML, Hales A, Reger M, Giza CC, Hovda DA. Repeat traumatic brain injury in the juvenile rat is associated with increased axonal injury and cognitive impairments. Dev Neurosci 2010;32:510–518.

[48] Abel EL. Football increases the risk for Lou Gehrig's disease, amyotrophic lateral sclerosis. Percept Mot Skills 2007;104(280):1251–2154.

[49] Seelen M, van Doormaal PT, Visser AE, Huisman MH, Roozekrans MH, de Jong SW, van der Kooi AJ, de Visser M, Voermans NC, Veldink JH, van den Berg LH. Prior medical conditions and the risk of amyotrophic lateral sclerosis. J Neurol. 2014 Oct; 261(10):1949-1956. doi: 10.1007/s00415-014-7445-1.

[50] Thomsen GM, Gowing G, Latter J, Chen M, Vit JP, Staggenborg K, Aalos P, Alkaslasi M, Ferraiuolo L, Likhites S, Kaspar BK, Svendsen CN. Delayed disease onset and extended survival in the SOD1G93A rat model of amyotrophic lateral sclerosis after suppression of mutant SOD1 in the motor cortex. J Neurosci 2014;34:15587–15600.

[51] Scarmeas N, Shih T, Stern Y, Ottman R, Rowland LP. Premorbid weight, body mass, and varsity athletics in ALS. Arch Neurol 2006;63(3):345–352. doi:10.1001/archneur.63.3.345.

[52] Pascuzzi RM. Shostakovich and amyotrophic lateral sclerosis. Semin Neurol 1999;19(Suppl 1):63–66.

[53] Campbell-Gilles V. Is rugby linked to motor neuron disease? http://ewn.co.za/2014/11/19/Motor-Neuron-Disease-associated-with-repeated-head-injury

[54] Drory VE, Goltsman E, Goldman Reznik J, Mosek A, Korczyn AD. The value of muscle exercise in patients with amyotrophic lateral sclerosis. J Neurol Sci 2001;191:133–137.

[55] Turner MR, Goldacre R, Ramagopalan S, Talbot K, Goldacre MJ. Autoimmune disease preceding amyotrophic lateral sclerosis. An epidemiologic study. Neurology 2013 Oct 1;81(14):1222–1225. doi: 10.1212/WNL.0b013e3182a6cc13.

[56] Harmon K. How Has Stephen Hawking Lived to 70 with ALS? January 7, 2012. Scientific American. 2012;7:7. Retrieved 23 March 2016. http://www.scientificamerican.com/article/stephen-hawking-als/

[57] Bosco DA, Morfini G, Karabacak NM, Song Y, Gros-Lows F, Pasinelli P, Goolaby H, Fontaine BA, Lemay N, McKenna-Yasek D, Frosch MP, Agar JN, Julien JP, Brady ST, Brown RH Jr, et al. Wild-type and mutant SOD1 share an aberrant conformation and a common pathogenic pathway in ALS. Nat Neurosci 2010;13(11):1396–1403. ISSN: 00223565.

[58] Kerman A, Liu HN, Croul S, et al. Amyotrophic lateral sclerosis is a nonamyloid disease in which extensive misfolding of SOD1 is unique to the familial form. Acta Neuropathol 2010;119(3):335–344, ISSN: 0001-6322.

[59] Liu JH, Yin F, Guo LX, Deng XH, Hu YH. Neuroprotection of geniposide against hydrogen peroxide induced PC12 cells injury: involvement of PI3 kinase signal pathway. Acta Pharmacol Sin 2009;30(2):159–165, ISSN: 16714083.

[60] Kolosova NG, Akulov AE, Stefanova NA, Moshkin MP, Savelov AA, Koptyug IV, Panov AV, Vavilin VA. Effect of malate on development of rotenoneinduced brain changes in Wistar and OXYS rats: an MRI study. Doklady Biol Sci 2011;437:1–4.

[61] Alexander Panov, Nury Steuerwald, Valentin Vavilin, Svetlana Dambinova and Herbert L. Bonkovsky (2012). Role of Neuronal Mitochondrial Metabolic Phenotype in Pathogenesis of ALS, Amyotrophic Lateral Sclerosis, Prof. Martin Maurer (Ed.), ISBN: 978-953-307-806-9, InTech, Available from: http://www.intechopen.com/books/amyotrophic-lateral-sclerosis/role-of-neuronal-mitochondrial-metabolicphenotype-in-pathogenesis-of-als

[62] David S. Shin, Ashley J. Pratt, Elizabeth D. Getzoff and J. Jefferson P. Perry (2011). Amyotrophic Lateral Sclerosis, Advanced Understanding of Neurodegenerative Diseases, Dr Raymond Chuen-Chung Chang (Ed.) ISBN: 978-953-307-529-7, InTech, Available from: http://www.intechopen.com/books/advanced-understanding-of-neurodegenerative-diseases/amyotrophic-lateral-sclerosis

[63] Maruyama H, Morino H, Ito H, Izumi Y, Kato H, Watanabe Y, Kinoshita Y, Kamada M, Nodera H, Suzuki H, Komure O, Matsuura S, Kobatake K, Morimoto N, Abe K, Suzuki N, Aoki M, Kawata A, Hirai T, Kato T, Ogasawara K, Hirano A, Takumi T, Kusaka H, Hagiwara K, Kaji R, Kawakami H. Mutations of optineurin in amyotrophic lateral sclerosis. Nature 2010;465(7295):223–226. ISSN 1476-4687.

[64] 20Yoshiaki Furukawa (2012). Protein Aggregates in Pathological Inclusions of Amyotrophic Lateral Sclerosis, Amyotrophic Lateral Sclerosis, Prof. Martin Maurer (Ed.), ISBN: 978-953-307-806-9, InTech, Available from: http://www.intechopen.com/books/amyotrophic-lateral-sclerosis/protein-aggregates-in-pathological-inclusions-of-amyotrophic-lateral-sclerosis

[65] Miller RG, Mitchell JD, Lyon M, Moore DH. Riluzole for amyotrophic lateral sclerosis (ALS)/motor neuron disease (MND). Cochrane Database Syst Rev 2007;1:CD001447.

[66] Paolo Bongioanni (2012). Communication Impairment in ALS Patients Assessment and Treatment, Amyotrophic Lateral Sclerosis, Prof. Martin Maurer (Ed.), InTech, DOI: 10.5772/30426. Available from: http://www.intechopen.com/books/amyotrophic-lateral-sclerosis/communication-impairment-in-als-patients-assessment-and-treatment

[67] Takeuchi S, Fujiwara N, Ido A, et al. Induction of protective immunity by vaccination with wild-type apo superoxide dismutase 1 in mutant SOD1 transgenic mice. J Neuropathol Exp Neurol 2010;69(10):1044–1056. ISSN: 00223069

[68] Lo Coco D, Marchese S, Corrao S, Pesco MC, La Bella V, Piccoli F, Lo Coco A. Development of chronic hypoventilation in Amyotrophic Lateral Sclerosis patients. Respir Med 2006;100:1028–1036.

[69] Lo Coco D, Marchese S, Pesco MC, La Bella V, Piccoli F, Lo Coco A. Noninvasive positive-pressure ventilation in ALS. Predictors of tolerance and survival. Neurology 2006;67:761–765.

[70] Lo Coco D, Marchese S, La Bella V, Piccoli T, Lo Coco A. The amyotrophic lateral sclerosis functional rating scale predicts survival time in amyotrophic lateral sclerosis patients on invasive mechanical ventilation. Chest 2007;132:64–69.

[71] Lo Coco D, Marchese S, Lo Coco A. Recent advances in respiratory care for Motor Neuron Disease. In: Motor Neuron Disease Research Progress, Mancini RL (Ed.), 253269, Nova Science Publishers, Inc., New York, U.S.A., 2008. ISBN 978-60456-155-5.

[72] Lo Coco D, Mattaliano P, Spataro R, Mattaliano A, La Bella V. Sleep-wake disturbances in patients with amyotrophic lateral sclerosis. J Neurol Neurosurg Psychiatry 2011;82:839–842.

[73] Daniele Lo Coco, Paolo Volanti, Domenico De Cicco, Antonio Spanevello, Gianluca Battaglia, Santino Marchese, Alfonsa Claudia Taiello, Rossella Spataro and Vincenzo La Bella (2012). Assessment and Management of Respiratory Dysfunction in Patients with Amyotrophic Lateral Sclerosis, Amyotrophic Lateral Sclerosis, Prof. Martin Maurer (Ed.), ISBN: 978-953-307-806-9, InTech, Available from: http://www.intechopen.com/books/amyotrophic-lateral-sclerosis/assessment-and-management-of-respiratorydysfunction-in-patients-with-amyotrophic-lateral-sclerosis

[74] Salim Surani (2011). Diaphragmatic Pacemaker, Modern Pacemakers - Present and Future, Prof. Mithilesh R Das (Ed.), ISBN: 978-953-307-214-2, InTech, Available from:

http://www.intechopen.com/books/modernpacemakers-present-and-future/diaphragmatic-pacemaker

[75] Moreno-Igoa M, Calvo AC, Penas C, Manzano R, Oliván S, et al. Fragment C of tetanus toxin, more than a carrier. Novel perspectives in non-viral ALS gene therapy. J Mol Med (Berl). 2010 Mar;88(3):297–308.

[76] Ahmad Al Mutairy, Khalaf Al Moutaery, Abdulrahman Al Asmari, Mohammed Arshaduddin and MohammadTariq (2012). An Overview of Target Specific Neuro-Protective and Neuro-Restorative Strategies, Neurodegeneration, Dr. L. Miguel Martins (Ed.), ISBN: 978-953-51-0502-2, InTech, Available from:http://www.intechopen.com/books/neurodegeneration/an-overview-of-target-specific-neuro-protective-and-neuro-restorative-strategies

[77] Masatoshi Suzuki, Chak Foon Tso and Michael G. Meyer (2012). Stem Cell Application for Amyotrophic Lateral Sclerosis: Growth Factor Delivery and Cell Therapy, Amyotrophic Lateral Sclerosis, Prof. Martin Maurer (Ed.), ISBN: 978-953-307-806-9, InTech, Available from: http://www.intechopen.com/books/amyotrophiclateral-sclerosis/stem-cell-application-for-amyotrophic-lateral-sclerosis-growth-factor-delivery-and-cell-therapy

[78] Jari Koistinaho and Gundars Goldsteins (2012). Mutant Cu/Zn-Superoxide Dismutase Induced Mitochondrial Dysfunction in Amyotrophic Lateral Sclerosis, Amyotrophic Lateral Sclerosis, Prof. Martin Maurer (Ed.), ISBN: 978-953-307-806-9, InTech, Available from: http://www.intechopen.com/books/amyotrophic-lateralsclerosis/mutant-cu-zn-superoxide-dismutase-induced-mitochondrial-dysfunction-in-amyotrophic-lateral-sclerosis

[79] Helen R. Broom, Heather A. Primmer, Jessica A.O. Rumfeldt, Peter B. Stathopulos, Kenrick A. Vassall, Young-Mi Hwang and Elizabeth M. Meiering (2012). Folding and Aggregation of Cu, Zn-Superoxide Dismutase, Amyotrophic Lateral Sclerosis, Prof. Martin Maurer (Ed.), ISBN: 978-953-307-806-9, InTech, Available from:http://www.intechopen.com/books/amyotrophic-lateral-sclerosis/folding-and-aggregation-of-cu-zn-superoxide-dismutase

[80] Sasaki S, Warita H, Abe K, Iwata M. Impairment of axonal transport in the axon hillock and the initial segment of anterior horn neurons in transgenic mice with a G93A mutant SOD1 gene. Acta Europathol 2005;110(1):4856. ISSN: 21527806.

[81] Luz Diana Santa-Cruz, Uri Nimrod Ramírez-Jarquín and Ricardo Tapia (2012). Role of Mitochondrial Dysfunction in Motor Neuron Degeneration in ALS, Amyotrophic Lateral Sclerosis, Prof. Martin Maurer (Ed.) ISBN: 978-953-307-806-9, InTech, Available from: http://www.intechopen.com/books/amyotrophic-lateral-sclerosis/role-of-mitochondrial-dysfunction-in-motor-neuron-degeneration-in-als

[82] Kiaei M, Kipiani K, Petri S, Choi MK, Chen J, Beal MF, Integrative role of Cpla WITH cox-2 and the effect of non-steriodal anti-inflammatory drugs in a transgenic mouse

model of amyotrophic lateral sclerosis. J Neurochem 2005;93(2):403–411, ISSN: 0022-3042.

[83] Ilse Gijselinck, Kristel Sleegers, Christine Van Broeckhoven and Marc Cruts (2012). A Major Genetic Factor at Chromosome 9p Implicated in Amyotrophic Lateral Sclerosis (ALS) and Frontotemporal Lobar Degeneration (FTLD), Amyotrophic Lateral Sclerosis, Prof. Martin Maurer (Ed.), ISBN: 978-953-307-806-9, InTech, Available from: http://www.intechopen.com/books/amyotrophic-lateral-sclerosis/a-major-genetic-factor-at-chromosome9p-implicated-in-amyotrophic-lateral-sclerosis-als-and-frontote

[84] Max Koppers, Michael van Es, Leonard H. van den Berg, Jan H. Veldink and R. Jeroen Pasterkamp (2012). Genetics of Amyotrophic Lateral Sclerosis, Amyotrophic Lateral Sclerosis, Prof. Martin Maurer (Ed.), ISBN:978-953-307-806-9, InTech, Available from: http://www.intechopen.com/books/amyotrophic-lateral-sclerosis/genetics-of-als

[85] Emily F. Goodall, Joanna J. Bury, Johnathan Cooper-Knock, Pamela J. Shaw and Janine Kirby (2012). Genetics of Familial Amyotrophic Lateral Sclerosis, Amyotrophic Lateral Sclerosis, Prof. Martin Maurer (Ed.),ISBN: 978-953-307-806-9, InTech, Available from: http://www.intechopen.com/books/amyotrophic-lateral-sclerosis/genetics-of-familial-als

[86] Amanda M. Haidet-Phillips and Nicholas J. Maragakis (2012). Glial Cells as Therapeutic Targets for ALS, Amyotrophic Lateral Sclerosis, Prof. Martin Maurer (Ed.), ISBN: 978-953-307-806-9, InTech, Available from:http://www.intechopen.com/books/amyotrophic-lateral-sclerosis/glial-cells-as-therapeutic-targets-for-als

[87] Kim Staats and Ludo Van Den Bosch (2012). The Astrocytic Contribution in ALS: Inflammation and Excitotoxicity, Amyotrophic Lateral Sclerosis, Prof. Martin Maurer (Ed.), ISBN: 978-953-307-806-9, InTech, Available from: http://www.intechopen.com/books/amyotrophic-lateral-sclerosis/the-astrocytic-contribution-in-als-inflammation-and-excitotoxicity

[88] George E. Barreto, Janneth Gonzalez, Francisco Capani and Ludis Morales (2011). Role of Astrocytes in Neurodegenerative Diseases, Neurodegenerative Diseases - Processes, Prevention, Protection and Monitoring, Dr Raymond Chuen-Chung Chang (Ed.), ISBN: 978-953-307-485-6, InTech, Available from: http://www.intechopen.com/books/neurodegenerative-diseases-processes-prevention-protection-andmonitoring/role-of-astrocytes-in-neurodegenerative-diseases

[89] Lulé Dorothée and Ludolph Albert Christian (2011). Degeneration of the Human Nervous System and Magnetic Resonance Neuroimaging, Neuroimaging for Clinicians - Combining Research and Practice, Dr. Julio F. P. Peres (Ed.), ISBN: 978-953-307-450-4, InTech, Available from:http://www.intechopen.com/books/neuroimaging-for-clinicians-combining-research-and-practice/degeneration-of-the-human-nervous-system-and-magnetic-resonance-neuroimaging

Chapter 2

PET Imaging in ALS

Bart Swinnen, Koen Van Laere and
Philip Van Damme

Additional information is available at the end of the chapter

http://dx.doi.org/10.5772/63545

Abstract

Amyotrophic lateral sclerosis is a neurodegenerative disorder that primarily affects the motor system, but extramotor involvement is common. Progressive muscle weakness and wasting, including bulbar and respiratory muscles, limit survival to 2–5 years after disease onset in most patients. The diagnosis is made on clinical grounds and is based on the presence of signs of upper and lower motor neuron loss in different body regions in the absence of other pathologies that can explain the symptoms and signs of the patient. Making an accurate diagnosis can be difficult in early disease stages. ALS is a heterogeneous disorder with variability in age at onset, in phenotypic presentation, in the extent of frontotemporal involvement and in the disease progression rate. There is a high unmet medical need for objective markers that aid in early diagnosis and in predicting disease outcome. In this chapter, the current knowledge about the diagnostic and prognostic value of ^{18}F 2-fluoro-2-deoxy-D-glucose-PET in ALS is discussed. The potential of other targets and PET tracers to visualize different aspects of ALS disease pathology is described.

Keywords: amyotrophic lateral sclerosis, frontotemporal dementia, extramotor involvement, FDG PET, neuroinflammation, imaging biomarker

1. Introduction

Amyotrophic lateral sclerosis (ALS) is a relentlessly progressive disorder, however, with considerable variability in phenotype, disease progression and aetiology. Reliable prognostication regarding unusually fast or slow progression is difficult in clinical practice. Since diagnosis is often delayed until patients are already a year into their disease, pharmacological treatment with riluzole is often postponed as well. Numerous therapeutic clinical trials

INTECH
open science | open minds

© 2016 The Author(s). Licensee InTech. This chapter is distributed under the terms of the Creative Commons Attribution License (http://creativecommons.org/licenses/by/3.0), which permits unrestricted use, distribution, and reproduction in any medium, provided the original work is properly cited.

using other drugs have failed to show any benefit. These problems highlight the high need for reliable biomarkers in ALS. Ideally, such a biomarker should be easily accessible and affordable, as well as very sensitive and specific for ALS [1]. It should also be of prognostic value and should change with disease progression making it suitable for treatment monitoring [1]. Besides peripheral biomarkers in blood and cerebrospinal fluid, several neuroimaging biomarkers have been proposed, of which several nuclear or molecular imaging targets seem to be very promising. Although radionuclide imaging is not commonly used in clinical practice for ALS, recent studies suggest that various aspects of ALS pathology can be visualized and quantified.

1.1. ALS and FTD: two overlapping disorders

In ALS, the motor system is primarily affected [2]. Degeneration of upper motor neurons (UMNs) in motor cortex and lower motor neurons (LMNs) in the brain stem and spinal cord results in a progressive weakness and wasting of limb, bulbar and respiratory muscles, limiting survival to 2–5 years after disease onset.

In frontotemporal dementia (FTD), the degenerative process starts in the frontal and/or anterior temporal cortex [3]. Depending on the neuroanatomical regions affected, disease presentations include behavioural variant FTD (with changes in behaviour with apathy, loss of empathy, hyperorality, repetitive behaviours or disinhibition and executive dysfunction) or language variants of FTD (such as primary non-fluent aphasia and semantic dementia). The disease progressively affects other cognitive functions. Survival after disease onset ranges from 5 to 8 years.

ALS and FTD are considered to be extremes of a disease spectrum [4]. In about 10% of patients, both diseases co-occur. In another 30–40%, there is some degree of overlap, with mild motor involvement in patients with FTD, or mild cognitive/behavioural impairment in patients with ALS. About 50% of patients have pure FTD or pure ALS.

The only approved therapy for ALS is riluzole, which extends survival by only a few months, whereas for FTD no disease modifying therapies are available. The cornerstone of the management of patients with FTD/ALS remains multidisciplinary care and supportive measures.

Ten percent of ALS patients and 40% of FTD patients have a positive family history. Mutations in a heterogeneous set of genes have been identified to cause this familial form of FTD/ALS [5]. The inheritance pattern usually is autosomal dominant. Mutations in *SOD1, TARDBP* and *FUS* cause ALS and sometimes ALS-FTD, and mutations in *GRN* and *MAPT* cause FTD, but rarely also ALS. However, by far the most common cause for ALS, FTD/ALS and FTD is the recently discovered mutation in *C9ORF72* [6, 7]. It underlies 30–50% of familial ALS (and ALS-FTD) and 20–25% of familial FTD [8].

At the neuropathological level, an overlap between ALS and FTD is present as well. Especially, cytoplasmic accumulations of TDP-43, the protein encoded by the *TARDBP* gene, are central to the overlap between ALS and FTD, as most patients with sporadic ALS and about half of patients with sporadic FTD have such pathology (FTD/ALS-TDP-43) [9]. In addition, several of the genetic forms of FTD/ALS have TDP-43 aggregates, including mutations in *TARDBP*,

C9ORF72 and *GRN*. TDP-43 is an RNA-binding protein with important functions in gene transcription, splicing, RNA transport and stress granule formation. Accumulations of FUS, another RNA-binding protein, with many structural and functional similarities to TDP-43, is also central to FTD/ALS as mutations in *FUS* cause ALS, rarely FTD, and FUS pathology is also observed in about 5% of sporadic FTD patients.

It has thus become clear that ALS is a neurodegenerative disease that primarily affects the motor system, but that a variable degree of extramotor involvement is present in most patients [4].

For treating physicians and for family members, it is important to uncover cognitive problems in ALS, but it is not always easy to perform extensive neuropsychological testing in patients with motor impairments. An imaging biomarker that reliably recognizes and measures both motor and extramotor involvement in ALS patients would be an important achievement for the management of ALS patients and for ALS research.

1.2. Need for an upper motor neuron marker

The diagnosis of ALS requires the presence of both UMN and LMN signs. LMN signs are often readily appreciated on clinical examination and electromyography (EMG) is a very sensitive method to confirm this and even detect subclinical LMN involvement. On the contrary, providing evidence of UMN involvement can be challenging. First, the clinical signs of UMN involvement (hyperreflexia, spasticity, pseudobulbar features, Hoffman's reflex and extensor plantar response) exhibit both a low sensitivity and interrater reliability. Second, there are no reliable tests to show that UMN involvement exists. This lack of a reliable method to detect UMN involvement and track the progressive loss of UMNs is an important blind spot in the ALS field.

Various markers of UMN involvement have been proposed so far. First, the appearance of the motor cortex on magnetic resonance imaging (MRI) has been shown to be altered in ALS patients. At the group level, the thickness of the motor cortex is decreased, especially on 7T MRI [10]. However, at the individual patient level, a clear atrophy can only be demonstrated in around 50% of ALS patients because of considerable overlap with healthy controls [11, 12]. Other parameters like T2 hypointensity and increased quantitative susceptibility mapping (QSM) are present in a high proportion of ALS patients. It probably reflects gliosis due to activated microglia, but still lacks convincing sensitivity and specificity [10, 13, 14]. Second, the appearance of the corticospinal tract (CST) on MRI has also been proposed as a potential UMN marker. T2 hyperintensity of the CST in the posterior limb of the internal capsule is present in almost 50% of ALS patients, while it is absent in other studies [14, 15]. Since only severe hyperintensity seems to be clearly related with ALS and this occurs only late in the disease course, it is of no value in the (early) diagnosis of ALS [16]. Diffusion tensor imaging (DTI) of the CST seemed to be very promising at first, but unfortunately also turned out to lack sensitivity and specificity [16–18]. Third, the functional assessment of the motor cortex and CST by means of transcranial magnetic stimulation (TMS), with motor evoked potentials (MEP) being the most important parameter, has been investigated as a potential UMN biomarker. Literature data are unfortunately discordant: while several studies reported a cortical hypoexcitability [19, 20], others found a clear hyperexcitablity [11, 21, 22]. Moreover, several studies showed that TMS cannot discriminate ALS patients from controls [18, 23], so better methods to detect UMN loss in ALS are needed.

1.3. Need for a (differential) diagnostic test

An early and certain diagnosis of ALS is of utmost importance for clinicians and patients. It allows an early initiation of riluzole therapy (as yet the only proven disease-modifying therapy for ALS), an accurate communication about the diagnosis and an early recruitment into clinical trials. Especially, in these early stages of the disease, the disease process may be amenable to therapy.

However, in daily clinical practice, the time between symptom onset and diagnosis (the diagnostic delay) is long, estimated to be 12–14 months in tertiary ALS referral centres [24]. There are various reasons for this delay, including patients-specific and doctor-specific delays. Aspecific presentations and phenotypic variability at onset contributes to the delay. Observation of patients, with repeat clinical examinations and electrodiagnostic testing is a reliable method to correctly identify ALS patients that present early with only mild and focal motor symptoms, but this approach increases the diagnostic delay. Some cases pose a differential diagnostic problem with certain ALS mimicking diseases, also adding significantly to the diagnostic delay. Since most of these diseases lack abnormalities on CT or MRI imaging, they can impossibly be excluded by conventional imaging. Only a tool that allows to make a positive diagnosis of ALS early in the disease course could solve this problem.

1.4. Need for a prognostic marker

ALS is a heterogeneous disorder. Not only the genetic causes and the age at onset, but also the disease progression is highly variable. The median survival after disease onset is only 33 months and most patients die 2–5 years after disease onset. However, numerous cases of extremely long and extremely short survival have been reported, making up the extreme ends of a wide prognostic spectrum [25]. Making a reliable prognostic estimation is pivotal for both patients and their families and neurologists likewise, but still largely impossible these days. A variety of prognostic factors has been identified, such as age of onset, site of onset, rate of symptom progression, comorbid frontotemporal involvement and nutritional and respiratory status [26–31]. Although they are clearly of value, they all reflect divergent clinical disease parameters and do not directly reflect the underlying disease process. The first prognostic models taking into account the different known prognostic factors are underway [32]. Other, more pathophysiologically relevant biomarkers, such as pNFH levels [33, 34], seem to be promising. But also imaging biomarkers that reliably reflect the extent of motor and extramotor involvement have the potential to become a reliable prognostic determinant.

1.5. Need for an in vivo marker of ALS pathophysiology

Conventional neuroimaging has only revealed gross pathological insights by showing atrophy of the motor cortex and alterations of the CST. These imaging modalities can reveal structural

http://dx.doi.org/10.5772/63545

changes in ALS at the group level with high spatial resolution. However, they lack the capacity to provide a reflection of the neuropathological process at the cellular or molecular level and are not applicable at the individual patient level. Imaging biomarkers that can visualize ALS disease pathology, such as neuroinflammation, neuronal death and ideally TDP-43 accumulation would greatly advance the field of ALS research. It would not only be valuable for diagnostic purposes, but would also be useful to monitor the evolution of disease over time and as a readout for treatment effects of disease-modifying therapies.

So far, positron emission tomography (PET) has not been commonly used in ALS. However, recent studies show that various radioligands have potential to be useful imaging biomarkers in ALS. These can be of value in the diagnosis, in predicting outcome and in imaging disease pathology in ALS. In this chapter, an overview of the PET studies in ALS is given and future perspectives on the use of PET in ALS are discussed. On overview of all tracers used in ALS

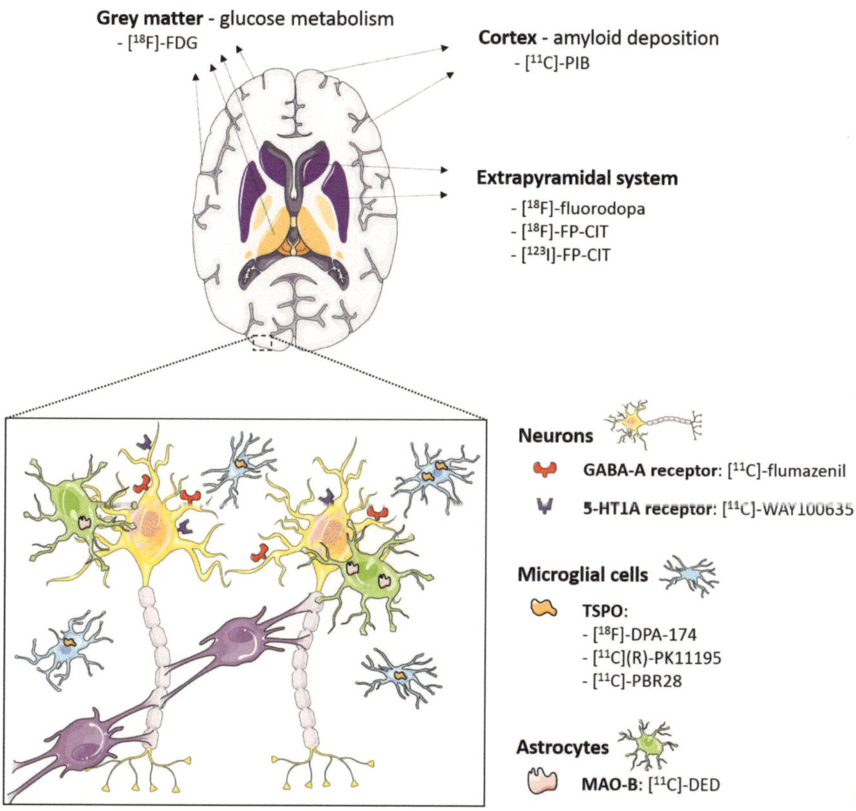

Figure 1. PET tracers used in ALS. Using PET imaging six different neurological systems or cell populations can be assessed using different tracers. General glucose metabolism in the grey matter is assessed by [^{18}F]-FDG. Cortical amyloid deposition can be assessed using [^{11}C]-PIB to distinguish ALS from Alzheimer's disease. The extrapyramidal system can be investigated using [^{18}F]-fluorodopa, [^{18}F]-FPCIT or [^{123}I]-FP-CIT. Neuronal integrity can be visualized using tracers for the GABA-A receptor ([^{11}C]-flumazenil) or the 5-HT1A receptor ([^{11}C]-WAY100635). Microglial cells can be highlighted using tracers targeting the translocator protein (TSPO), like [^{18}F]-DPA-174, [^{11}C]-(R)-PK11195 or [^{11}C]-PBR28. Astrocytes are visualized by tracers for the MAO-B enzyme ([^{11}C]-DED).

so far is provided in **Figure 1**. Apart from the commonly used tracers for indirect neuronal functioning, such as glucose metabolism ([^{18}F]-FDG) and perfusion, more specific receptor or protein deposition tracers used in other neurodegenerative diseases, like Parkinson's disease ([^{18}F]-FP-CIT) and Alzheimer's disease ([^{11}C]-PIB), have also been investigated in ALS patients. Recently, tracers with an affinity for specific cell types, like neurons ([11C]-flumazenil, [11C]-WAY100635), microglial cells (TSPO ligands) and astrocytes ([11C]-DED), can also highlight specific pathophysiological processes of ALS.

2. FDG PET imaging in ALS

2.1. Early FDG PET and perfusion SPECT studies revealed widespread cortical abnormalities

In the 1980s and 1990s of the previous century a mere handful of studies investigated a small number of ALS patients using ^{18}F-2-fluoro-2-deoxy-D-glucose PET (FDG PET) imaging. The common denominator of their findings was a generalized cerebral hypometabolism [35–37]. Despite the low spatial resolution of the PET scanners at the time, some studies did reveal a predominance for the motor cortex [36] and even provided preliminary evidence for frontal hypometabolism [37, 38] which was even related to clinical cognitive impairment in one study. A few studies assessing cerebral perfusion using SPECT imaging confirmed a predominant involvement of the motor cortex with extensive frontal hypoperfusion, often related to cognitive impairment [39–41]. These pilot studies were instrumental in redirecting the view of ALS as a disease exclusively affecting motor neurons towards a multisystem neurodegenerative disease as generally accepted nowadays.

2.2. Regions involved on recent FDG PET imaging

More recent FDG PET studies in ALS patients, using the next-generation PET scanners with higher spatial resolution, could confirm the presence of hypometabolism in the primary motor cortex, which is hence thought to be the signature of ALS on FDG PET imaging [42–44]. Besides the primary motor cortex, other peri-Rolandic regions like the premotor cortex and primary sensory cortex have been found to be affected on FDG PET [42–45]. In keeping with the clinical and pathophysiological overlap with FTD, several prefrontal (dorsolateral prefrontal cortex, orbitofrontal cortex, anterior frontal cortex) and temporal (anterior temporal lobe, fusiform gyrus) regions frequently display hypometabolism in ALS patients [42–45]. Some studies even report hypometabolism of primary and associative visual cortices in ALS patients [42, 45]. Examples of typical FDG PET patterns seen in ALS are given in **Figure 2**. Patient 1 is an example of an ALS patient with modest hypometabolism in the peri-Rolandic areas on FDG PET. In patient 2, extensive hypometabolism in the motor cortex can be noted. In about 10% of patients, extensive regions of hypometabolism are also present in the frontal and/or anterior temporal lobes. Patient 3 is an example of an ALS patients with extensive areas of hypometabolism in the frontal areas. Patient 4 has pronounced anterior temporal hypometabolism.

http://dx.doi.org/10.5772/63545

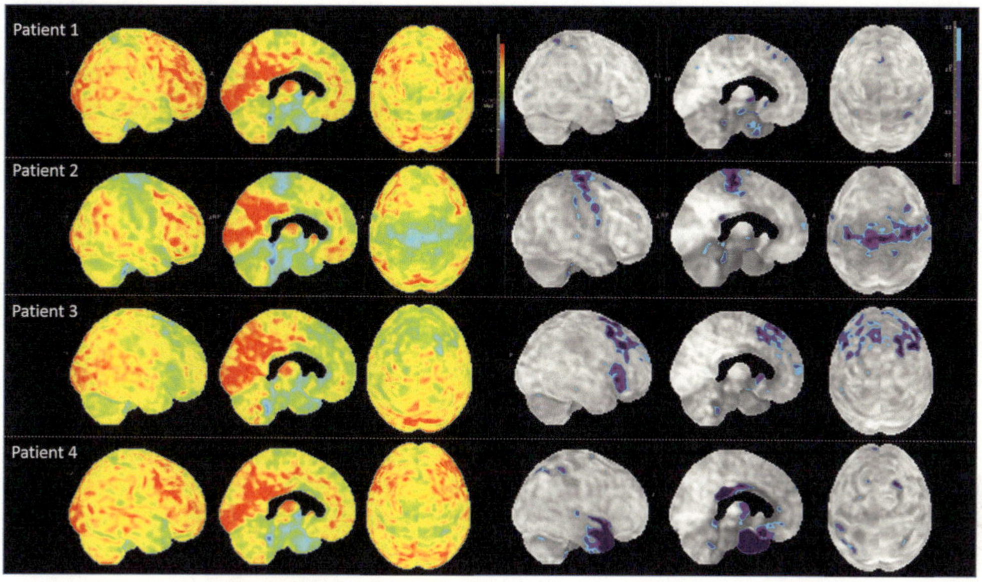

Figure 2. Commonly affected regions on FDG PET in ALS patients. Three regions frequently and typically display hypometabolism on FDG PET in ALS patients; motor cortex, prefrontal cortex and anterior temporal lobe. The three left images depict the stereotactic surface projections of brain FDG PET uptake. The three images on the right show the corresponding Z-score images (comparing patient to healthy volunteers). In patient 1 and 2, hypometabolism in the Rolandic area (including parts of the motor cortex) is noted. While this is only mild in patient 1, patient 2 has extensive hypometabolism. In patient 3, an obvious hypometabolism in the prefrontal cortex is noted. In patient 4, extensive hypometabolism of the anterior temporal lobe is noted.

Recently, several studies also reported the presence of (relative) hypermetabolism on FDG PET in certain regions. Hypermetabolism in ALS patients seems to be most obvious in the infratentorial region, like midbrain, pons and cerebellum [44–46]. This hypermetabolism is thought to be the reflection of increased astrocytosis along the course of the CST [45]. Also, hypermetabolism in mesial temporal structures, like hippocampus and amygdala, has been reported [44, 45].

2.3. Detection of frontotemporal involvement on FDG PET

As explained above, a clear link between ALS and FTD has been established over the last years. This is also backed up by the early studies showing frontotemporal hypometabolism using FDG PET and rCBF measures [37, 38]. Based on the extent of frontotemporal versus motor neuron involvement, patients across the ALS-FTD spectrum can be divided into five categories [47]. Pure ALS (without any evident cognitive abnormality) and pure FTD (without any obvious motor abnormality) are located at the opposite ends of this spectrum. Patients who meet diagnostic criteria for both ALS as FTD are considered to have 'ALS-FTD'. ALS patients with mild behavioural dysfunction are classified as having ALS with behavioural impairment ('ALSbi'), whereas patients with mild executive and language dysfunction are said to have ALS with cognitive impairment ('ALSci'). Patients with a diagnosis of FTD and some motor neuron involvement are said to have 'FTD-MND'.

The signature of frontotemporal involvement on PET imaging constitutes hypometabolism mainly focused on the prefrontal cortex, often extending to the entire frontal cortex and anterior temporal cortex and even to the thalamus [48, 49]. Contrary to FTD patients, this frontotemporal hypometabolism is often more symmetric in ALS-FTD patients [49]. Importantly, this hypometabolism is often already present in otherwise normal frontotemporal lobes on MRI, leading to the general view that hypometabolism precedes atrophy [50]. This makes FDG PET a very sensitive tool to detect frontotemporal involvement even in a very early clinical stage. Hence, frontotemporal hypometabolism on FDG PET has extensive potential to become an important diagnostic marker, and this independently from hypometabolism in the primary motor cortex.

Several studies performing both PET imaging as neuropsychological testing in ALS patients found a correlation between extent of frontotemporal hypometabolism and neuropsychological performance [37, 38, 43]. A recent large study indeed confirmed that ALS patients with mild cognitive impairment ('ALSci') exhibit moderate frontotemporal hypometabolism, which is clearly more pronounced in real 'ALS-FTD' patients and less pronounced to even absent in 'pure ALS' patients [48]. So, when patients are stratified along the ALS-FTD spectrum, there seems to be a proportionate correlation between clinical cognitive involvement and frontotemporal hypometabolism on PET imaging.

Frontotemporal hypometabolism on PET not only has the potential to become a diagnostic marker, it has also been shown to provide important prognostic information. In a considerably large study of ALS patients, extensive prefrontal hypometabolism was associated with significantly shorter survival [51].

2.4. FDG PET as a (differential) diagnostic marker

Extensive studies demonstrating high diagnostic accuracy are a prerequisite for any imaging biomarker to become incorporated into the diagnostic criteria of ALS. Recently, four large studies assessed the sensitivity and specificity of FDG PET in ALS patients compared to healthy controls. The first study made use of a 'region of interest method' [42]. When all brain regions were taken into account, FDG PET was able to discriminate ALS patients from controls with a sensitivity of 89% and specificity of 82.5%. When only a specific set of regions was used, an even higher sensitivity (95%) with the same specificity (82.5%) could be obtained. The second study analysed FDG PET images using a method evaluating disease-specific spatial patterns on a voxel-based manner, trying to disclose the networks with the highest diagnostic value [52]. When all relevant networks were taken into account an astonishing accuracy of 99.0% was achieved. Remarkably, when only the most discriminating network (i.e. bilateral cerebellum and midbrain) was used, accuracy was still 96.3%. The third study reported an accuracy of 89.7% using a VOI-based discriminant analysis, further increasing to 95% if a discriminant analysis based on a support vector machine (SVM) approach was used [44]. In the fourth study, a prospective validation of the diagnostic algorithm based on SVM was carried out in 105 novel cases and a sensitivity and specificity of 100% was obtained [51]. All these studies suggest that FDG PET is a very sensitive marker of ALS pathology that can be used in a clinical setting.

http://dx.doi.org/10.5772/63545

There is, however, one major limitation of these studies. While these studies report a high sensitivity using healthy controls, it is clear specificity may be lower since ALS patients need to be discriminated from patients with ALS mimicking diseases. Unfortunately, no large studies using FDG PET in such disease mimics exist. A study performing FDG PET in ten patients with Kennedy's disease even surprisingly revealed the presence of frontal hypometabolism [53]. This means that FDG PET may be insufficient to discriminate ALS from certain ALS mimicking diseases.

2.5. FDG PET as a prognostic marker

Besides its capacities as a diagnostic marker, FDG PET is increasingly proposed as a potential marker for prognosis. So far, only two studies assessed the value of FDG PET in predicting the prognosis of ALS [44]. Assessing 70 ALS patients, extensive prefrontal hypometabolism was associated with a significantly shorter survival. This is in line with previous studies that reported concomitant clinical FTD or cognitive/behavioural impairment with a worse prognosis [4]. More recently, a larger prospectively collected cohort of 175 (including the initial 70 patients) was studied [51]. It was confirmed with longer follow-up that extensive hypometabolism in the prefrontal or anterior temporal lobe was associated with a shorter survival. In a Cox regression, taking into account other prognostic factors, such as age of onset, site of onset, diagnostic delay, FVC and slope in the ALS FRS-R, extensive frontotemporal hypometabolism was significantly correlated with shortened survival (**Figure 3**).

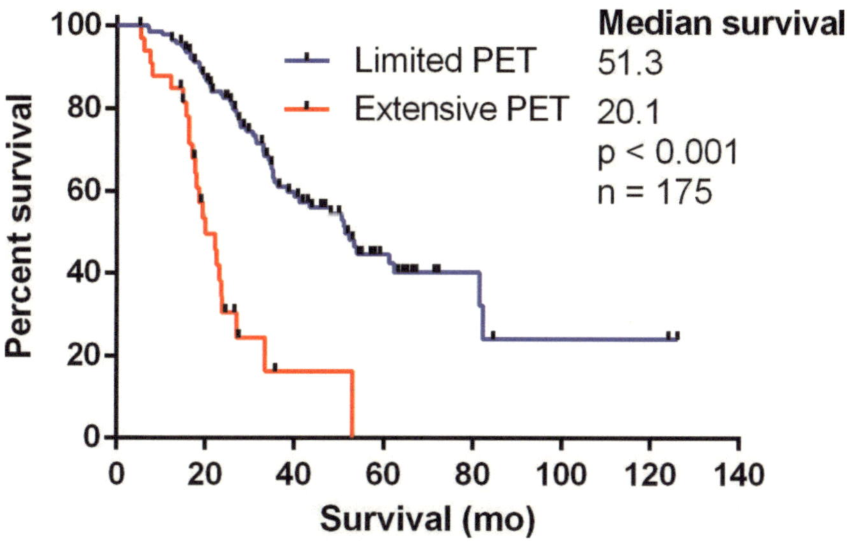

Figure 3. Relation of ALS survival with degree of frontotemporal hypometabolism. Kaplan-Meier survival plot of all ALS patients (ALS group 1 + ALS group 2) with (red line, n = 34) and without (blue line, n = 141) extensive hypometabolism in the frontal and/or temporal cortex (n = 175, p < 0.001) (This research was originally published in *JNM*. Van Weehaege et al. prospective validation of 18F-FDG brain PET discriminant analysis methods in the diagnosis of amyotrophic lateral sclerosis. *J Nucl Med*. 2016;vol:pp-pp. © by the Society of Nuclear Medicine and Molecular Imaging, Inc.) [51].

3. Other tracers

3.1. Tracers assessing the extrapyramidal system

The exact role of the extrapyramidal system in the pathophysiology of ALS is still under debate. Although several large clinical studies reported the increased presence of extrapyramidal symptoms and signs (increased tonus, postural instability and backward falls) in ALS patients [54, 55], others even reported an increased incidence of Parkinson's disease in the ALS population [56]. The presence of extrapyramidal symptoms in ALS is correlated with the presence of a hexanucleotide repeat expansion in *C9orf72* in many patients [57, 58]. PET studies have tried to make a significant contribution in elucidating a possible link between ALS and extrapyramidal symptoms.

[^{18}F]-fluorodopa was one of the first radioligands used to assess the integrity of the nigrostriatal tract with PET by quantifying dopadecarboxylase activity presynaptically, while nowadays dopamine transporter imaging due to its better access using [^{123}I]-FP-CIT SPECT is the most widely used method to assess the extrapyramidal system. More novel and specific tracers such as [^{18}F]-PE2I for PET dopamine transporters are already in use at several centres worldwide [59].

Literature data regarding extrapyramidal radionuclide imaging in ALS patients is still sporadic and seems to be discordant. While two earlier studies reported a dopaminergic deficit in sporadic and familial ALS patients without clinical extrapyramidal disease [60, 61], this was contradicted in a more recent small study investigating ALS patients with concomitant clinical parkinsonism ('ALS-parkinsonism') [62]. Another study did report dopaminergic deficits in two ALS-parkinsonism patients assessed by [^{18}F]-FP-CIT PET [63]. These discrepancies are believed to be due to the heterogeneity of ALS-parkinsonism, and larger datasets are needed.

While in some cases the extrapyramidal signs are thought to be caused by true degeneration of the extrapyramidal system, in other cases, they are believed to be the result of cortical lesions. The latter concept is confirmed by a more recent study investigating UMN-ALS patients using [^{123}I]-FP-CIT SPECT [64]. While a dopaminergic deficit was indeed evident in the majority of patients which even correlated with disease duration, there was no correlation with functional extrapyramidal scores (like UPDRS). This means that, although the neuropathological process in ALS extends towards the extrapyramidal system, some of the extrapyramidal signs noted in ALS patients are probably due to spasticity, which is a typical UMN feature.

3.2. Tracers for neuroinflammation

Neurons rely on several supportive cells, commonly named glial cells, to survive and exert their normal function. These glial cells, including astrocytes, microglia and oligodendrocytes, provide nutritional and trophic support to neurons, especially motor neurons. ALS is characterized by a neuroinflammatory reaction consisting of an activation of astrocytes and microglia. Several studies using ALS animal models have taught us that dysfunction of these cell types significantly contributes to motor neuron death, independent of intrinsic motor neuron dysfunction, leading to the view of ALS as a non-cell autonomous disease [65].

Two targets have been used to visualize this 'neuroinflammation' in ALS patients using radionuclide imaging. [^{11}C]-DED, a deprenyl derivative, selectively binds the MAO-B enzyme which is primarily though not exclusively located in astrocytes. Because of the high background activity of this ligand and newer derivatives, they are limited to research applications. The second, more frequently used target is the activated microglial cell, the macrophages of the central nervous system [66]. One of the most studied targets for activated microglia is the translocator protein (TSPO), a mitochondrial protein that is highly overexpressed in activated microglia [67]. Several radioligands such as [^{11}C]-(R)-PK11195, [^{18}F]-DPA-174 and [^{11}C]-PBR28 can be used to quantify TSPO binding.

The major finding in TSPO PET studies in ALS is an increased binding in the motor cortex, highlighting this region as the primary focus of neuropathology [68–70]. The degree of neuroinflammation in the motor cortex is positively correlated with clinical UMN scores and probably negatively correlated with ALS-FRS. Other frequently involved regions are the prefrontal cortex, thalamus, pons and CST [68–71]. The latter two probably reflect the secondary neuroinflammation due to degeneration of the CST. Interestingly, some studies have shown that the inflammation can be detected on the individual patient level.

Thus, PET imaging assessing neuroinflammation has a high potential to become a specific UMN marker which can be used at the single patient level. Moreover, it could be an interesting method to monitor the effect of treatment selectively targeting the neuroinflammatory process.

3.3. Tracers reflecting neuronal loss and/or dysfunction

Although the neurodegenerative process in ALS is non-cell autonomous, markers of selective motor neuron death would be of significant value. FDG PET assesses glucose metabolism in general, hence encompassing various processes like neuronal dysfunction, atrophy, microgliosis and astrocytosis. Therefore, the capabilities of FDG PET to selectively assess motor neuron degeneration are limited.

Two tracers have been used so far to specifically assess neuronal loss and/or dysfunction. [^{11}C]-flumazenil, which selectively binds GABA-A receptors expressed by neurons, is the most widely used. It is, however, unclear whether this ligand primarily visualizes pyramidal neurons (like motor neurons) or interneurons. Although an early study reported an almost generalized decreased signal in the cortex [72], more recent studies revealed a more selected involvement of primary motor and motor association cortices, which was even correlated with a clinical UMN score [73, 74]. One study used the radioligand [^{11}C]-WAY100635 targeting the 5-HT1A serotonin receptor which is expressed in pyramidal neurons [75]. They also reported a generalized cortical decrease, which was most pronounced in the motor cortex and frontotemporal regions.

So, these neuronal radioligands seem to be able to specifically highlight the primary pathophysiological process of ALS, which is degeneration and dysfunction of the UMNs. Hence, it seems promising to further investigate the diagnostic and prognostic value of these potential UMN markers.

4. Correlation with phenotype

4.1. ALS subtypes

The pattern of motor neuron involvement in ALS is highly heterogeneous. Depending on the relative upper and LMN involvement and depending on the neuroanatomical region within the motor system with the most extensive pathology, different subtypes of motor neuron degeneration have been defined. While in some patients UMN features (spasticity, hyperreflexia) dominate the clinical picture, LMN features prevail in other patients. It remains unclear if the pure UMN disorder, PLS (primary lateral sclerosis), and the pure LMN disorder, progressive muscular atrophy (PMA), should be regarded as separate disease entities or merely as the extreme ends of the ALS spectrum [25]. Similarly, the site of onset is also highly variable, with onset in a limb ('spinal onset') being more frequent than onset in the bulbar musculature ('bulbar onset') [25]. The neuroimaging signature of these subtypes has not yet been extensively studied using PET. The challenge will be to find commonalities and differential representations of the different endophenotypes.

4.1.1. PLS and Mills' syndrome

PLS is a variant of ALS with selective UMN signs for several years [76]. Mills' syndrome is an unusual unilateral variant of PLS, which eventually spreads to the contralateral side after a variable time period [25]. On postmortem examination, there is no difference in the essential pathological processes (e.g. TDP-43 positive intraneuronal inclusions) [77]. However, to explain this phenotypic variability, there must be a difference in the focal initiation and spreading pattern of the neurodegeneration. PET imaging has several advantages to assess this question, like in vivo usability and availability of specific tracers. Unfortunately, since no large studies investigating PET in PLS/Mills' patients have been undertaken so far, we need to rely on a handful of small case series. Four studies in PLS patients performed either FDG PET or [^{11}C]-flumazenil PET and mainly found similar abnormalities as seen in ALS patients [44, 51, 78, 79]. However, in one study involvement of the primary motor cortex seemed to be more severe than in pure ALS [79]. On the other hand, some specific regions like the prefrontal cortex and posterior cingulate seem to be spared in PLS [44, 78]. So, based on these PET findings, neuropathology in PLS may be more restricted to the motor cortex.

Only five cases of Mills' patients with PET imaging have been reported so far. While one patient had an asymmetric involvement of the motor cortices, an almost unilateral pattern of hypometabolism (FDG PET) or hypercaptation (TSPO radioligand) has been noticed in the four remaining patients [80–82]. So, compared to PLS, neuropathology in Mills' syndrome seems to be focused even more on one unilateral motor cortex, suggesting a more restricted contiguous spread of disease in this endophenotype.

4.1.2. PMA

PMA is a motor neuron disease with selective involvement of the LMN, and probably has to be seen as an unusual variant of ALS [25]. Literature regarding FDG PET in PMA patients is very limited. Only two early studies performing FDG PET in ALS patients performed a subanalysis in patients with only LMN signs. In keeping with the clinical absence of UMN signs, no to only very mild cerebral hypometabolism is present in these patients [35, 36]. Larger studies are required to establish if peri-Rolandic hypometabolism is present in a proportion of PMA patients and if this predicts progression to ALS or disease outcome.

In comparison, a few MRI-based imaging studies investigating UMN involvement in PMA remained inconclusive as well. One study found no evidence for thinning of the motor cortex on high-resolution MRI [83]. While one study found modest though clear abnormalities of the CST on DTI imaging [84], this was contradicted by another earlier study [85]. Finally, an fMRI study revealed modest prefrontal activation abnormalities in PMA patients [86].

So based on several imaging modalities, it is so far unclear whether significant measurable UMN involvement is present in all PMA patients.

4.1.3. Spinal versus bulbar

In most ALS patients, the disease starts with asymmetric weakness of a limb, and hence, this classical form of ALS is called 'spinal onset ALS'. In about 20% of ALS patients, however, weakness starts in the bulbar muscles, this form is called 'bulbar onset ALS' [25]. While both endophenotypes clearly have a distinct disease initiation and disease course, they eventually converge into a common phenotype of generalized weakness. The pathological substrates underlying these initial differences are largely not understood. PET imaging has tried to elucidate some aspects of this enigma.

While one study using FDG PET suggested a differential pattern of involvement between spinal and bulbar onset ALS in frontal and parietal regions [45], this was not confirmed by others [42]. A study investigating perfusion (regional cerebral blood flow, rCBF) in ALS patients reported a significantly lower rCBF of the frontal lobe in bulbar onset patients compared to spinal onset [87]. Based on TSPO PET imaging, one study found evidence for increased neuroinflammation in the brainstem of bulbar onset ALS patients, whereas neuroinflammation in the motor cortex seemed to be less pronounced [70]. So, the specific functional imaging correlate of these two endophenotypes has not been clearly established yet.

4.2. Severity of disease

An independent objective marker for severity and spreading pattern of disease pathology is highly needed. None of the imaging biomarkers so far has been able to reflect local disease severity and disease spreading in a longitudinal fashion. A limited amount of studies investigated the link between PET imaging and clinical scores. First, although several FDG PET studies in ALS patients found no correlation with parameters of disease severity in general, one study did reveal a correlation of prefrontal hypometabolism with a reduced ALS-FRS R (ALS functional rating scale revised version) [44]. Second, PET imaging of microglia, via TSPO radioligands, was not correlated with ALS-FRS R in two studies [68, 69]. However, one of these studies found a relation with clinical burden of UMN signs [68]. Third, abnormalities on [^{11}C]-flumazenil PET in one study was not correlated with ALS-FRS, whereas it was associated with the UMN score [74]. So in general, findings with the currently available PET targets show very little, if any, clear correlation with clinical severity of disease. Longitudinal studies are required to find out if PET imaging is of value in tracking disease progression.

5. Correlation with genotype

While most cases of ALS are sporadic, about 10% are caused by a variety of genetic deficits, with alterations in the *C9orf72* and *SOD1* gene being the most frequent and most studied [88]. A few PET studies have been performed in genetic subtypes of ALS.

5.1. C9orf72

Two recent studies investigated 26 patients in total with *C9orf72*-related ALS using FDG PET and found in general more severe hypometabolism [44, 46]. Remarkably, both studies also reported hypometabolism in the thalamus and parts of the limbic system to be present almost uniquely in *C9orf72* patients. An example of FDG PET findings in a *C9orf72* ALS patient is

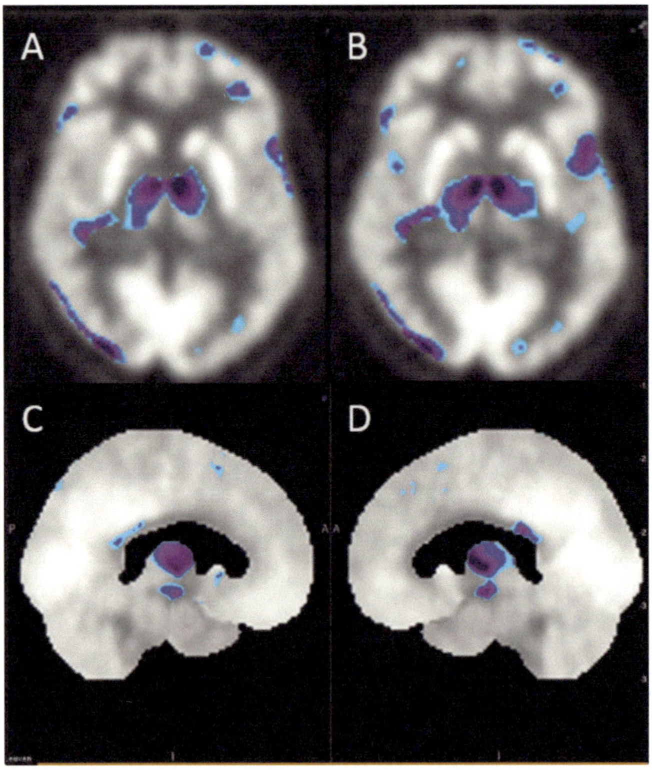

Figure 4. PET abnormalities in a C9orf72 ALS patient. Example of Z-score images of FDG PET imaging of a *C9orf72* patient with ALS revealing a remarkable hypometabolism of the thalamus, as noted on axial (A and B) and sagittal (C and D) sections.

provided in **Figure 4**. This involvement of thalamus, extrapyramidal system and limbic system is probably the neuroanatomical correlate of the increased incidence of phenocopies of several other neurodegenerative diseases in *C9orf72* mutation carriers. Among others, phenocopies of Parkinson's disease, Huntington's disease, corticobasal degeneration, Alzheimer's disease and several neuropsychiatric diseases (psychosis, schizophrenia) have been reported in *C9orf72* mutation carriers [57].

5.2. SOD1 (D90A)

Worldwide, the D90A is the most common *SOD1* mutation, although it is not the most studied one [89]. This mutation can be inherited in an autosomal recessive or dominant way, which is quite unusual in ALS. Two studies performing [^{11}C]-Flumazenil-PET in a total of 21 D90A patients revealed that these patients showed a specific pattern of reduced tracer binding confined to the left frontotemporal junction and anterior cingulate gyrus, without involvement of the motor and premotor cortices [73, 74]. Larger studies on other *SOD1* mutations or other genetic subtypes of ALS are largely lacking.

6. Future perspectives

More than a decade PET imaging has seen a revival in the ALS field using either new hardware and software technologies or novel tracers. In the near future, PET will hopefully find applications in both clinical practices, namely clinical trials and neurobiological research.

First, PET imaging could become of value in the ALS diagnosis in the future. Although conventional imaging (e.g. MRI) is only intended to rule out other diseases, FDG PET has the potential to be used as a positive argument to make a diagnosis of ALS at the single patient level. Both hypometabolism in the motor cortex as in the frontotemporal cortex will be of diagnostic value and could be considered to incorporate in clinical criteria for ALS, similar to the inclusion of frontotemporal hypometabolism in the diagnostic criteria of FTD [90]. However, additional research comparing ALS patients with ALS mimicking diseases is needed to reliably assess the sensitivity and especially the specificity in the real-life clinical setting of early diagnosis.

Second, PET imaging will be further investigated as a biomarker of disease. More studies assessing the correlation with severity of disease need to be undertaken. Similarly, more longitudinal studies are needed to relate early PET abnormalities with clinical course, hopefully fulfilling the high need for a prognostic marker in the clinic.

Third, PET imaging could become valuable in clinical trials of ALS patients. By increasing the diagnostic yield, especially early in the disease, it will be possible to include patients early after disease onset, hence increasing the power to obtain positive results in pharmaceutical trials. Additionally, several tracers (neuroinflammation, neuronal loss …) could be used as a read out to demonstrate target engagement or even to assess the effect of treatments. Of particular interest, a tracer for TDP-43 would revolutionize the field, as PET detection and quantification of misfolded proteins have done in Alzheimer's disease with beta-amyloid and tau imaging.

Fourth, tracers assessing neuroinflammation will be further investigated, and aside from TSPO other targets such as type 2 cannabinoid receptors, the purinergic receptor P2X7, and matrix metalloproteinases are investigated currently. The power of protein or receptor tracers mainly lies in the selectivity of their target, that is they selectively reflect one aspect of ALS pathogenesis which increases with disease progression. Hence, in contrast to FDG PET which reflects general glucose metabolism, these tracers have the potential to be used as 'positive tracers' for disease severity and progression. They are also of high interest to gain insight in the pathophysiology of ALS. Probably, several tracers assessing other aspects of ALS pathology will be developed and investigated as well.

Author details

Bart Swinnen[1,2], Koen Van Laere[3] and Philip Van Damme[1,2*]

*Address all correspondence to: philip.vandamme@uzleuven.be

1 KU Leuven – University of Leuven, Department of Neurosciences, VIB – Vesalius Research Center, Experimental Neurology – Laboratory of Neurobiology, Leuven, Belgium

2 University Hospitals Leuven, Department of Neurology, Leuven, Belgium

3 University Hospitals Leuven, Department of Nuclear Medicine, Leuven, Belgium

References

[1] Turner MR, Kiernan MC, Leigh PN, Talbot K. Biomarkers in amyotrophic lateral sclerosis. Lancet Neurol 2009;8:94–109. doi:10.1016/S1474-4422(08)70293-X.

[2] Rowland LP. Amyotrophic lateral sclerosis. NEJM 2001;344:1688–700.

[3] Neary D, Snowden J, Mann D. Frontotemporal dementia. Lancet Neurol 2005;4:771–80. doi:10.1016/S1474-4422(05)70223-4.

[4] Phukan J, Pender NP, Hardiman O. Cognitive impairment in amyotrophic lateral sclerosis. Lancet Neurol 2007;6:994–1003.

[5] Al-Chalabi A, Jones A, Troakes C, King A, Al-Sarraj S, van den Berg LH. The genetics and neuropathology of amyotrophic lateral sclerosis. Acta Neuropathol 2012;124:339–52. doi:10.1007/s00401-012-1022-4.

[6] DeJesus-Hernandez M, Mackenzie IR, Boeve BF, Boxer AL, Baker M, Rutherford NJ, et al. Expanded GGGGCC hexanucleotide repeat in noncoding region of C9ORF72 causes

chromosome 9p-linked FTD and ALS. Neuron 2011;72:245–56. doi:10.1016/j.neuron.2011.09.011.

[7] Renton AE, Majounie E, Waite A, Simón-sánchez J, Rollinson S, Gibbs JR, et al. A hexanucleotide repeat expansion in C9ORF72 is the cause of chromosome 9p21-linked ALS-FTD. Neuron 2011;72:257–68. doi:10.1016/j.neuron.2011.09.010.A.

[8] Majounie E, Renton AE, Mok K, Dopper EGP, Waite A, Rollinson S, et al. Frequency of the C9orf72 hexanucleotide repeat expansion in patients with amyotrophic lateral sclerosis and frontotemporal dementia: a cross-sectional study. Lancet Neurol 2012;11:323–30. doi:10.1016/S1474-4422(12)70043-1.

[9] Neumann M, Sampathu DM, Kwong LK, Truax AC, Micsenyi MC, Chou TT, et al. Ubiquitinated TDP-43 in frontotemporal lobar degeneration and amyotrophic lateral sclerosis. Science 2006;314:130–3. doi:10.1126/science.1134108.

[10] Cosottini XM, Donatelli XG, Costagli XM, Ienco XEC, Frosini XD, Pesaresi XI, et al. High-resolution 7T MR imaging of the motor cortex in amyotrophic lateral sclerosis. Am J Neuroradiol 2016;37:1–7. doi:10.3174/ajnr.A4562.

[11] Grieve SM, Menon P, Korgaonkar MS, Gomes L, Foster S, Kiernan MC, et al. Potential structural and functional biomarkers of upper motor neuron dysfunction in ALS. Amyotroph Lateral Scler Front Degener 2015;8421:1–8. doi: 10.3109/21678421.2015.1074707.

[12] Walhout R, Westeneng H-J, Verstraete E, Hendrikse J, Veldink JH, van den Heuvel MP, et al. Cortical thickness in ALS: towards a marker for upper motor neuron involvement. J Neurol Neurosurg Psychiatry 2014;86:1–7. doi:10.1136/jnnp-2013-306839.

[13] Schweitzer AD, Liu T, Zheng K, Seedial S, Gupta A, Shtilbans A, et al. Quantitative Susceptibility Mapping (QSM) for characterization of the motor cortex in amyotrophic lateral sclerosis (ALS) and other motor neuron diseases. 2nd Int Work MRI Phase Contrast Quant Susceptibility Mapp 2013:154–7. doi:10.2214/AJR.14.13459.

[14] Cervo A, Cocozza S, Saccà F, Giorgio S, Morra V, Tedeschi E, et al. The combined use of conventional MRI and MR spectroscopic imaging increases the diagnostic accuracy in amyotrophic lateral sclerosis. Eur J Radiol 2015;84:151–7.

[15] Kono Y, Sengoku R, Mitsumura H, Bono K, Sakuta K, Yamasaki M, et al. Clinical characteristics associated with corticospinal tract hyperintensity on magnetic resonance imaging in patients with amyotrophic lateral sclerosis. Clin Neurol Neurosurg 2014;127:1–4.

[16] Protogerou G, Ralli S, Tsougos I, Patramani I, Hadjigeorgiou G, Fezoulidis I, et al. T2 FLAIR increased signal intensity at the posterior limb of the internal capsule: clinical significance in ALS patients. Neuroradiol J 2011;24:226–34.

[17] Rajagopalan V, Allexandre D, Yue G, Pioro E. Diffusion tensor imaging evaluation of corticospinal tract hyperintensity in upper motor neuron-predominant als patients. J Aging Res 2011.

[18] Furtula J, Johnsen B, Frandsen J, Rodell A, Christensen PB, Pugdahl K, et al. Upper motor neuron involvement in amyotrophic lateral sclerosis evaluated by triple stimulation technique and diffusion tensor MRI. J Neurol 2013;260:1535–44. doi: 10.1007/s00415-012-6824-8.

[19] Khedr EM, Ahmed MA, Hamdy A, Shawky OA. Cortical excitability of amyotrophic lateral sclerosis: transcranial magnetic stimulation study. Neurophysiol Clin 2011;41:73–9. doi:10.1016/j.neucli.2011.03.001.

[20] Osei-Lah AD, Mills KR. Optimising the detection of upper motor neuron function dysfunction in amyotrophic lateral sclerosis – a transcranial magnetic stimulation study. J Neurol 2004;251:1364–9. doi:10.1007/s00415-004-0545-6.

[21] Menon P, Kiernan MC, Vucic S. Cortical hyperexcitability precedes lower motor neuron dysfunction in ALS. Clin Neurophysiol 2015;126:803–9. doi:10.1016/j.clinph. 2014.04.023.

[22] Vucic S, Cheah BC, Yiannikas C, Kiernan MC. Cortical excitability distinguishes ALS from mimic disorders. Clin Neurophysiol 2011;122:1860–6. doi:10.1016/j.clinph. 2010.12.062.

[23] De Carvalho M, Turkman A, Swash M. Motor responses evoked by transcranial magnetic stimulation and peripheral nerve stimulation in the ulnar innervation in amyotrophic lateral sclerosis: the effect of upper and lower motor neuron lesion. J Neurol Sci 2003;210:83–90. doi:10.1016/S0022-510X(03)00024-8.

[24] Chiò A. ISIS Survey: an international study on the diagnostic process and its implications in amyotrophic lateral sclerosis. J Neurol 1999;246:III1–I5. doi:10.1007/ BF03161081.

[25] Swinnen B, Robberecht W. The phenotypic variability of amyotrophic lateral sclerosis. Nat Rev Neurol 2014;10:661–70. doi:10.1038/nrneurol.2014.184.

[26] Kollewe K, Mauss U, Krampfl K, Petri S, Dengler R, Mohammadi B. ALSFRS-R score and its ratio: a useful predictor for ALS-progression. J Neurol Sci 2008;275:69–73.

[27] Chiò A, Logroscino G, Hardiman O, Swingler R, Mitchell D, Beghi E, et al. Prognostic factors in ALS: a critical review. Amyotroph Lateral Scler 2009;10:310–23.

[28] Elamin M, Phukan J, Bede P, Jordan N, Byrne S, Pender N, et al. Executive dysfunction is a negative prognostic indicator in patients with ALS without dementia. Neurology 2011;76:1263–9. doi:10.1212/WNL.0b013e318214359f.

[29] Wolf J, Safer A, Wöhrle J, Palm F, Nix W, Maschke M, et al. Factors predicting one-year mortality in amyotrophic lateral sclerosis patients – data from a population-based registry. BMC Neurol 2014;14:197.

[30] Watanabe H, Atsuta N, Nakamuran R, Hirakawa A, Ito M, Senda J, et al. Factors affecting longitudinal functional decline and survival in amyotrophic lateral sclerosis patients. Amyotroph Lateral Scler Front Degener 2015;16:230–6.

[31] Lunetta C, Lizio A, Melazzini M, Maestri E, Sansone V. Amyotrophic Lateral Sclerosis Survival Score (ALS-SS): a simple scoring system for early prediction of patient survival. Amyotroph Lateral Scler Front Degener 2015;17:1–8.

[32] Elamin M, Bede P, Montuschi A, Pender N, Chio A, Hardiman O. Predicting prognosis in amyotrophic lateral sclerosis: a simple algorithm. J Neurol 2015;262:1447–54. doi: 10.1007/s00415-015-7731-6.

[33] Boylan K, Glass J, Crook J, Yang C, Thomas C, Desaro P, et al. Phosphorylated neurofilament heavy subunit (pNF-H) in peripheral blood and CSF as a potential prognostic biomarker in amyotrophic lateral sclerosis. J Neurol Neurosurg Psychiatry 2013;84:467–72.

[34] Lehnert S, Costa J, de Carvalho M, Kirby J, Kuzma-Kozakiewicz M, Morelli C, et al. Multicentre quality control evaluation of different biomarker candidates for amyotrophic lateral sclerosis. Amyotroph Lateral Scler Frontotemporal Degener 2014;8421:1–7. doi:10.3109/21678421.2014.884592.

[35] Dalakas M, Hatazawa J, Brooks R, Di Chiro G. Lowered cerebral glucose utilization in amyotrophic lateral sclerosis. Ann Neurol 1987;22:580–6. doi:10.1002/ana.21369.

[36] Hatazawa J, Brooks R, Dalakas M, Mansi L, Di Chiro G. Cortical motor-sensory hypometabolism in amyotrophic lateral sclerosis: a PET study. J Comput Assist Tomogr 1988;12:630–6. doi:10.1097/RCT.0b013e31828583c8.

[37] Ludolph A, Langen K, Regard M, Herzog H, Kemper B, Kuwert T, et al. Frontal lobe function in amyotrophic lateral sclerosis: a neuropsychologic and positron emission tomography study. Acta Neurol Scand 1992;85:81–9.

[38] Abrahams S, Leigh PN, Kew JJ, Goldstein LH, Lloyd CM, Brooks DJ. A positron emission tomography study of frontal lobe function (verbal fluency) in amyotrophic lateral sclerosis. J Neurol Sci 1995;129 Suppl:44–6.

[39] Kew J, Leigh P, Playford E, Passingham R, Goldstein L, Frackowiak R, et al. Cortical function in amyotrophic lateral sclerosis. A positron emission tomography study. Brain 1993;116:655–80.

[40] Liu W, Ikeda Y, Hishikawa N, Yamashita T, Deguchi K, Abe K. Characteristic RNA foci of the abnormal hexanucleotide GGCCUG repeat expansion in spinocerebellar ataxia type 36 (Asidan). Eur J Neurol 2014;21:1377–86. doi:10.1111/ene.12491.

[41] Abrahams S, Goldstein L, Kew J, Brooks D, Lloyd C, Frith C, et al. Frontal lobe dysfunction in amyotrophic lateral sclerosis: a PET study. Brain 1996;119:2105–20.

[42] Pagani M, Chiò A, Valentini MC, Öberg J, Nobili F, Calvo A, et al. Functional pattern of brain FDG-PET in amyotrophic lateral sclerosis. Neurology 2014;83:1067–74. doi: 10.1212/WNL.0000000000000792.

[43] Renard D, Collombier L, Castelnovo G, Fourcade G, Kotzki P, LaBauge P. Brain FDG-PET changes in ALS and ALS-FTD. Acta Neurol Belgica 2011;111:306–9.

[44] Van Laere K, Vanhee A, Verschueren J, De Coster L, Driesen A, Dupont P, et al. Value of 18fluorodeoxyglucose-positron-emission tomography in amyotrophic lateral sclerosis: a prospective study. JAMA Neurol 2014;71:553–61. doi:10.1001/jamaneurol. 2014.62.

[45] Cistaro A, Valentini MC, Chiò A, Nobili F, Calvo A, Moglia C, et al. Brain hypermetabolism in amyotrophic lateral sclerosis: a FDG PET study in ALS of spinal and bulbar onset. Eur J Nucl Med Mol Imaging 2012;39:251–9. doi:10.1007/s00259-011-1979-6.

[46] Cistaro A, Pagani M, Montuschi A, Calvo A, Moglia C, Canosa A, et al. The metabolic signature of C9ORF72-related ALS: FDG PET comparison with nonmutated patients. Eur J Nucl Med Mol Imaging 2014;41:844–52. doi:10.1007/s00259-013-2667-5.

[47] Strong MJ, Grace GM, Freedman M, Lomen-Hoerth C, Woolley S, Goldstein LH, et al. Consensus criteria for the diagnosis of frontotemporal cognitive and behavioural syndromes in amyotrophic lateral sclerosis. Amyotroph Lateral Scler 2009;10:131–46. pii: 907462414. doi:10.1080/17482960802654364.

[48] Canosa A, Pagani M, Cistaro A, Montuschi A, Iazzolino B, Fania P, et al. 18F-FDG-PET correlates of cognitive impairment in ALS. Neurology 2016;86:44–9.

[49] Jeong Y, Park KC, Cho SS, Kim EJ, Kang SJ, Kim SE, et al. Pattern of glucose hypometabolism in frontotemporal dementia with motor neuron disease. Neurology 2005;64:734–6. doi:10.1212/01.WNL.0000152047.58767.9D.

[50] Rajagopalan V, Pioro EP. Comparing brain structural MRI and metabolic FDG-PET changes in patients with ALS-FTD: "the chicken or the egg?" question. J Neurol Neurosurg Psychiatry 2014;86:952–8. doi:10.1136/jnnp-2014-308239.

[51] Van Weehaege D, Ceccarini J, Delva A, Robberecht W, Van Damme P, Van Laere K. Prospective validation of 18 F-FDG brain PET discriminant analysis methods in the diagnosis of amyotrophic lateral sclerosis. J Nucl Med 2016. doi:10.2967/jnumed. 115.166272.

[52] Pagani M, Öberg J, De Carli F, Calvo A, Moglia C, Canosa A, et al. Metabolic spatial connectivity in amyotrophic lateral sclerosis as revealed by independent component analysis. Hum Brain Mapp 2015;37(3):942–53. doi:10.1002/hbm.23078.

[53] Lai T-H, Liu R-S, Yang B-H, Wang P-S, Lin K-P, Lee Y-C, et al. Cerebral involvement in spinal and bulbar muscular atrophy (Kennedy's disease): a pilot study of PET. J Neurol Sci 2013;335:139–44. doi:10.1016/j.jns.2013.09.016.

[54] Desai J, Swash M. Extrapyramidal involvement in amyotrophic lateral sclerosis: backward falls and retropulsion. J Neurol Neurosurg Psychiatry 1999;67:214–6.

[55] Manno C, Lipari A, Bono V, Taiello AC, La Bella V. Sporadic Parkinson disease and amyotrophic lateral sclerosis complex (Brait-Fahn-Schwartz disease). J Neurol Sci 2013;326:104–6. doi:10.1016/j.jns.2013.01.009.

[56] Gilbert RMW, Fahn S, Mitsumoto H, Rowland LP. Parkinsonism and motor neuron diseases: twenty-seven patients with diverse overlap syndromes. Mov Disord 2010;25:1868–75. doi:10.1002/mds.23200.

[57] Cooper-Knock J, Shaw PJ, Kirby J. The widening spectrum of C9ORF72-related disease; genotype/phenotype correlations and potential modifiers of clinical phenotype. Acta Neuropathol 2014;127:333–45. doi:10.1007/s00401-014-1251-9.

[58] Boeve B, Boylan K. Characterization of frontotemporal dementia and/or amyotrophic lateral sclerosis associated with the GGGGCC repeat expansion in C9ORF72. Brain 2012;March:765–83. doi:10.1093/brain/aws004.

[59] Appel L, Jonasson M, Danfors T, Nyholm D, Askmark H, Lubberink M, et al. Use of 11C-PE2I PET in differential diagnosis of parkinsonian disorders. J Nucl Med 2015;56:234–42. doi:10.2967/jnumed.114.148619.

[60] Takahashi H, Snow B, Bhatt M, Peppard R, Eisen A, Calne D. Evidence for a dopaminergic deficit in sporadic amyotrophic lateral sclerosis on positron emission scanning. Lancet 1993;342:1016–8.

[61] Przedborski S, Dhawan V, Donaldson D, Murphy P, McKenna-Yasek D, Mandel F, et al. Nigrostriatal dopaminergic function in familial amyotrophic lateral sclerosis patients with and without copper/zinc superoxide dismutase mutations. Neurology 1996;47:1546–51.

[62] Hideyama T, Momose T, Shimizu J, Tsuji S, Kwak S. A positron emission tomography study on the role of nigral lesions in parkinsonism in patients with amyotrophic lateral sclerosis. Arch Neurol 2006;63:1719–22. doi:10.1001/archneur.63.12.1719.

[63] Park HK, Lim Y-M, Kim JS, Lee MC, Kim SM, Kim BJ, et al. Nigrostriatal dysfunction in patients with amyotrophic lateral sclerosis and parkinsonism. J Neurol Sci 2011;301:12–3. doi:10.1016/j.jns.2010.11.017.

[64] D'Ascenzo C, Cecchin D, Santelli L, Palmieri A, Gaiani A, Querin G, et al. Parkinson-like features in ALS with predominant upper motor neuron involvement. Amyotroph Lateral Scler 2012;13:137–43. doi:10.3109/17482968.2011.603732.

[65] Philips T, Rothstein JD. Glial cells in amyotrophic lateral sclerosis. Exp Neurol 2014;262PB:111–20. doi:10.1016/j.expneurol.2014.05.015.

[66] Jacobs AH, Tavitian B. Noninvasive molecular imaging of neuroinflammation. J Cereb Blood Flow Metab 2012;32:1393–415. doi:10.1038/jcbfm.2012.53.

[67] Lavisse S, Guillermier M, Herard A-S, Petit F, Delahaye M, Van Camp N, et al. Reactive astrocytes overexpress TSPO and are detected by TSPO positron emission tomography imaging. J Neurosci 2012;32:10809–18. doi:10.1523/JNEUROSCI.1487-12.2012.

[68] Turner M, Cagnin A, Turkheimer F, Miller CC, Shaw C, Brooks D, et al. Evidence of widespread cerebral microglial activation in amyotrophic lateral sclerosis: an [11C](R)-PK11195 positron emission tomography study. Neurobiol Dis 2004;15:601–9. doi: 10.1016/j.nbd.2003.12.012.

[69] Corcia P, Tauber C, Vercoullie J, Arlicot N, Prunier C, Praline J, et al. Molecular imaging of microglial activation in amyotrophic lateral sclerosis. PLoS One 2012;7:e52941. doi: 10.1371/journal.pone.0052941.

[70] Zürcher NR, Loggia ML, Lawson R, Chonde DB, Izquierdo-Garcia D, Yasek JE, et al. Increased in vivo glial activation in patients with amyotrophic lateral sclerosis: assessed with [11C]-PBR28. NeuroImage Clin 2015;7:409–14. doi:10.1016/j.nicl.2015.01.009.

[71] Johansson A, Engler H, Blomquist G, Scott B, Wall A, Aquilonius SM, et al. Evidence for astrocytosis in ALS demonstrated by [11C](l)-deprenyl-D2 PET. J Neurol Sci 2007;255:17–22. doi:10.1016/j.jns.2007.01.057.

[72] Lloyd CM, Richardson MP, Brooks DJ, Al-Chalabi A, Leigh PN. Extramotor involvement in ALS: PET studies with the GABA-A ligand [11C]flumazenil. Brain 2000;123:2289–96. doi:10.1093/brain/123.11.2289.

[73] Turner MR, Osei-Lah AD, Hammers A, Al-Chalabi A, Shaw CE, Andersen PM, et al. Abnormal cortical excitability in sporadic but not homozygous D90A SOD1 ALS. J Neurol Neurosurg Psychiatry 2005;76:1279–85. doi:10.1136/jnnp.2004.054429.

[74] Turner MR, HammersA, Al-ChalabiA, Shaw CE, Andersen PM, Brooks DJ, et al. Distinct cerebral lesions in sporadic and "D90A" SOD1 ALS: studies with [11C]flumazenil PET. Brain 2005;128:1323–9. doi:10.1093/brain/awh509.

[75] Turner MR, Rabiner EA, Hammers A, Al-Chalabi A, Grasby PM, Shaw CE, et al. [11C]-WAY100635 PET demonstrates marked 5-HT1A receptor changes in sporadic ALS. Brain 2005;128:896–905. doi:10.1093/brain/awh428.

[76] Gordon PH, Cheng B, Katz IB, Pinto M, Hays AP, Mitsumoto H, et al. The natural history of primary lateral sclerosis. Neurology 2006;66:647–53. doi:10.1212/01.wnl.0000200962.94777.71.

[77] D'amico E, Pasmantier M, Lee Y-W. Clinical evolution of pure upper motor neuron disease/dysfunction (PUMND). Muscle Nerve 2013;47:28–32. doi:10.1002/mus.23496.Clinical.

[78] Turner MR, Hammers A, Al-Chalabi A, Shaw CE, Andersen PM, Brooks DJ, et al. Cortical involvement in four cases of primary lateral sclerosis using [11C]-flumazenil PET. J Neurol 2007;254:1033–6. doi:10.1007/s00415-006-0482-7.

[79] Claassen D, Josephs K, Peller P. The stripe of primary lateral sclerosis: focal primary motor cortex hypometabolism seen on fluorodeoxyglucose F18 positron emission tomography. Arch Neurol 2010;67:122–5.

[80] Scialò C, Morbelli S, Girtler N, Mandich P, Mancardi GL, Caponnetto C, et al. Bilateral motor and premotor cortex hypometabolism in a case of Mills syndrome. Amyotroph Lateral Scler Frontotemporal Degener 2015;16:414–7. doi: 10.3109/21678421.2015.1026828.

[81] Turner MR, GerhardA, Al-Chalabi A, Shaw CE, Hughes RAC, Banati RB, et al. Mills' and other isolated upper motor neurone syndromes: in vivo study with 11C-(R)-PK11195 PET. J Neurol Neurosurg Psychiatry 2005;76:871–4. doi:10.1136/jnnp.2004.047902.

[82] Van Laere K, Wilms G, Van Damme P. FDG-PET findings in three cases of Mills' syndrome. J Neurol Neurosurg Psychiatry 2016;87:222–3. doi:10.1136/jnnp-2014-309952.

[83] Schuster C, Kasper E, Machts J, Bittner D, Kaufmann J, Benecke R, et al. Focal thinning of the motor cortex mirrors clinical features of amyotrophic lateral sclerosis and their phenotypes: a neuroimaging study. J Neurol 2013;260:2856–64. doi:10.1007/s00415-013-7083-z.

[84] Van der Graaff MM, Sage CA, Caan MWA, Akkerman EM, Lavini C, Majoie CB, et al. Upper and extra-motoneuron involvement in early motoneuron disease: a diffusion tensor imaging study. Brain 2011;134:1211–28. doi:10.1093/brain/awr016.

[85] Cosottini M, Giannelli M, Siciliano G, Lazzarotti G, Michelassi MC, Del Corona A, et al. Diffusion-tensor MR imaging of corticospinal tract in amyotrophic lateral sclerosis and progressive muscular atrophy. Radiology 2005;237:258–64. doi:10.1148/radiol.2371041506.

[86] Raaphorst J, van Tol M-J, Groot PFC, Altena E, van der Werf YD, Majoie CB, et al. Prefrontal involvement related to cognitive impairment in progressive muscular atrophy. Neurology 2014;83:818–25. doi:10.1212/WNL.0000000000000745.

[87] Morimoto N, Kurata T, Sato K, Ikeda Y, Sato S, Abe K. Frontal dysfunctions of ALS-PBP patients in relation to their bulbar symptoms and rCBF decline. J Neurol Sci 2012;319:96–101. doi:10.1016/j.jns.2012.04.020.

[88] Renton AE, Chiò A, Traynor BJ. State of play in amyotrophic lateral sclerosis genetics. Nat Neurosci 2014;17:17–23. doi:10.1038/nn.3584.

[89] Kaur SJ, McKeown S, Rashid S. Mutant SOD1 mediated pathogenesis of amyotrophic lateral sclerosis. Gene 2015;577:109–18. doi:10.1016/j.gene.2015.11.049.

[90] Rascovsky K, Hodges JR, Knopman D, Mendez MF, Kramer JH, Neuhaus J, et al. Sensitivity of revised diagnostic criteria for the behavioural variant of frontotemporal dementia. Brain 2011;134:2456–77. doi:10.1093/brain/awr179.

Chapter 3

Motor Cortex Hyperexcitability, Neuroplasticity, and Degeneration in Amyotrophic Lateral Sclerosis

Ilya S. Bakulin, Alexander V. Chervyakov,
Natalia A. Suponeva, Maria N. Zakharova and
Michael A. Piradov

Additional information is available at the end of the chapter

http://dx.doi.org/10.5772/63310

Abstract

Neuronal hyperexcitability is a well-known phenomenon in amyotrophic lateral sclerosis and other neurodegenerative diseases. The use of transcranial magnetic stimulation in clinical and research practice has recently made it possible to detect motor cortex hyperexcitability under clinical conditions. Despite numerous studies, the mechanisms and sequelae of the development of hyperexcitability still have not been completely elucidated. In this chapter, we discuss the possibilities for detecting motor cortex hyperexcitability in patients with amyotrophic lateral sclerosis using transcranial magnetic stimulation. The potential relationship between hyperexcitability and neuronal degeneration or neuroplasticity processes is discussed using the data obtained by navigated transcranial magnetic stimulation and neuroimaging data, as well as the data of experimental studies.

Keywords: transcranial magnetic stimulation, amyotrophic lateral sclerosis, hyperexcitability, excitotoxicity, neuroplasticity

1. Introduction

Amyotrophic lateral sclerosis (ALS) is a fatal neurodegenerative disease affecting the upper and lower motor neurons. Despite the significant advance in molecular biology and genetics over the past years, many aspects of etiology and pathogenesis of ALS remain unstudied; neither biomarkers of the disease nor effective treatment methods have been designed [1].

INTECH
open science | open minds

© 2016 The Author(s). Licensee InTech. This chapter is distributed under the terms of the Creative Commons Attribution License (http://creativecommons.org/licenses/by/3.0), which permits unrestricted use, distribution, and reproduction in any medium, provided the original work is properly cited.

A significant advance in understanding the pathophysiological mechanisms of the development of the neurodegenerative process of ALS has been made over the past years after novel neurophysiological and neuroimaging techniques were introduced into the research and clinical practice [2–4]. Transcranial magnetic stimulation (TMS) is a noninvasive brain stimulation method that is used to evaluate the functional status of the upper motor neuron in ALS patients. It has been shown in the recent studies that different TMS parameters are altered in ALS patients [4]. TMS is currently viewed as a valuable research and diagnostic tool in ALS.

Development of hyperexcitability of the primary motor cortex and the entire motor system is a well-studied phenomenon in ALS. Motor cortex hyperexcitability can be determined using TMS as reduced resting motor threshold and increased motor evoked potential (MEP) amplitude, decreased silent period, reduced effectiveness of short-interval intracortical inhibition (SICI), and increased intracortical facilitation (ICF) (see review [4]). Most authors attribute motor cortex hyperexcitability in ALS patients to enhanced glutamatergic neurotransmission in the neocortex and reduced gamma-aminobutyric acid (GABA)ergic inhibitory neurotransmission, thus suggesting that hyperexcitability provokes degeneration of motor neurons [5–7]. However, no direct evidence has been obtained yet that would unambiguously demonstrate the relationship between motor cortex hyperexcitability in ALS patients and its degeneration. There is an alternative opinion that hyperexcitability can potentially be related to neuroplasticity processes taking place in the motor cortex and compensation for the lost function.

We would like to discuss the potential relationship of motor cortex hyperexcitability with motor neuron degeneration and neuroplasticity in ALS patients, as well as the possible methods to solve this problem using modern neurophysiological and neuroimaging methods.

2. Motor cortex hyperexcitability in ALS

Although the term 'hyperexcitability' is widely used, it still does not have a commonly accepted definition. According to Bae et al. (2013), it 'means an increased or exaggerated response to a stimulus, which may usually have been expected to evoke a normal response' [7]. We deem that hyperexcitability is discussed in modern TMS studies more broadly: as the ability to respond to stimuli that normally do not evoke any response and, speaking more generally, as the predominance of excitation over inhibition.

Hyperexcitability in ALS patients can be determined using various methods at different levels of the motor system. It can be detected at the level of individual neurons and ion channels in cell cultures in transgenic animals, clinically (presenting as the well-known phenomena, such as fasciculation or cramps) or using the modern neurophysiological techniques such as electromyography (EMG) and TMS [7].

Motor cortex excitability is a complex integral parameter that depends on numerous factors. Hence, the hyperexcitability phenomenon is also a complex and multifactorial process that

http://dx.doi.org/10.5772/63310

depends on glutamate synthesis and release, its reuptake and degradation, expression and functional status of several types of glutamate receptors, excitable properties of neuronal membranes, and the status of inhibitory GABAergic neurotransmission. A number of experimental studies demonstrated that all the aforementioned processes are disturbed in ALS [8, 9]. **Table 1** summarizes the results of some key studies.

Mechanism	Supporting facts
Decreased Glutamate reuptake	• A 70-80% decrease in expression of high-affinity astroglial glutamate transporter EAAT2 (excitatory amino acid transporter) in the motor cortex and spinal cord in ALS patients as a result of posttranslational modifications, oxidative stress, and other factors [10, 11]
	• Early reduction of glutamate transporter expression in mSOD1 transgenic animals [12]
	• Degeneration of motor neurons in the motor cortex and spinal cord as glutamate reuptake is inhibited *in vitro* in an organotypic cell culture [13]
	• The absence of compensatory increase in glutamate transporter expression by glial cells under excitotoxic conditions and oxidative stress [14]
Dysfunction of inhibitory GABAergic neurotransmission	• Degeneration of inhibitory interneurons in the motor cortex and spinal cord in ALS patients according to pathomorphological and animal model studies [15–17]
	• Decreased GABA level in the motor cortex according to the MR spectroscopy [18] and reduced ^{11}C-flumazenil binding according to the PET data [19]
	• Decreased level of mRNA of GABA(A) receptor subunits in a postmortem study [20]
Changes in excitability of motor neuron membranes	• Increased density and excitability of voltage-gated sodium channels in SOD1 transgenic animals [21, 22]
	• Decreased conductance of potassium channels Kv 1.2
	• Hyperexcitability of individual motor neurons in a cell culture [23, 24]
Changes in expression and functions of glutamate receptors	• Decreased expression of the GluR2 subunit blocking calcium delivery to the cell in ALS patients with transgenic animals [25]
	• Disturbance of posttranslational modification of GluR2 subunit increasing permeability to calcium ions [25]

Table 1. Potential mechanisms of development of motor neuron hyperexcitability in ALS patients.

Today, TMS is the key and actually the only method for clinical investigation of motor cortex excitability. The use of the entire range of TMS parameters allows one to perform a relatively differentiated study of various factors contributing to motor cortex excitation [26]. TMS can be employed for assessing the functional status of the corticospinal tract due to the ability to excite motor cortex neurons by induced electrical current followed by propagation of excitation to alpha motor neurons of spinal cord. This causes contraction of muscle fibers within a certain motor unit, which can be recorded by cutaneous electrodes as a MEP [27]. TMS assesses the functional status of neuronal contours of the motor cortex [28].

Motor threshold is the key parameter used to assess motor cortex excitability. The motor threshold represents the density of corticospinal projections and can be regarded as a biomarker of neuronal membrane excitability [26]. Decreased motor threshold is considered to be one of the key signs of motor cortex hyperexcitability.

According to most studies, the motor threshold in ALS patients is increased, probably being indicative of degeneration of cortical motor neurons [29–35]. Meanwhile, a paradoxical decrease in the motor threshold when examining patients at the onset of the disease was shown in some studies [36–39]. The motor threshold is likely to decrease at the onset of ALS, probably until clinical signs appear, and subsequently increases as motor neurons die. A statistically significant direct correlation between the motor threshold and disease duration was demonstrated in some studies [29, 40].

Physiologically, the motor threshold is primarily determined by rapid AMPA receptor (AMPAR)-mediated glutamatergic neurotransmission in the neocortex and excitability of motor neuron membranes that depends on voltage-gated sodium channels [41]. In ALS, AMPA receptor-mediated glutamatergic neurotransmission increases and properties of sodium channels change (presenting as increased conductance) [23, 24, 42, 43]. Alteration in functional properties of potential-gated sodium channels has been revealed: more rapid recovery after inactivation, increased permeability to sodium, and increased density of ion channels [21]. Pieri et al. demonstrated a decrease in the action potential threshold, an increase in pulse frequency, and an increase in persistent sodium current in cortical motor neurons isolated in G93A mutant mice [22].

MEP amplitude is determined by the number of reduced motor units and the number of activated alpha motor neurons in the spinal cord. Increased stimulation intensity enhances MEP amplitude due to superimposition of late I-waves and I1-wave [28, 44]. Like the motor threshold, MEP amplitude is determined by the density of corticospinal projections. Meanwhile, MEP amplitude to a greater extent represents the function of neurons with lower excitability or those located farther from the stimulation site [4]. GABAergic drugs reduce MEP amplitude, which results from the scheme of generation of late I-waves modulated by inserted inhibitory GABAergic interneurons [41]. Noteworthy, the motor threshold and MEP amplitude are modulated by drugs belonging to different pharmacological classes, thus emphasizing the difference between the mechanisms of their formation.

Identically to the motor threshold, MEP amplitude in ALS patients changes in opposite directions depending on stage of the disease. MEP amplitude decreases in most cases, being accompanied by increased motor threshold and representing a decrease in motor neuron number and reduction of density of corticospinal projections [4]. On the contrary, some patients with the reduced motor threshold may have increased MEP amplitude and the ratio between MEP amplitude and M-response amplitude [45, 46]. The increased slope ratio of the amplitude vs intensity curve is additional evidence to motor cortex hyperexcitability in ALS patients as it demonstrates a more pronounced amplitude increment with increasing stimulation intensity compared to the norm. The increase in MEP amplitude and the slope ratio of the amplitude vs intensity curve in ALS patients is probably related to both enhanced glutamatergic and reduced inhibitory GABAergic neurotransmission in the neocortex [4].

The *cortical silent period* (cSP) represents inhibition of voluntary muscular activity during a certain period after a magnetic stimulus was applied [47]. It has been demonstrated that the first one-third of cSP is mostly controlled by inhibitory mechanisms at the spinal cord level, while the remaining two thirds are of cortical origin and are related to inhibitory neurotransmission through GABA(B) receptors [27].

It was demonstrated in most studies that patients with sporadic and familial ALS had either decreased cSP or no cSP at all, which is regarded as significant evidence attesting to intracortical inhibitory dysfunction in ALS patients [48–50].

Paired pulse stimulation is used to assess intracortical inhibition and excitation processes. The method involves sequential generation of two pulses: the conditioning (S1) and testing (S2) pulses. The physiological effects of paired pulse stimulation are determined by the intensity of S1 and the interval between S1 and S2 pulses. Application of the sub-threshold S1 pulse 1–6 ms before the supra-threshold S2 pulse reduces MEP amplitude compared to isolated application of a supra-threshold stimulus [51]. This phenomenon is known as SICI. Contrariwise, an increase of the interstimulus interval to 8–20 ms rises the amplitude of MEP to the testing pulse (ICF). Several protocols have been proposed where the conditioning pulse has the supra- and sub-threshold intensity. MEP amplitude increases at the long interstimulus interval (long-interval intracortical inhibition, LICI) and decreases at the short interval (short-interval intracortical facilitation, SICF) [27].

The neurophysiological mechanisms of formation of these phenomena remain insufficiently studied; however, it has been demonstrated rather convincingly that they have the predominantly intracortical origin. Thus, SICI and LICI protocols cause suppression of amplitude and the number of late descending waves [51, 52]. Intracortical inhibition processes are assumed to be caused by activation of neocortical inhibitory interneurons under the action of the conditioning pulse; SICI being mediated by inhibition through GABA(A) receptors and LICI, through GABA(B) receptors. The ICF phenomenon is presumably caused by activation of glutamatergic neurotransmission through NMDA glutamate receptors [26].

Disruption of intracortical inhibition and facilitation under paired-pulse stimulation is currently believed to be the most convincing evidence that motor cortex hyperexcitability develops in ALS patients and has been detected in numerous studies [6, 53, 54, 55]. It should be mentioned that a decrease in efficiency of SICI is revealed at the earliest stages of the disease, including asymptomatic SOD1 mutation carriers, and correlates with axonal degeneration of peripheral motor neurons [45]. Assessment of the disruptions of intracortical inhibition using the new threshold tracking technique is considered to be a potential diagnostic tool in ALS demonstrating high sensitivity and specificity [56, 57].

The role of inhibitory interneurons dysfunction in pathogenesis of ALS has been actively studied over the past years [58–60]. Degeneration of inhibitory interneurons both in the spinal cord and in the motor cortex was demonstrated in several pathomorphological studies carried out in the 1990s. Nihei et al. (1993) reported a reduced amount of parvalbumin-positive interneurons in the motor cortex in ALS patients [61]. In addition, Petri et al. (2003) demonstrated that the level of GABA(A) receptor alpha-1 subunit mRNA decreases in ALS patients

[20]. Dysfunction of inhibitory neurotransmission in the neocortex has also been confirmed in neuroimaging studies presenting as a decrease in GABA amount according to magnetic resonance spectroscopy [18] and decreased ^{11}C-flumazenil binding as shown by PET [19].

The TMS data additionally confirm that inhibitory neurotransmission in the neocortex is disrupted in ALS patients. It should be mentioned that TMS has been used to show the disturbance of inhibition in the motor cortex both mediated by GABA(A) (decreased SICI) and by GABA(B) receptors (decreased LICI and sCP), being indicative of degeneration of interneurons or GABA metabolism disruption rather than dysfunction of receptors of this mediator in the postsynaptic membrane.

Other factors that cause SICI disruption in ALS patients are being discussed. Thus, riluzole was reported to induce partial recovery of SICI in ALS patients, which gives grounds for suggesting that enhancement of glutamatergic neurotransmission plays a role in disturbance of intracortical inhibition in ALS patients. NMDA receptor antagonists, memantine and amantadine, were shown to increase SICI and decrease ICF in several pharmaco-TMS studies [41]. These data suggest that decreased intracortical inhibition in ALS patients can be related not only to reduction of inhibitory GABAergic neurotransmission but also to enhancement of glutamatergic neurotransmission through NMDAR.

Increased intracortical facilitation is another evidence for involvement of NMDAR in pathogenesis of ALS. This phenomenon is currently predominantly attributed to glutamatergic neurotransmission through NMDAR, which is confirmed, in particular, by its reduction due to antagonists of these receptors [41].

Hence, a large body of data attesting to the development of motor cortex hyperexcitability in ALS patients can currently be obtained by TMS. Signs attesting to degeneration of the upper motor neuron are detected simultaneously (**Table 2**). Importantly, some TMS parameters (MEP threshold and amplitude) can change in opposite directions and attest to motor cortex hyperexcitability at onset of the disease and degeneration as the disease progresses. Meanwhile, such signs of hyperexcitability as decreased cSP and efficiency of SICI are detected even in patients with pronounced degeneration of motor neurons. This phenomenon in ALS patients was referred to as 'dying but overactive' [7]; it can cause difficulties for interpretation of TMS results in a specific patient.

Hyperexcitability	Degeneration
• Resting motor threshold decreased	• Resting motor threshold increased
• MEP amplitude increased	• CMCT increased
• SICI reduced and ICF increased	• MEP amplitude decreased
• SP decreased	• Central conduction failure (triple stimulation technique)

Table 2. Motor cortex hyperexcitability and degeneration in ALS: TMS findings.

http://dx.doi.org/10.5772/63310

Table 3 summarizes the TMS data on the potential mechanisms responsible for the signs of motor cortex hyperexcitability in ALS patients. It should be mentioned that the variety of TMS procedures makes it possible not only to reveal the dysfunction of individual mediator systems but also to perform differentiated evaluation of neurotransmission through different types of glutamate and GABA receptors in ALS patients.

Sign	Mechanism
Decreased motor threshold	• Increased glutamatergic neurotransmission through AMPAR • Increased sodium current due to an increase in density and/or alteration in functional properties of sodium channels
Increased MER amplitude	• Increased glutamatergic neurotransmission through AMPAR • Decreased inhibitory GABAergic neurotransmission
Decreased silent period	• Decreased inhibitory GABAergic neurotransmission through GABA(B) receptors
Decreased SICI	• Decreased inhibitory GABAergic neurotransmission through GABA(A) receptors • Increased glutamatergic neurotransmission through NMDAR
Increased ICF	• Increased glutamatergic neurotransmission through NMDAR

Table 3. Potential mechanisms of formation of TMS signs of motor cortex hyperexcitability in ALS.

Based on TMS findings, it is rather promising and reasonable to suggest that motor cortex hyperexcitability and the underlying molecular events (e.g., excitotoxicity) cause degeneration of motor neurons in ALS patients. We attempt to discuss the specific potential mechanisms underlying motor cortex hyperexcitability in ALS and present the evidence for its pathogenetic relationship with degeneration of motor neuron.

3. What does motor cortex hyperexcitability mean?

3.1. Is hyperexcitability bad?

The evidence that motor cortex hyperexcitability plays a role in pathogenesis of ALS is still rather sparse [62]. Hyperexcitability is registered at different stages of the disease, including the pre-symptomatic ones [23, 45]. However, this fact tells nothing about its role in pathogenesis of the disease. It is still unclear when true onset of neurodegeneration occurs; however, the results of studies using transgenic animals demonstrate that the pathological process in ALS may start at the earliest stages of embryogenesis (e.g., at the stage when neural networks are formed) [63]. In this situation, all the objectively detectable alterations may be either primary or secondary (i.e., emerge as one of nonspecific stages of neurodegeneration or via the compensatory mechanism).

The enhancement of excitatory glutamatergic neurotransmission and reduction of inhibitory GABAergic neurotransmission in the neocortex, which underlie hyperexcitability in ALS patients, are believed to damage motor neurons via the excitotoxicity mechanism [4, 7]. The role of excitotoxicity as one of the universal mechanisms causing neuronal death in various nervous system diseases has currently been demonstrated [8, 9, 64]. High sensitivity of motor neurons to excitotoxicity can be related to high expression of glutamate receptors and low expression of calcium-binding proteins [9].

An important argument in favor of the role of hyperexcitability and the underlying molecular processes in ALS pathogenesis is that this phenomenon can be early detected using TMS in asymptomatic SOD1 mutation carriers. Vucic et al. (2008) demonstrated a decrease in SICI in three SOD1 mutation carriers who were asymptomatic at the time the study was performed but developed clinical signs of the disease during a prospective study within 3 years. It is interesting that no neurophysiological signs of motor cortex excitability were revealed in 14 other asymptomatic carriers and they did not present with any clinical manifestations of the disease within the entire study period [45]. Early development of signs of hyperexcitability of neurons of the motor cortex, spinal cord, and even the extramotor areas such as hippocampus (e.g., see [23]) were demonstrated in a large series of experimental studies using a culture of neurons isolated from transgenic animals. Additional evidence is that signs of motor cortex hyperexcitability in ALS patients can be detected before the pyramidal pathways are affected and EMG signs of degeneration of the lower motor neuron emerge. A recent study carried out by Menon et al. (2015) showed that 24 patients with ALS had a statistically significant decrease in motor threshold, duration of cSP and intracortical inhibition, while simultaneously having an increased MER amplitude and intracortical facilitation at onset of the disease [5]. No signs of alterations in central motor conduction time (CMCT) were detected in these patients, thus attesting to the fact that the conduction function of the pyramidal pathway was retained and there were signs of denervation and reinnervation process according to the EMG data. The results of this study demonstrated that motor cortex hyperexcitability precedes degeneration of both the upper and the lower motor neurons and is the earliest neurophysiological signs of neurodegeneration. This supports the hypothesis proposed by Charkot back in 1869 that the upper motor neuron is the first one to be affected in ALS patients ('dying-forward') [65].

The certain effectiveness of riluzole in treating ALS also indirectly confirms the pathogenetic role of hyperexcitability and excitotoxicity. Despite the diversity of its mechanisms of action, riluzole is primarily considered to be a medication reducing excitotoxicity [66]. It has been demonstrated that riluzole can partially normalize SICI and reduce excitability of peripheral nerve axons in ALS patients [67].

The indirect evidence to the pathogenetic role of excitotoxicity was also obtained in studies on using therapeutic repetitive magnetic stimulation in ALS. High-frequency repetitive TMS increases neuronal excitability in the stimulated area (see reviews [68] and [69]). It has been demonstrated in a small study conducted by Di Lazzaro et al. (2004) that high-frequency stimulation may accelerate onset of the disease, while low-frequency stimulation may inhibit it [70]. Hence, high-frequency stimulation may increase excitotoxic degeneration of motor neurons and motor cortex excitability, having an unfavorable effect on the course of the disease.

3.2. Is hyperexcitability good?

Excitotoxicity and hyperexcitability have been for a long time regarded only as damaging phenomena facilitating neuronal death. However, findings obtained in a number of studies suggest that hyperexcitability can also have a compensatory effect, at least at early stages. Furthermore, molecular alterations that accompany excitotoxicity are similar to the processes taking place when neuroplasticity is ensured. We present the results of some studies confirming the validity of this alternative view of the hyperexcitability problem in patients with ALS and other neurodegenerative diseases.

3.2.1. Motor cortex excitability and neuroplasticity

The term 'neuroplasticity' means brain's ability to alter structurally and functionally in response to internal and external factors. This ability is currently attributed both to strengthening or weakening of the existing neural connections and to the formation of new connections or destruction of the old ones [71]. Starting with the first description of cellular mechanisms of neuroplasticity, this universal property of neural tissue is inseparably associated with alteration in neuronal excitability. Long-term potentiation was shown to be predominantly of postsynaptic origin and is mostly connected to the glutamatergic system [72–74].

A series of studies have shown the alteration in motor cortex excitability and reorganization of the cortical representation of muscles after motor learning and acquisition of new skills [75, 76]. The TMS data confirmed that there is a relationship between neuroplastic alterations and an increase in motor cortex excitability [77–79]. Thus, Tyč and Boyadjian (2011) performed TMS mapping of cortical representation of the deltoid and brachioradialis muscles in healthy volunteers before and after a 6-week training (playing darts three to four times a week). The boundaries of cortical representation of the muscles under study were expanded after training, which was accompanied by an increase in the slope ratio of the amplitude-intensity curve, being indicative of the increase in motor cortex excitability [80]. According to Perez et al. (2004), a 32-minute training causes statistically significant increase in the slope ratio of the amplitude-intensity curve and a decrease in intracortical inhibition [81]. Increased motor cortex excitability presenting as increased MER amplitude and reduced motor threshold is observed in healthy volunteers not only after actual training but also after they had imagined the movements [82]. Professional sportsmen and musicians were found to have increased motor cortex excitability and increased ability of the motor cortex to undergo plastic alterations [83, 84].

To sum up, the aforementioned facts indicate that motor cortex excitability and glutamatergic neurotransmission increase during neuroplastic alterations.

3.2.2. Hyperexcitability and neuroplasticity in pathology

The most forcible evidence for the possible relationship between hyperexcitability and neuroplasticity was observed in patients with Alzheimer's disease (AD). Neurodegeneration in this disease is not limited to the structures involved in the cognitive function and affects other brain regions as well, including the primary motor cortex. At the late stages of the disease, AD patients often have motor disorders, including spasticity and pathologic plantar responses, attesting to involvement of the upper motor neuron [85]. Furthermore, lesions of the motor cortex, predominantly giant pyramidal cells of Betz, were detected in AD patients in pathomorphological studies [86]. In this connection, investigation of the structural and functional status of the motor cortex in AD patients is of interest as a model of clinically asymptomatic neurodegeneration of the motor cortex.

In AD patients, identically to those with ALS, motor cortex hyperexcitability can be recorded using TMS. It has been demonstrated in many studies that the motor threshold decreases in AD patients. Decreased intracortical inhibition and short cSP duration were also detected in some studies (although not all of them) (see reviews [87, 88]). There is controversy in data on disrupted inhibitory neurotransmission in AD patients; however, decreased SICI in AD is most probably not associated with dysfunction of the GABAergic system [89]. The enhanced glutamatergic neurotransmission is currently the predominant conception of the development of motor cortex hyperexcitability in AD patients.

It is interesting to mention that motor cortex hyperexcitability in AD patients is predominantly attributed to neuroplasticity processes. Hyperexcitability is believed to develop via the compensatory mechanism as a response to disruption of associative connections [90].

Motor cortex hyperexcitability in AD patients is accompanied by reorganization of the cortical representation of muscles according to TMS mapping presenting as displacement of the center of gravity of the cortical representation in the frontomedial direction with respect to localization of hot spots in patients without motor disorders [90]. Ferreri et al. (2011) believe that this may attest to plastic brain alterations aimed at maintaining normal motor activity as the neuron number decreases progressively [91]. fMRI studies in patients at early stages of AD, identically to those with ALS, showed areas with increased activation, which is also regarded as a result of compensatory changes [92]. In their recent study, Guerra et al. (2015) demonstrated the relationship between motor cortex hyperexcitability and neuroplasticity. Examination of seven patients with vascular dementia and nine AD patients showed a statistically significant decrease in motor threshold compared to healthy volunteers of comparable age. Parameters related to motor cortex excitability (the area of cortical representation of muscles and the area of active cortical points) showed a statistically significant correlation with neuroplastic reorganization of the motor cortex assessed based on the distance between the center of gravity of the maps and hot spot localization. The authors drew a conclusion that motor cortex hyperexcitability may promote neuroplasticity [93].

As opposed of the cortical motor zones, most AD patients at the dementia stage have decreased connectivity and activation of the hippocampus, medial temporal, and prefronal cortex when performing cognitive tasks involving short-term memory [94]. Meanwhile, activity of these areas is increased in AD patients at the moderate cognitive impairment stage and in asymptomatic carriers of mutations in the presenilin-1 gene [95–97]. This is believed to result from turning on of the compensatory mechanisms. It should be mentioned that transgenic animals at the presymptomatic stage and stage of initial manifestations (which approximately corresponds to the moderate cognitive impairment stage in humans) showed an increased expression of a number of genes promoting synaptic plasticity [98]. In particular, transgenic mice showed enhanced expression of the AMPAR subunit genes at the early stages of the pathological process [99]. Furthermore, experimental studies revealed an increase in synaptic plasticity and hyperexcitability in hippocampal neurons, which preceded β-amyloid deposition [100, 101]. Schneider et al. (2001) reported that hippocampal neurons in transgenic mice with presenilin mutation are characterized not only by hyperexcitability and reduced threshold to excitotoxic damage but also by facilitation of long-term synaptic potentiation [102]. In their pathomorphological study, Bell et al. (2007) showed that patients with moderate cognitive impairments had increased density of presynaptic boutons in glutamatergic synapses, while the density of presynaptic boutons in AD patients was reduced [103]. On the contrary, expression of the genes involved in synaptic plasticity and energy exchange was shown to decrease at the late stages of the disease [98, 104]. These data give grounds for assuming that the increase in neuronal excitability in AD patients at early stages of the disease may occur via the compensatory mechanism.

3.2.3. Compensatory hyperexcitability in ALS: evidence from fundamental research

Several recently published studies using transgenic animals expressing mSOD1 have compromised the conception of the pathological role of excitability of motor neurons in ALS. Saxena et al. (2013) demonstrated that hyperexcitability can be a defense mechanism preventing degeneration of motor neurons. Thus, reduced excitability of motor neurons decreased accumulation of mutant SOD1, whereas increased excitability was accompanied by the greater number of intracellular aggregates and quicker death of motor neurons. It was also demonstrated that mutant protein accumulation increases after AMPAR blockade and decreases when AMPA is introduced. Stronger excitatory stimulation may contribute to the decrease in severity of endoplasmic stress and accumulation of abnormal proteins, thus exhibiting protective properties. Interestingly, mutant SOD1 accumulation was first detected in the least excitable fast fatiguing (FF) motor neurons of the spinal cord [105]. Leroy et al. (2014) studied the excitability of various populations of spinal cord motor neurons isolated from G93A mutant mice [106]. In this study, the electrophysiological signs of hyperexcitability were revealed only in degeneration-resistant motor neurons. The authors believe that their findings indicate that hyperexcitability does not cause degeneration; instead, it can be a defense mechanism [106].

3.2.4. Neuroplasticity in ALS: evidence from fMRI studies

Nowadays, fMRI is the key method for studying neuroplasticity in ALS patients. Numerous studies have revealed the changes in activation patterns of various brain regions in ALS both in rest and using various paradigms [2]. In this publication, the changes in activation patterns in ALS patients performing motor tasks are of special interest.

In the study performed by Konrad et al. (2002), ALS patients and healthy volunteers underwent fMRI as they performed a motor paradigm (bending fingers) [107]. Significant changes in the patterns of cortex activation were observed: a forward displacement of the activation cluster, into the supplementary motor area, and an increase in its volume. Activation volume in the inferior frontal gyrus (Brodmann area 6) in the contralateral hemisphere and parietal lobes increased bilaterally. The authors have put forward a hypothesis that these changes represent the structural and functional rearrangement of the motor system induced by degeneration of the upper and lower motor neuron [107]. Lule et al. (2007) reported that an increase in activation of the primary motor and premotor cortex in ALS patients is revealed not only when performing the movement but also when imaging it [108]. Stanton et al. (2007) detected that activation in the sensorimotor cortex (Brodmann areas 1, 2, and 4), the inferior parietal lobule, and the superior temporal gyrus increased when the ALS patients performed a motor task, while activation in the dorsolateral prefrontal cortex decreased [109]. It is noteworthy that these changes were observed when comparing ALS patients not only to healthy volunteers but also to patients with peripheral nerve disorders [109]. This confirms that involvement of the upper motor neuron plays a crucial role in development of these changes and does not give grounds for considering them as just a response to the development of muscle fatigue.

Thus, an analysis of the results of fMRI with the motor paradigm in ALS patients demonstrates that the activation areas expand when a motor task is being performed. Interestingly, the changes in activation during fMRI can have a prognostic value. Poujois et al. (2013) reported that activation in the somatosensory and parietal cortex increases in ALS patients performing a simple motor task compared to the control group. The dynamic follow-up for 1 year has shown that activity of the contralateral parietal lobe has a statistically significant negative correlation with the rate of disease progression ($p = 0.001$) [110].

These findings give grounds for suggesting that expansion of activation areas as an ALS patient performs a motor task has the compensatory mechanism and is probably aimed at maintaining the motor function in response to progressive degeneration of cortical motor neurons. Meanwhile, certain researchers believe that the activation areas can increase due to degeneration of inhibitory interneurons [2]. The relationship between alterations in activation patterns in ALS patients according to fMRI data and changes in motor cortex excitability according to TMS data has not been studied yet. It should be mentioned that the positive prognostic significance of neuroplastic alterations demonstrated by Poujois et al. (2013) is in contrast with the views about the negative role of hyperexcitability in this disease.

4. Navigated TMS mapping in ALS

Navigated TMS (nTMS) is today considered to be the most promising method to answer the question about the relationship between hyperexcitability and neuroplastic alterations in the motor cortex under kinetic conditions. On the one hand, nTMS is a neuroimaging technique and allows visualization of the location of cortical representation of certain muscles on individual MR images and provides an opportunity to assess the changes in their size and displacement with respect to anatomical landmarks. On the other hand, nTMS is a neurophysiological method that allows one to assess various parameters showing the excitability and degeneration of the motor cortex. The nTMS method uses the brain of a person being examined as a landmark when applying stimuli for an individual MR model; the stimuli can be accurately applied to a certain area with allowance for the area of interest, the individual anatomy, and topography of the gyri [111].

In our recent study, we mapped the cortical representation of m. abductor pollicis brevis (APB) in 30 ALS patients and 24 healthy volunteers [29]. It was demonstrated that ALS patients exhibit a statistically significant increase in the resting motor threshold and a decrease in the MEPs amplitude, as well as a statistically significant reduction of the volume of cortical representation of APB ($p < 0.001$). The latter observation agrees with the results of the findings of Carvalho et al. (1999) who demonstrated a progressive decrease in size of the cortical representation in ALS patients [112]. This phenomenon is probably based on the neurodegenerative process that reduces motor cortex excitability and decreases the number of cortical motor neurons. According to our data, the volume of cortical representation statistically significantly correlates with disease duration and negatively correlates with strength of the corresponding muscle and disease severity according to ALS Functional Rating Scale Revised (ALS FRS-R). These data give grounds for hypothesizing that the size of cortical representation can be regarded as a neurophysiological marker of disease severity, which opens new avenues for using it both in fundamental research and in clinical trials of new therapy methods. Further studies are needed to determine the sensitivity and specificity of this marker compared to other neurophysiological parameters and to determine its diagnostic significance.

The capabilities of navigated TMS made it possible not only to determine the size of cortical representation but also to accurately localize the maps within the anatomic landmarks. In most ALS patients, the maps were localized within the precentral gyrus (Brodmann area 4); some active sites, similar to those in healthy volunteers, were detected within the postcentral gyrus (Brodmann area 1) and the premotor cortex.

Meanwhile, we detected expanded boundaries of individual maps of the APB in some ALS patients, usually presenting as a displacement of the greatest portion of the map toward the postcentral gyrus. It was found by analyzing these cases that the aforementioned reorganization is mostly typical of patients at onset of the disease or when the disease course is relatively benign (**Figures 1** and **2**). It is important to mention that the motor threshold in these cases remained within the normal values or was decreased.

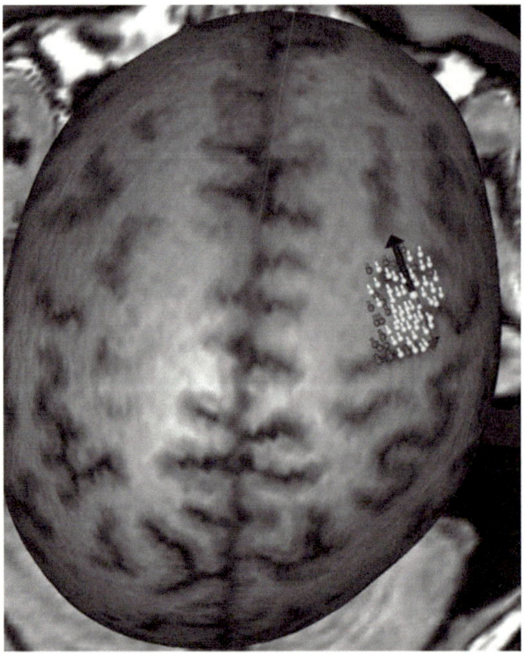

Figure 1. Map of cortical representation of the APB in a healthy volunteer (28 years old, motor threshold—43%). Here and in other figures, the points whose stimulation provides MEPs with amplitude over 50 μV from the contralateral APB are shown in white.

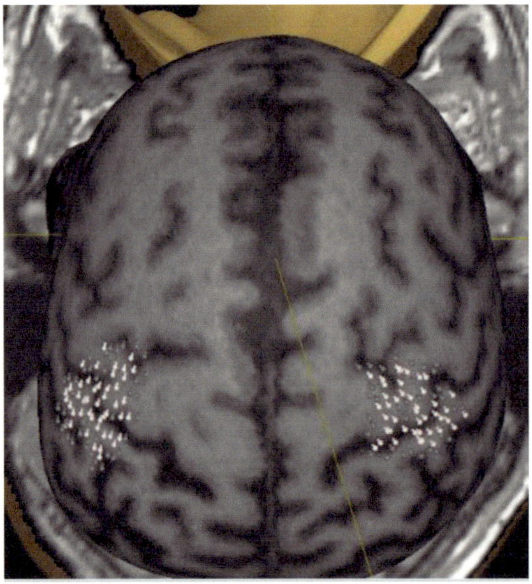

Figure 2. Maps of cortical representation of the APB in ALS patient with the relatively benign course of the disease (54 years old, right-side motor threshold—31%, left-side motor threshold—35%, duration of the disease—25 months, APB strength is bilaterally reduced to MRC score 4).

http://dx.doi.org/10.5772/63310

Although we have not performed mathematical analysis of the relationship between motor cortex excitability and reorganization of cortical representation, we suppose that hyperexcitability can be one of the mechanisms of the aforementioned neuroplastic alterations. Thus, a statistically significant relationship between the passive threshold as an excitability marker and the volume of cortical representation has been revealed. So the largest cortical representation was revealed in patients with lower thresholds. This made it possible to rule out the possible role of higher-intensity stimuli in expansion of the map boundaries in ALS patients compared to the control group. Indeed, the motor threshold in some patients was 100% and we used this intensity in mapping. However, only single MEPs were detected in the aforementioned cases and the size of cortical representation was very small (**Figure 3**).

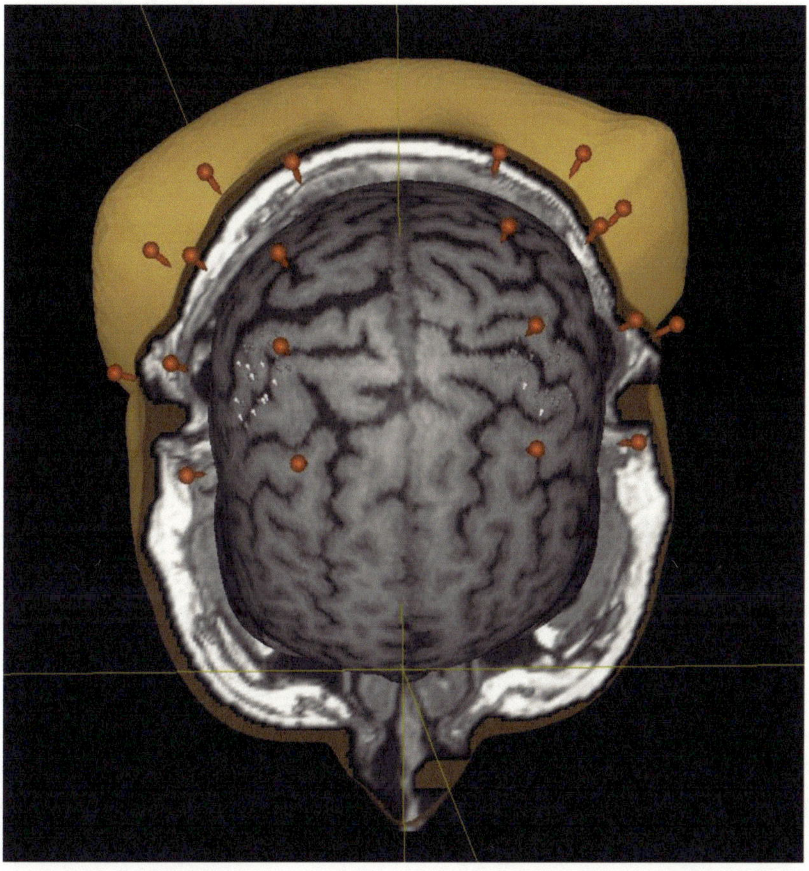

Figure 3. Maps of cortical representation of the APB in a 62-year-old female patient with ALS. Upper-limb form of the disease; disease duration—8 months. ALS-FRS-R—38. APB strength is bilaterally reduced to MRC score 2. Motor threshold on the right and left sides—100%. The volume of cortical representation is significantly decreased.

Our findings agree with the fMRI data described above that attest to expansion of the activation areas in ALS patients performing a motor task. Like fMRI, visual assessment of nTMS mapping data allows one to detect displacement of cortical representation. Our preliminary data demonstrate that displacement of the boundaries of cortical representation as a result of neuroplastic alterations can be caused by decreased motor cortex excitability. Hence, the phenomenon of motor cortex hyperexcitability can have the compensatory function in ALS patients.

5. Conclusions and future perspectives

Motor cortex hyperexcitability in ALS patients is a well-studied phenomenon that can be of significant interest as a biomarker of neurodegeneration. However, despite the large number of studies, the reasons and sequelae currently remain poorly studied. Since motor cortex hyperexcitability in ALS patients was first described, this phenomenon has been attributed to the development of excitotoxicity and weakening of inhibitory neurotransmission in the neocortex, thus ensuring its pathogenetic role in the development of neurodegeneration. However, no direct evidence to the fact that motor cortex hyperexcitability in ALS patients attests to development of excitotoxicity and precedes its degeneration has been obtained yet. Meanwhile, hyperexcitability can be one of the mechanisms of neuroplastic alterations, thus having the compensatory (sanogenetic) rather than pathogenetic value. This theory has been supported by the data on interaction between decreased motor cortex excitability and neuroplasticity in the norm and in some pathologic conditions such as Alzheimer's disease and vascular dementia. Furthermore, expansion of the cortical representation of certain muscles was demonstrated for ALS patients in fMRI and nTMS studies, which can be a manifestation of neuroplasticity and related to increased motor cortex excitability.

It should be mentioned that hyperexcitability is not a specific sign of ALS and is also revealed in other neurodegenerative diseases. More and more data supporting the similarity between pathophysiology of neurodegeneration in various diseases and its relationship with intracellular accumulation of abnormal proteins have been obtained. This may result in dysfunction of synaptic connections and a compensatory increase in expression of the genes ensuring increased excitability and synaptic plasticity.

A hypothesis can be put forward based on these data that hyperexcitability plays different roles at different stages of the disease (**Figure 4**). At onset of the disease, this phenomenon can develop via the compensatory mechanism in response to reduced number of functioning motor neurons and disruption of synaptic connections. Hence, increased hyperexcitability can be regarded as a method for maintaining functioning of the system as the number of its components decreases. In addition, hyperexcitability can have a protective effect at the cellular level as it prevents accumulation of pathologically altered proteins. As the disease progresses, hyperexcitability may start to have a pathological effect and induce excitotoxicity. Does this mean that our effect on motor cortex excitability in ALS patients needs to be differentiated depending on disease stage? Further research involving various methods and focusing on patients at different stages of the disease needs to be carried out to answer this question.

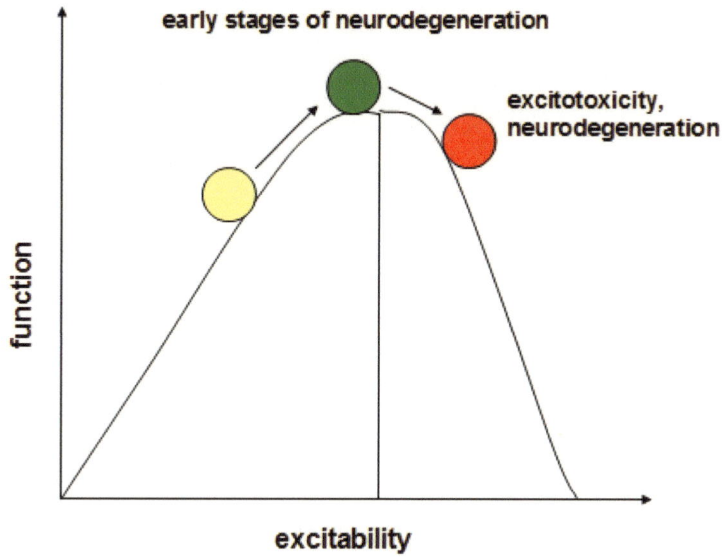

Figure 4. A link between excitability and function.

Author details

Ilya S. Bakulin, Alexander V. Chervyakov*, Natalia A. Suponeva, Maria N. Zakharova and Michael A. Piradov

*Address all correspondence to: tchervyakovav@gmail.com

Research Center of Neurology, Moscow, Russia

References

[1] Turner MR, Bowser R, Bruijn L, Dupuis L, Ludolph A, McGrath M. Mechanisms, models and biomarkers in amyotrophic lateral sclerosis. Amyotroph Lateral Scler Frontotemporal Degener. 2013;14(1):19–32. DOI: 10.3109/21678421.2013.778554.

[2] Chiò A, Pagani M, Agosta F, Calvo A, Cistaro A, Filippi M. Neuroimaging in amyotrophic lateral sclerosis: insights into structural and functional changes. Lancet Neurol. 2014;13(12):1228–40. DOI: 10.1016/S1474-4422(14)70167-X.

[3] Bede P, Hardiman O. Lessons of ALS imaging: Pitfalls and future directions - A critical review. Neuroimage Clin. 2014; 27(4):436–43. DOI: 10.1016/j.nicl.2014.02.011.

[4] Vucic S, Ziemann U, Eisen A, Hallett M, Kiernan MC. Transcranial magnetic stimulation and amyotrophic lateral sclerosis: pathophysiological insights. J Neurol Neurosurg Psychiatry. 2013;84(10):1161–70. DOI: 10.1136/jnnp-2012-304019.

[5] Menon P, Kiernan MC, Vucic S. Cortical hyperexcitability precedes lower motor neuron dysfunction in ALS. Clin Neurophysiol. 2015;126(4):803–9. DOI: 10.1016/j.clinph.2014.04.023.

[6] Zanette G, Tamburin S, Manganotti P, Refatti N, Forgione A, Rizzuto N. Different mechanisms contribute to motor cortex hyperexcitability in amyotrophic lateral sclerosis. Clin Neurophysiol. 2002;113(11):1688–97.

[7] Bae JS, Simon NG, Menon P, Vucic S, Kiernan MC. The puzzling case of hyperexcitability in amyotrophic lateral sclerosis. J Clin Neurol. 2013;9(2):65–74. DOI: 10.3988/jcn.2013.9.2.65.

[8] King AE, Woodhouse A, Kirkcaldie MT, Vickers JC. Excitotoxicity in ALS: Overstimulation, or overreaction? Exp Neurol. 2016;275(1):162–71. DOI: 10.1016/j.expneurol.2015.09.019.

[9] Blasco H, Mavel S, Corcia P, Gordon PH. The glutamate hypothesis in ALS: pathophysiology and drug development. Curr Med Chem. 2014;21(31):3551–75.

[10] Fray AE, Ince, PG, Banner SJ, Milton ID, Usher PA, Cookson MR, Shaw PJ. The expression of the glial glutamate transporter protein EAAT2 in motor neuron disease: an immunohistochemical study. Eur. J. Neurosci. 1998;10(8):2481–2489.

[11] Sasaki S, Komori T, Iwata M. Excitatory amino acid transporter 1 and 2 immunoreactivity in the spinal cord in amyotrophic lateral sclerosis. Acta Neuropathol. 2000;100(2):138–44.

[12] Howland DS, Liu J, She Y, Goad B, Maragakis NJ, Kim B, Erickson J, Kulik J, DeVito L, Psaltis G, DeGennaro LJ, Cleveland DW, Rothstein JD. Focal loss of the glutamate transporter EAAT2 in a transgenic rat model of SOD1 mutant-mediated amyotrophic lateral sclerosis (ALS). Proc. Natl. Acad. Sci. U. S. A. 2002;99(3):1604–1609.

[13] Velasco I, Tapia R, Massieu L. Inhibition of glutamate uptake induces progressive accumulation of extracellular glutamate and neuronal damage in rat cortical cultures. J. Neurosci. Res. 1996;44(6):551–561.

[14] Benkler C, Ben-Zur T, Barhum Y, Offen D. Altered astrocytic response to activation in SOD1(G93A) mice and its implications on amyotrophic lateral sclerosis pathogenesis. Glia. 2013;61(3):312–326. DOI: 10.1002/glia.22428.

[15] Ince P, Stout N, Shaw P, Slade J, Hunziker W, Heizmann CW, Baimbridge KG. Parvalbumin and calbindin D-28k in the human motor system and in motor neuron disease. Neuropathol. Appl. Neurobiol. 1993;19(4):291–299.

[16] Stephens B, Guiloff RJ, Navarrete R, Newman P, Nikhar N, Lewis P. Widespread loss of neuronal populations in the spinal ventral horn in sporadic motor neuron disease. A morphometric study. J. Neurol. Sci. 2006;244(1-2):41–58.

[17] McGown A, McDearmid JR, Panagiotaki N, Tong H, Al Mashhadi S, Redhead N, Lyon AN, Beattie CE, Shaw PJ, Ramesh TM. Early interneuron dysfunction in ALS: insights from a mutant sod1 zebrafish model. Ann. Neurol. 2013;73(2):246–258. DOI: 10.1002/ana.23780.

[18] Foerster BR, Callaghan BC, Petrou M, Edden RA, Chenevert TL, Feldman EL. Decreased motor cortex γ-aminobutyric acid in amyotrophic lateral sclerosis. Neurology. 2012;78(20):1596–600. DOI: 10.1212/WNL.0b013e3182563b57.

[19] Turner MR, Hammers A, Al-Chalabi A, Shaw CE, Andersen PM, Brooks DJ, Leigh PN. Distinct cerebral lesions in sporadic and 'D90A' SOD1 ALS: studies with [11C]flumazenil PET. Brain. 2005;128(Pt 6):1323–9.

[20] Petri S, Krampfl K, Hashemi F, Grothe C, Hori A, Dengler R, Bufler J. Distribution of GABAA receptor mRNA in the motor cortex of ALS patients. J Neuropathol Exp Neurol. 2003;62(10):1041–51.

[21] Kuo JJ, Siddique T, Fu R, Heckman CJ. Increased persistent Na(+) current and its effect on excitability in motoneurones cultured from mutant SOD1 mice. J Physiol. 2005; 563(3):843–854.

[22] Pieri M, Carunchio I, Curcio L, Mercuri NB, Zona C. Increased persistent sodium current determines cortical hyperexcitability in a genetic model of familial amyotrophic lateral sclerosis. Exp Neurol. 2009;215(2):368–379. DOI: 10.1016/j.expneurol.2008.11.002.

[23] van Zundert B, Peuscher MH, Hynynen M, Chen A, Neve RL, Brown RH, Jr, Constantine-Paton M, Bellingham MC. Neonatal neuronal circuitry shows hyperexcitable disturbance in a mouse model of the adult-onset neurodegenerative disease amyotrophic lateral sclerosis. J Neurosci. 2008;28(43):10864–10874. DOI: 10.1523/JNEUROSCI.1340-08.2008.

[24] Pambo-Pambo A, Durand J, Gueritaud J-P. Early excitability changes in lumbar motoneurons of transgenic $SOD1^{G85R}$ and $S0D1^{G93A\text{-}Low}$ mice. J Neurophysiol. 2009;102(6):3627–3642. DOI:10.1152/jn.00482.2009.

[25] Kawahara Y, Ito K, Sun H, Aizawa H, Kanazawa I, Kwak S. Glutamate receptors: RNA editing and death of motor neurons. Nature. 2004;427(6977):801.

[26] Di Lazzaro V, Ziemann U. The contribution of transcranial magnetic stimulation in the functional evaluation of microcircuits in human motor cortex. Front Neural Circuits. 2013;13(7):18. DOI: 10.3389/fncir.2013.00018.

[27] Rossini PM, Burke D, Chen R, Cohen LG, Daskalakis Z, Di Iorio R et al. Non-invasive electrical and magnetic stimulation of the brain, spinal cord, roots and peripheral

nerves: basic principles and procedures for routine clinical and research application. An updated report from an I.F.C.N. Committee. Clin Neurophysiol. 2015;126(6):1071–107. DOI: 10.1016/j.clinph.2015.02.001.

[28] Di Lazzaro V. Biological effects of non-invasive brain stimulation. Handb Clin Neurol. 2013;2013(116):367-74. DOI: 10.1016/B978-0-444-53497-2.00030-9.

[29] Chervyakov AV, Bakulin IS, Savitskaya NG, Arkhipov IV, Gavrilov AV, Zakharova MN, Piradov MA. Navigated transcranial magnetic stimulation in amyotrophic lateral sclerosis. Muscle Nerve. 2015;51(1):125–31. DOI: 10.1002/mus.24345.

[30] de Carvalho M, Turkman A, Swash M. Motor responses evoked by transcranial magnetic stimulation and peripheral nerve stimulation in the ulnar innervation in amyotrophic lateral sclerosis: the effect of upper and lower motor neuron lesion. J Neurol Sci. 2003;210(1–2):83–90.

[31] Miscio G, Pisano F, Mora G, Mazzini L. Motor neuron disease: usefulness of transcranial magnetic stimulation in improving the diagnosis. Clin Neurophysiol. 1999;110(5):975–81.

[32] Eisen A, Shytbel W, Murphy K, Hoirch M. Cortical magnetic stimulation in amyotrophic lateral sclerosis. Muscle Nerve. 1990;13(2):146–51.

[33] Mills KR. The natural history of central motor abnormalities in amyotrophic lateral sclerosis. Brain. 2003;126(Pt 11):2558–66.

[34] Triggs WJ, Menkes D, Onorato J, Yan RS, Young MS, Newell K et al. Transcranial magnetic stimulation identifies upper motor neuron involvement in motor neuron disease. Neurology. 1999;53(3):605–11.

[35] Urban PP, Wicht S, Hopf HC. Sensitivity of transcranial magnetic stimulation of cortico-bulbar vs. cortico-spinal tract involvement in Amyotrophic Lateral Sclerosis (ALS). J Neurol. 2001;248(10):850–5.

[36] Vucic S, Cheah BC, Kiernan MC. Defining the mechanisms that underlie cortical hyperexcitability in amyotrophic lateral sclerosis. Exp Neurol. 2009;220(1):177–82. DOI: 10.1016/j.expneurol.2009.08.017.

[37] Caramia MD, Cicinelli P, Paradiso C, Mariorenzi R, Zarola F, Bernardi G, Rossini PM. Excitability changes of muscular responses to magnetic brain stimulation in patients with central motor disorders. Electroencephalogr Clin Neurophysiol. 1991;81(4):243–50.

[38] Vucic S, Kiernan MC. Novel threshold tracking techniques suggest that cortical hyperexcitability is an early feature of motor neuron disease. Brain. 2006;129(Pt 9):2436–46.

[39] Mills KR, Nithi KA. Corticomotor threshold is reduced in early sporadic amyotrophic lateral sclerosis. Muscle Nerve. 1997;20(9):1137–41.

[40] Khedr EM, Ahmed MA, Hamdy A, Shawky OA. Cortical excitability of amyotrophic lateral sclerosis: transcranial magnetic stimulation study. Neurophysiol Clin. 2011;41(2):73–9. DOI: 10.1016/j.neucli.2011.03.001.

[41] Ziemann U, Reis J, Schwenkreis P, Rosanova M, Strafella A, Badawy R, Müller-Dahlhaus F. TMS and drugs revisited 2014. Clin Neurophysiol. 2015;126(10):1847–68. DOI: 10.1016/j.clinph.2014.08.028.

[42] Carriedo SG, Sensi SL, Yin HZ, Weiss JH. AMPA exposures induce mitochondrial Ca(2+) overload and ROS generation in spinal motor neurons in vitro. J Neurosci. 2000;20(1):240–50.

[43] Saba L, Viscomi MT, Caioli S, Pignataro A, Bisicchia E, Pieri M, Molinari M, Ammassari-Teule M, Zona C. Altered Functionality, Morphology, and Vesicular Glutamate Transporter Expression of Cortical Motor Neurons from a Presymptomatic Mouse Model of Amyotrophic Lateral Sclerosis. Cereb Cortex. 2016;26(4):1512-28. pii: bhu317.

[44] Paulus W, Classen J, Cohen LG, Large CH, Di Lazzaro V, Nitsche M, Pascual-Leone A, Rosenow F, Rothwell JC, Ziemann U. State of the art: pharmacologic effects on cortical excitability measures tested by transcranial magnetic stimulation. Brain Stimul. 2008;1(3):151–63. DOI: 10.1016/j.brs.2008.06.002.

[45] Vucic S, Nicholson GA, Kiernan MC. Cortical hyperexcitability may precede the onset of familial amyotrophic lateral sclerosis. Brain. 2008;131(6):1540-50. DOI: 10.1093/brain/awn071.

[46] Vucic S, Kiernan MC. Cortical excitability testing distinguishes Kennedy's disease from amyotrophic lateral sclerosis. Clin Neurophysiol. 2008;119(5):1088–96. DOI: 10.1016/j.clinph.2008.01.011.

[47] Wilson SA, Lockwood RJ, Thickbroom GW, Mastaglia FL. The muscle silent period following transcranial magnetic cortical stimulation. J Neurol Sci. 1993;114(2):216–22.

[48] Zanette G, Tamburin S, Manganotti P, Refatti N, Forgione A, Rizzuto N. Changes in motor cortex inhibition over time in patients with amyotrophic lateral sclerosis. J Neurol. 2002;249(12):1723–8.

[49] Siciliano G, Manca ML, Sagliocco L, Pastorini E, Pellegrinetti A, Sartucci F et al. Cortical silent period in patients with amyotrophic lateral sclerosis. J Neurol Sci. 1999;169(1–2):93–7.

[50] Prout AJ, Eisen AA. The cortical silent period and amyotrophic lateral sclerosis. Muscle Nerve. 1994;17(2):217–23.

[51] Kujirai T, Caramia MD, Rothwell JC, Day BL, Thompson PD, Ferbert A et al. Cortico-cortical inhibition in human motor cortex. J Physiol. 1993;471(1):501-19.

[52] Nakamura H, Kitagawa H, Kawaguchi Y, Tsuji H. Intracortical facilitation and inhibition after transcranial magnetic stimulation in conscious humans. J Physiol. 1997;498 (Pt 3):817–23.

[53] Vucic S, Cheah BC, Yiannikas C, Kiernan MC. Cortical excitability distinguishes ALS from mimic disorders. Clin Neurophysiol. 2011;122(9):1860–6. DOI: 10.1016/j.clinph.2010.12.062.

[54] Ziemann U, Winter M, Reimers CD, Reimers K, Tergau F, Paulus W. Impaired motor cortex inhibition in patients with amyotrophic lateral sclerosis. Evidence from paired transcranial magnetic stimulation. Neurology. 1997;49(5):1292–8.

[55] Yokota T, Yoshino A, Inaba A, Saito Y. Double cortical stimulation in amyotrophic lateral sclerosis. J Neurol Neurosurg Psychiatry. 1996;61(6):596–600.

[56] Menon P, Geevasinga N, Yiannikas C, Howells J, Kiernan MC, Vucic S. Sensitivity and specificity of threshold tracking transcranial magnetic stimulation for diagnosis of amyotrophic lateral sclerosis: a prospective study. Lancet Neurol. 2015;14(5):478–84. DOI: 10.1016/S1474-4422(15)00014-9.

[57] Geevasinga N, Menon P, Yiannikas C, Kiernan MC, Vucic S. Diagnostic utility of cortical excitability studies in amyotrophic lateral sclerosis. Eur J Neurol. 2014;21(12): 1451–7. DOI: 10.1111/ene.12422.

[58] Clark R, Blizzard C, Dickson T. Inhibitory dysfunction in amyotrophic lateral sclerosis: future therapeutic opportunities. Neurodegener Dis Manag. 2015;5(6):511–25. DOI: 10.2217/nmt.15.49.

[59] Martin LJ, Chang Q. Inhibitory synaptic regulation of motoneurons: a new target of disease mechanisms in amyotrophic lateral sclerosis. Mol Neurobiol. 2012;45(1):30–42. DOI: 10.1007/s12035-011-8217-x.

[60] Turner MR, Kiernan MC. Does interneuronal dysfunction contribute to neurodegeneration in amyotrophic lateral sclerosis? Amyotroph Lateral Scler 2012;13(3):245–50. DOI: 10.3109/17482968.2011.636050.

[61] Nihei K, McKee AC, Kowall NW. Patterns of neuronal degeneration in the motor cortex of amyotrophic lateral sclerosis patients. Acta Neuropathol. (Berl.) 1993;86(1):55–64.

[62] Leroy F, Zytnicki D. Is hyperexcitability really guilty in amyotrophic lateral sclerosis? Neural Regen Res. 2015;10(9):1413–5. DOI: 10.4103/1673-5374.165308.

[63] van Zundert B, Izaurieta P, Fritz E, Alvarez FJ. Early pathogenesis in the adult-onset neurodegenerative disease amyotrophic lateral sclerosis. J Cell Biochem. 2012;113(11): 3301–12. DOI: 10.1002/jcb.24234.

[64] Jia M, Njapo SA, Rastogi V, Hedna VS. Taming glutamate excitotoxicity: strategic pathway modulation for neuroprotection CNS Drugs. 2015;29(2):153–62. DOI: 10.1007/s40263-015-0225-3.

[65] Bromberg MB. The cart or the horse first? Did Charcot have it right? Clin Neurophysiol. 2015;126(4):647–8. DOI: 10.1016/j.clinph.2014.07.019.

[66] Bellingham MC. A review of the neural mechanisms of action and clinical efficiency of riluzole in treating amyotrophic lateral sclerosis: what have we learned in the last decade? CNS Neurosci Ther. 2011;17(1):4–31. DOI: 10.1111/j.1755-5949.2009.00116.x.

[67] Vucic S, Lin CS, Cheah BC, Murray J, Menon P, Krishnan AV, Kiernan MC. Riluzole exerts central and peripheral modulating effects in amyotrophic lateral sclerosis. Brain. 2013;136(Pt 5):1361–70. DOI: 10.1093/brain/awt085.

[68] Chervyakov AV, Chernyavsky AY, Sinitsyn DO, Piradov MA. Possible mechanisms underlying the therapeutic effects of transcranial magnetic stimulation. Front Hum Neurosci. 2015;9:303. DOI: 10.3389/fnhum.2015.00303.

[69] Tang A, Thickbroom G, Rodger J. Repetitive Transcranial Magnetic Stimulation of the Brain: Mechanisms from Animal and Experimental Models. Neuroscientist. [Epub ahead of print]. pii: 1073858415618897.

[70] Di Lazzaro V, Oliviero A, Saturno E, Pilato F, Dileone M, Sabatelli M, Tonali PA. Motor cortex stimulation for amyotrophic lateral sclerosis. Time for a therapeutic trial? Clin Neurophysiol. 2004;115(6):1479–85.

[71] Nitsche MA, Müller-Dahlhaus F, Paulus W, Ziemann U. The pharmacology of neuroplasticity induced by non-invasive brain stimulation: building models for the clinical use of CNS active drugs. J Physiol. 2012;590(Pt 19):4641–62. DOI: 10.1113/jphysiol.2012.232975.

[72] Malenka RC, Kauer JA, Zucker RS, Nicoll RA. Postsynaptic calcium is sufficient for potentiation of hippocampal synaptic transmission. Science. 1988;242(4875):81–84.

[73] Malinow R, Malenka RC. AMPA receptor trafficking and synaptic plasticity. Annu Rev Neurosci. 2002;25(1):103–126.

[74] Liao D, Hessler NA, Malinow R. Activation of postsynaptically silent synapses during pairing-induced LTP in CA1 region of hippocampal slice. Nature. 1995;375(6530):400–404.

[75] Chernikova LA, Kremneva EI, Cherviakov AV, Saenko IV, Konovalov RN, Piramidov MA, Kozlovskaia IB. New approaches in the study of neuroplasticity process in patients with central nervous system lesion Fiziol Cheloveka. 2013;39(3):54–60. Russian.

[76] Bezzola L., Merillat S., Jäncke L. Motor training-induced neuroplasticity. The Journal of Gerontopsychology and Geriatric Psychiatry. 2012;25(4):189–197.

[77] Koeneke S, Lutz K, Herwig U, Ziemann U, Jäncke L. Extensive training of elementary finger tapping movements changes the pattern of motor cortex excitability. Exp Brain Res. 2006;174(2):199–209.

[78] Svensson P, Romaniello A, Wang K, Arendt-Nielsen L, Sessle BJ. One hour of tongue-task training is associated with plasticity in corticomotor control of the human tongue musculature. Exp Brain Res. 2006;173(1):165–73.

[79] Classen J, Liepert J, Hallett M, Cohen L. Plasticity of movement representation in the human motor cortex. Electroencephalogr Clin Neurophysiol Suppl. 1999;51(1):162–73.

[80] Tyč F, Boyadjian A. Plasticity of motor cortex induced by coordination and training. Clin Neurophysiol. 2011;122(1):153–62. DOI: 10.1016/j.clinph.2010.05.022.

[81] Perez MA, Lungholt BK, Nyborg K, Nielsen JB. Motor skill training induces changes in the excitability of the leg cortical area in healthy humans. Exp Brain Res. 2004;159(2): 197–205.

[82] Mokienko OA, Chervyakov AV, Kulikova SN, Bobrov PD, Chernikova LA, Frolov AA, Piradov MA. Increased motor cortex excitability during motor imagery in brain-computer interface trained subjects. Front Comput Neurosci. 2013;7:168. DOI: 10.3389/fncom.2013.00168.

[83] Rosenkranz K, Williamon A, Rothwell JC. Motorcortical excitability and synaptic plasticity is enhanced in professional musicians. J Neurosci. 2007;27(19):5200–6.

[84] Pearce AJ, Thickbroom GW, Byrnes ML, Mastaglia FL. Functional reorganisation of the corticomotor projection to the hand in skilled racquet players. Exp Brain Res. 2000;130(2):238–43.

[85] Funkenstein HH, Albert MS, Cook NR, West CG, Scherr PA, Chown MJ, Pilgrim D, Evans DA. Extrapyramidal signs and other neurological findings in clinically diagnosed Alzheimer's disease. Arch Neurol. 1993;50(1):51–6.

[86] Rogers J, Morrison JH. Quantitative morphology and regional and laminar distribution of senile plaques in Alzheimer's disease. J Neurosci. 1985;5(10):2801–8.

[87] Pennisi G, Ferri R, Lanza G, Cantone M, Pennisi M, Puglisi V, Malaguarnera G, Bella R. Transcranial magnetic stimulation in Alzheimer's disease: a neurophysiological marker of cortical hyperexcitability. J Neural Transm (Vienna). 2011;118(4):587–98. DOI: 10.1007/s00702-010-0554-9.

[88] Guerra A, Assenza F, Bressi F, Scrascia F, Del Duca M, Ursini F, Vollaro S, Trotta L, Tombini M, Chisari C, Ferreri F. Transcranial magnetic stimulation studies in Alzheimer's disease. Int J Alzheimers Dis. 2011; 2011:263817. DOI: 10.4061/2011/263817.

[89] Di Lazzaro V, Oliviero A, Pilato F, Saturno E, Dileone M, Marra C, Daniele A, Ghirlanda S, Gainotti G, Tonali PA. Motor cortex hyperexcitability to transcranial magnetic stimulation in Alzheimer's disease. J Neurol Neurosurg Psychiatry. 2004; 75(4):555–9.

[90] Ferreri F, Pauri F, Pasqualetti P, Fini R, Dal Forno G, Rossini PM. Motor cortex excitability in Alzheimer's disease: a transcranial magnetic stimulation study. Ann Neurol. 2003;53(1):102–8.

[91] Ferreri F, Pasqualetti P, Määttä S, Ponzo D, Guerra A, Bressi F, Chiovenda P, Del Duca M, Giambattistelli F, Ursini F, Tombini M, Vernieri F, Rossini PM. Motor cortex excitability in Alzheimer's disease: a transcranial magnetic stimulation follow-up study. Neurosci Lett. 2011;492(2):94–8. DOI: 10.1016/j.neulet.2011.01.064.

[92] Vidoni ED, Thomas GP, Honea RA, Loskutova N, Burns JM. Evidence of altered corticomotor system connectivity in early-stage Alzheimer's disease. J Neurol Phys Ther. 2012;36(1):8–16. DOI: 10.1097/NPT.0b013e3182462ea6.

[93] Guerra A, Petrichella S, Vollero L, Ponzo D, Pasqualetti P, Määttä S et al. Neurophysiological features of motor cortex excitability and plasticity in Subcortical Ischemic Vascular Dementia: a TMS mapping study. Clin Neurophysiol. 2015; 126(5):906–13. DOI: 10.1016/j.clinph.2014.07.036.

[94] Dickerson BC, Sperling RA. Large-scale functional brain network abnormalities in Alzheimer's disease: insights from functional neuroimaging. Behav. Neurol. 2009;21(1): 63–75. DOI: 10.3233/BEN-2009-0227.

[95] Dickerson BC, Salat DH, Greve DN, Chua EF, Rand-Giovannetti E, Rentz DM, Bertram L, Mullin K, Tanzi RE, Blacker D, Albert MS, Sperling RA. Increased hippocampal activation in mild cognitive impairment compared to normal aging and AD. Neurology. 2005;65(3):404–411.

[96] Hamalainen A, Pihlajamaki M, Tanila H, Hanninen T, Niskanen E, Tervo S, Karjalainen PA, Vanninen RL, Soininen H. Increased fMRI responses during encoding in mild cognitive impairment. Neurobiol Aging. 2007;28(12):1889–1903.

[97] Kircher TT, Weis S, Freymann K, Erb M, Jessen F, Grodd W, Heun R, Leube DT. Hippocampal activation in patients with mild cognitive impairment is necessary for successful memory encoding. J. Neurol. Neurosurg. Psychiatry 2007;78(8):812–818.

[98] Saura CA, Parra Damas A, Enriquez-Barreto L. Gene expression parallels synaptic excitability and plasticity changes in Alzheimer's disease. Front Cell Neurosci. 2015;9:318. DOI: 10.3389/fncel.2015.00318.

[99] Palop JJ, Chin J, Roberson ED, Wang J, Thwin MT, Bien-Ly N, Yoo J, Ho KO, Yu GQ, Kreitzer A, Finkbeiner S, Noebels JL, Mucke L. Aberrant excitatory neuronal activity and compensatory remodeling of inhibitory hippocampal circuits in mouse models of Alzheimer's disease. Neuron. 2007;55(5):697–711.

[100] Busche MA, Eichhoff G, Adelsberger H, Abramowski D, Wiederhold KH, Haass C, Staufenbiel M, Konnerth A, Garaschuk O. Clusters of hyperactive neurons near amyloid plaques in a mouse model of Alzheimer's disease. Science. 2008;321(5896): 1686–1689. DOI: 10.1126/science.1162844.

[101] Jolas T, Zhang XS, Zhang Q, Wong G, Del Vecchio R, Gold L, Priestley T. Long-term potentiation is increased in the CA1 area of the hippocampus of APP (swe/ind) CRND8 mice. Neurobiol. Dis. 2002;11(3):394–409.

[102] Schneider I, Reverse D, Dewachter I, Ris L, Caluwaerts N, Kuiperi C, Gilis M, Geerts H, Kretzschmar H, Godaux E, Moechars D, Van Leuven F, Herms J. Mutant presenilins disturb neuronal calcium homeostasis in the brain of transgenic mice, decreasing the threshold for excitotoxicity and facilitating long-term potentiation. J Biol Chem. 2001;276(15):11539–44.

[103] Bell KF, Bennett DA, Cuello AC. Paradoxical upregulation of glutamatergic presynaptic boutons during mild cognitive impairment. J Neurosci. 2007;27(40):10810–7.

[104] Cantanelli P, Sperduti S, Ciavardelli D, Stuppia L, Gatta V, Sensi SL. Age-dependent modifications of AMPA receptor subunit expression levels and related cognitive effects in 3xTg-AD mice. Front Aging Neurosci. 2014;6:200. DOI: 10.3389/fnagi.2014.00200.

[105] Saxena S, Roselli F, Singh K, Leptien K, Julien JP, Gros-Louis F, Caroni P. Neuroprotection through excitability and mTOR required in ALS motoneurons to delay disease and extend survival. Neuron. 2013;80(1):80–96. DOI: 10.1016/j.neuron.2013.07.027.

[106] Leroy F, Lamotte d'Incamps B, Imhoff-Manuel RD, Zytnicki D. Early intrinsic hyperexcitability does not contribute to motoneuron degeneration in amyotrophic lateral sclerosis. Elife. 2014;3: e04046. doi: 10.7554/eLife.04046.

[107] Konrad C, Henningsen H, Bremer J, Mock B, Deppe M, Buchinger C et al. Pattern of cortical reorganization in amyotrophic lateral sclerosis: a functional magnetic resonance imaging study. Exp Brain Res. 2002;143(1):51–6.

[108] Lulé D, Diekmann V, Kassubek J, Kurt A, Birbaumer N, Ludolph AC, Kraft E. Cortical plasticity in amyotrophic lateral sclerosis: motor imagery and function. Neurorehabil Neural Repair. 2007;21(6):518–26.

[109] Stanton BR, Williams VC, Leigh PN, Williams SC, Blain CR, Jarosz JM, Simmons A. Altered cortical activation during a motor task in ALS. Evidence for involvement of central pathways. J Neurol. 2007;254(9):1260–7.

[110] Poujois A, Schneider FC, Faillenot I, Camdessanché JP, Vandenberghe N, Thomas-Antérion C, Antoine JC. Brain plasticity in the motor network is correlated with disease progression in amyotrophic lateral sclerosis. Hum Brain Mapp. 2013; 34(10):2391–401. DOI: 10.1002/hbm.22070.

[111] Ruohonen J, Karhu J. Navigated transcranial magnetic stimulation. Neurophysiol Clin. 2010;40(1):7–17. DOI: 10.1016/j.neucli.2010.01.006.

[112] de Carvalho M, Miranda PC, Luís ML, Ducla-Soares E. Cortical muscle representation in amyotrophic lateral sclerosis patients: changes with disease evolution. Muscle Nerve. 1999;22(12):1684–92.

Chapter 4

SOD1, from Bench to Bed: New Role for the Oldest Protein Implicated in ALS

Diamanti Luca, Zucchi Elisabetta, Pansarasa Orietta,
Ceroni Mauro and Cereda Crisitna

Additional information is available at the end of the chapter

http://dx.doi.org/10.5772/63307

Abstract

In 1993, the first superoxide dismutase 1 (SOD1) mutation in amyotrophic lateral sclerosis (ALS) patients has been described by Rosen et al. successively, the scientific literature focused on the role of SOD1 in the pathogenesis of ALS. While a clear genetic scenario has been presented, heterogeneous data have been formulated regarding transcriptional and post-transcriptional regulation of SOD1 so far. In particular, the dilemma concerns the SOD1 protein expression, in the direction of a loss of function of the wild-type SOD1 or a toxic gain of function of the altered SOD1, both in FALS (mutant-SOD1) and in SALS (misfolded-SOD1). In this chapter, we focus on the evolution of scientific knowledge about SOD1 protein in ALS patients, reviewing in detail the results obtained using peripheral blood cells in this research field. To conclude, we propose a brief summary of the described clinical correlation and discuss the possible SOD1 implication as a biomarker of ALS.

Keywords: trascriptional regulation, post-trascriptional regulation, amyotrophic lateral sclerosis (ALS), superoxide dismutase 1 (SOD1), biomarkers, protein aggregation

1. Introduction

Cu/Zn superoxide dismutase (SOD1) is a 32-KDa homodimeric enzyme that assumes a pivotal role in the scavenging process of the toxic superoxide radicals in the cells [1]. SOD1 is highly expressed in the cytoplasm, but in the 1980s, Chang and colleagues identified SOD1 in other sub-cellular compartments, such as nucleus, lysosomes, and mitochondria [2]. In the 1990s, the scientific literature focused on the genetic and biochemical characterization of SOD1, and in

INTECH
open science | open minds

© 2016 The Author(s). Licensee InTech. This chapter is distributed under the terms of the Creative Commons Attribution License (http://creativecommons.org/licenses/by/3.0), which permits unrestricted use, distribution, and reproduction in any medium, provided the original work is properly cited.

1993, Rosen et al. [3] described the first SOD1 gene mutation associated with amyotrophic lateral sclerosis (ALS) [3]. ALS is an adult-onset neurodegenerative disease that affects selectively cortical, bulbar, and spinal motor neurons, leading invariably to a fatal prognosis. The majority of ALS cases (90–95%) are sporadic (SALS), whereas 5–10% are familial (FALS), with genetic mutations dominantly inherited. Among these, more than 150 SOD1 mutations have been reported that are responsible for 20% of FALS, but also 1% of SALS [4]. During the last 20 years, many studies were focused on SOD1 protein in the pathogenesis of ALS, both for FALS and for SALS. Hitherto, some aspects remain unclear: (1) SOD1 alterations give selective loss of motor neurons, even though the enzyme is ubiquitous in every cell; (2) mutations confer SOD1 enzyme's loss of function reducing antioxidant activity but, in some way, mutated enzyme can acquire toxicity; (3) the ALS phenotype doesn't reflect the common presentation of the loss-of-function-related diseases, in terms of age of onset, clinical spreading, and evolution. In this chapter, we would like to pass through the recent understandings about SOD1 protein in the pathogenesis of ALS, in particular focusing on its aggregation in peripheral blood cells and its transcriptional/post-transcriptional regulation.

2. SOD1 and ALS models

2.1. Investigating SOD1-mediated pathogenesis in different cellular models

The SOD1 gene is located on chromosome 21q22.11 (**Figure 1**), and more than 150 mutations have been discovered since 1993, all of them proving to be causative of ALS.

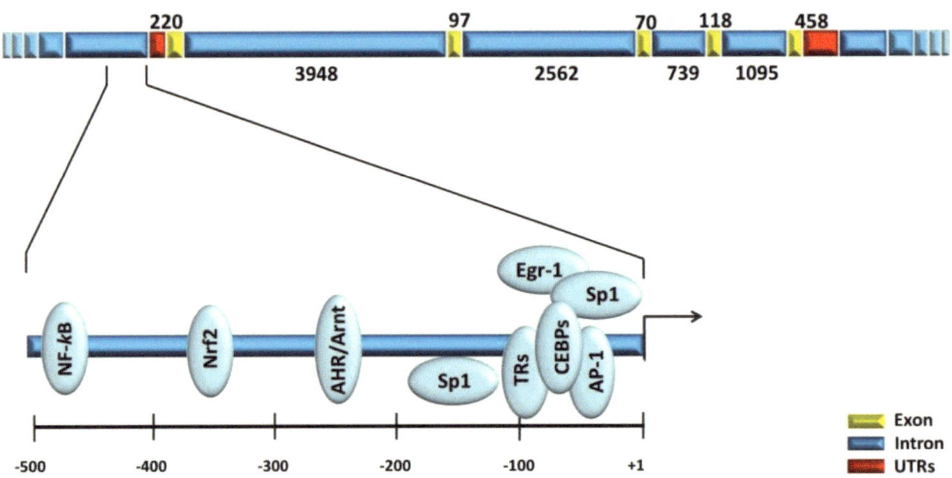

Figure 1. Structure of SOD1 gene.

The discovery of SOD1 mutations in ALS patients allowed the possibility to create transgenic models of the pathology. As familial and sporadic forms of ALS demonstrated to be clinically undistinguishable, in the 1990s SOD1-G93A mouse model was realized and allowed for an in-depth stepwise exploration of the neurodegenerative process occurring in ALS.

Conversely, a different scientific approach applies to the understanding of the mechanisms of disease directly in humans. The major limitation is represented indeed by the scarce availability of samples in sufficient quality and high relevance for ALS [5], being spinal cord, brain stem, motor cortex, and muscles as the primary targets of the disease process. The first criticality towards the use of post-mortem tissues is that they represent the end stage of the disease. In second place, the quality of tissues may be compromised by the interval after death and protein alterations occurring independently of ALS that may affect the specificity of the finding [6]. Thus, the proximity of the tissue to the disease pathogenic process, and thus the possibility to uncover a biologically meaningful, highly specific, marker of disease progression, is at the expenses of the accessibility of the given tissues and the opportunity to sample them more than once.

Regarding muscle biopsy, one of the advantages is the shorter processing time compared to post-mortem tissues, but at present there are no sufficient data to support this method of analysis. The presence of neurogenic atrophy is peculiar, but non-disease specific, of ALS. Besides that, these alterations are known to occur late during disease course and they could be measured less invasively with electrodiagnostic testing [6, 7]. As a last consideration, most of the changes observed at the muscle sample are not acknowledged to belong to some specific biochemical pathways or to be just a mere consequence of the denervation process [7, 8].

Because of the large feasibility for repeated testing and the presence of standard operating procedures, blood and cerebrospinal fluid (CSF) have become the most popular biofluids deployed for ALS research [7]. Indeed, these features allow for longitudinal sample collection at high quality and minimal inter-assay differences. On the contrary, both matrices will contain only diluted concentrations of the protein of interest, which can turn into an advantage if the disease process for which the biomarker is released occurs at multiple scattered points within central nervous system (CNS) impossible to be sampled [5]. Furthermore, there is a massive dynamic range of proteins within these two fluids that is present at several orders of magnitude above the candidate biomarkers and could interfere with their detection. CSF is the closest of the two to the CNS compartment, and thus it is more likely to reflect pathological processes occurring within it; in contrast, blood-brain barrier is narrowing the amount of biomarkers possibly circulating in serum or plasma, even though recent studies revealed an impaired function of the latter [9]. On the clinical ground, lumbar puncture is definitely more invasive than venopuncture and subject to an increasing number of variables, such as the possibility of contamination with blood at the side of the puncture and the heterogeneity of sampled volume. Serum or plasma collection is much more accessible, and patients are more compliant to multiple sampling [10]. Both these biofluids can be influenced by multiple systemic phenomena at the time, such as inflammation, dysmetabolism, or damage at the neuromuscular level, which could increase the sensitivity and also act as confounding factors in the interpretation of the source of these candidate biomarkers [5].

Considering the ubiquitous nature of SOD1, and the aforementioned privilege of multiple blood sampling for the research of this highly progressive, severely disabling disease, SOD1-

mediated pathogenesis of ALS has been extensively investigated through the use of blood cells. Moreover, damaged metabolism of lymphocytes was studied in other neurodegenerative diseases, confirming the pertinence of these cells as an appealing tool in understanding the pathogenesis of neurodegeneration [11].

2.2. SOD1 aggregation

In the 1990s, early studies on erythrocytes and lymphocytes of mutated SOD1 FALS proved decreased concentrations and altered the activity of the enzyme years before the onset of pathology [12–14]. However, this modification was restricted to mutated SOD1 ALS patients. In the last years, a growing body of studies showed peripheral blood mononuclear cells (PBMC) of ALS patients and, regardless of the genetic basis, displayed distinctive traits compared to healthy and neurological controls. These alterations mainly concern an aberrant antioxidant response reflected by mitochondrial and calcium-dysregulated metabolism [15] and decreased Bcl-2 and SOD1 expression in peripheral lymphocytes [16, 17] accompanied by the inability to down-regulate these proteins under oxidative stress [16].

In 2010, while investigating mRNA SOD1 expression in lymphocytes from SALS patients as a potential explanation for the decreased levels of SOD1 protein, Gagliardi et al. [18] found that there is increased transcription of SOD1 in the lymphocytes of SALS (compared to healthy and neurological controls). Similar enhanced expression of SOD1 mRNA was found in selected sections of motor spinal cord and brain stem of ALS patients as well, though this phenomenon was absent from cerebellum and non-motor areas of the same patients. At the same time, SOD1 protein levels in the disease-affected tissues from SALS patients did not show any statistical difference compared to controls [18]. These observations imply that SOD1 increased transcription and the decreased protein expressions are disease-specific cellular events, which are apparent, and thus possible to study, at peripheral level. This gap of knowledge between mRNA and protein levels of SOD1 in ALS patients opened a new scenario, in which the study of sub-cellular compartments was pivotal. Initially, a conformational modified SOD1 was observed both in SALS and FALS (misfolded SOD1 and mutant SOD1 respectively), instead of wild-type SOD1 [19]. The pathogenic role of misfolded SOD1 was first hypothesized by Gruzman et al. [20], and additional evidence was subsequently provided by other authors [21, 22]. Specifically, Forsberg et al. [22–23] found similar misfolded SOD1-Bcl2 aggregations in SALS and Pasinelli et al. [24] described it in FALS (mutant SOD1-Bcl2) [23, 24]. Given that, the hypothesis was that wild-type SOD1, under many environmental triggers, became misfolded SOD1 with reduced antioxidant activity (loss of function) and acquired toxic property as mutant SOD1 has [25]. Cereda and co-workers [26] demonstrated a bigger total amount of SOD1 in PBMCs of SALS patients than in cells of healthy controls or Alzheimer patients [26]. Curiously, the SOD1 distribution allowed to distinguish two different categories of patients: the first group had perinuclear SOD1 aggregates and the second one higher nuclear SOD1. In addition, Cereda [26] observed that patients with more perinuclear SOD1 expressed a major amount of insoluble proteins while the other group, characterized by predominant nuclear SOD1, had especially soluble fractions. Eventually, the authors tested whether these findings had clinical correlates (see **Table 1** for general characteristics of patient cohort). Indeed, longer disease durations from onset to time of sampling and from onset to last visit were found in patients with larger amount of soluble nuclear SOD1 (**Figure 2, A, B,** $p < 0.05$). In contrast, no significant correlation was observed between nuclear SOD1 ratio and duration from time of sampling to last visit (data not shown). At the same time, a mild increasing trend was found between patients with high nuclear SOD1 and early ALS stage as assessed by ALSFRS-r score at sampling (**Figure 2C,** $p > 0.05$). If these data were confirmed in larger cohorts followed-up longitudinally and employing specific antibodies against misfolded SOD1, this hallmark could be a useful biomarker for stratifying patients according to the pace of progression of the disease.

Clinimetrics	Patients
Gender	7/12
Female/male	
Age of onset (years)	61.2 ± 2.75
Mean ± SEM	
Diagnostic latency (months)	14.8 ± 4.38
Mean ± SEM	
Site of onset	9/10
Bulbar/limb	
Disease duration at sampling (months)	25.4 ± 7.26
Mean ± SEM	
ALS-FRS_r at visit	38.7 ± 2.11
Mean ± SEM	
Progression rate at baseline (PRB)	0.55 ± 0.23
Mean ± SEM	
Disease duration from baseline to last visit/death (months)	50.2 ± 11.18
Mean ± SEM	
UMN/LMN dominance	1/1/6/6/5
Exclusive UMN/dominant UMN/both UMN-LMN/dominant LMN/exclusive LMN	
Cognitive involvement	3/16
Yes/no	
Respiratory involvement	11/8
Yes/no	
SOD1 localization	13/6
High nuclear fraction/low nuclear fraction	

PRB, progression rate at baseline that is calculated as (48-ALSFRS-r score at baseline)/timeline between onset of disease and baseline visit; PRB values <0.5 between 0.5–1 and >1 imply patients are slow, intermediate, or fast progressors, respectively.

Table 1. Characteristics of patients.

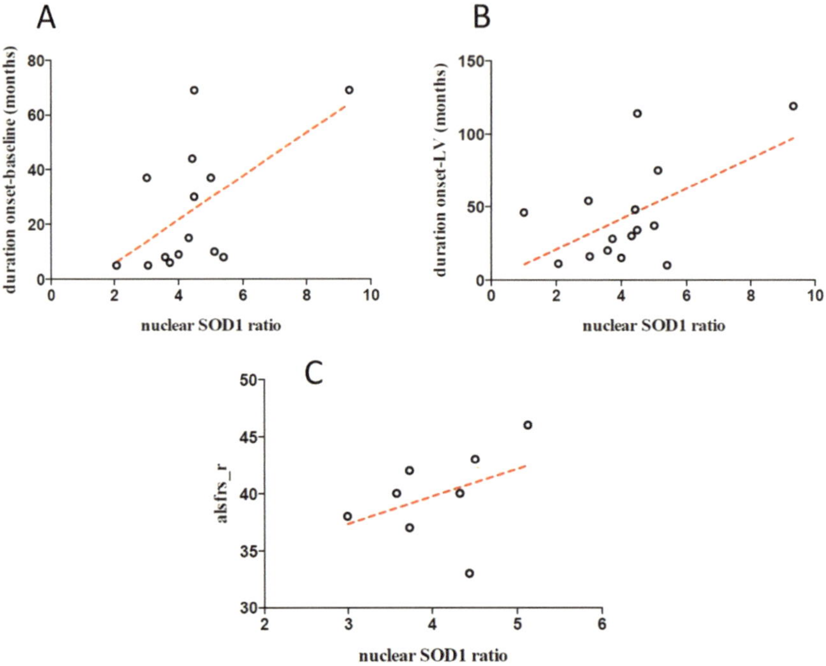

Figure 2. Correlations between nuclear SOD1 and clinimetrics.

Furthermore, this mechanism of pathogenesis could be present in other neurodegenerative disease (such as Parkinson's disease, Alzheimer dementia) and in different conditions, such as prion disease or amyloidosis, possibly unifying all these pathologies under the term 'proteinopathies', where an aberrantly fold protein becomes the 'seeding template' for other normally constituted proteins to misfold and aggregate in intra- and extra-neuronal beta-strand structures, conferring toxicity to selected populations of neurons. Interestingly, recent studies have attempted to unravel the mechanism of spreading the abnormally fold proteins from one neuron to the other. One of the main hypothesis scientific literature is testing now is that extracellular vesicles, which are small plasma membrane-derived spheres containing RNAs, enzymes, signal transduction factors, etc., and acting as transporters of these substances [27], may be the vehicles of toxic proteins, explaining how the disease seeds from very distant sites to others with certain degrees of selectivity.

3. SOD1 protein

3.1. Transcriptional regulation

SOD1 has high and ubiquitous expression; its induction is fine-tuned and modulated by complex intracellular events which probably engage multiple positive and negative regulatory elements acting altogether [28]. Different transcriptional factors were involved in SOD1 constitutive and inducible expression. Among these, the C/EBPs (CCAAT/enhancer-binding proteins) have been demonstrated to be necessary for SOD1 constitutive expression. C/EBP consensus element partially overlaps the Sp1/Egr1 sequence, suggesting that these transcription factors may act in the control of SOD1 gene expression regulation [29]. Furthermore, also the transcription factor CCAAT/enhancer-binding protein delta is involved in the regulation of human SOD1 transcription [30]: In particular, it enhances SOD1 mRNA expression in cisplatin-treated human urothelial carcinoma cell line (NTUB1) via a direct promoter transactivation. The over-expression of Sp1 (Specificity Protein 1) enhances SOD1 basal promoter activity [31].

It has also been demonstrated that cytokines and stress signals (radiation, injury, and oxidative or mechanical stress) can induce the expression of early growth response-1 (Egr1), a nuclear phosphoprotein regulator of transcription. Minc and co-workers [32] demonstrated that SOD1 mRNA level rapidly increased after phorbol-12-myristate-13-acetate (PMA) treatment in HeLa cells, and the region between nucleotides −59 and −48 presents noncanonical consensus recognition sequences for Sp1 and Egr1, and it is bound by Egr1 in response to PMA exposure.

It has been demonstrated that activating protein 1 (AP1) represses SOD1 transcription by sequestrating essential coactivators such as Sp1 [31]. Furthermore, neuronal nitric oxide synthase (nNOS) over-expression causes SOD1 down-regulation of mRNA, protein, and activity levels [33], and that this seems to be caused by both the decreased binding of Sp1 to SOD1 promoter, caused by nNOS interaction with Sp1, and a concomitant increased binding activity of AP1 to the same site.

An increased expression of SOD1 mRNA and protein was reported after the exposure of human HepG2 and HeLa cells to the 2,3,7,8-tetrachlorodibenzo-pdioxin (TCDD), an environmental contaminant and interacting with aryl hydrocarbon receptor (AHR) [34]. They also identified the presence of a xenobiotic responsive element (XRE) in the 5′ -flanking region of human SOD1 gene (between −255 and −238 from the transcription start site), which is responsible for the induction by TCDD. A thyroid hormone (TR) inhibitory element was identified between −157 and +17 of the human SOD1 promoter, and T3 exposure reverses the induction of SOD1 transcription caused by the ROS-producing paraquat and PMA agents [35]. Also, SOD1 promoter is significantly up-regulated by unliganded TRs.

NF-κB was one of the first transcription factors shown redox regulated [36, 37]. Moreover, cell treatment with H_2O_2 triggers the PI3K/Akt cascade, which participates in NF-κB activation and in consequent SOD1 transcriptional induction. Thus, a p65-NF-κB-binding site in the human SOD1 promoter (GGTAAGTCCC) was identified, and Akt-activated NF-κB presents an increased binding to this sequence, mediating the up-regulation of SOD1 expression [38].

Dell'Orco et al. [39] investigated if SOD1 over-expression could be related to transcriptional regulation; in particular, they consider the relationship between the nuclear factor E2-related factor 2 (Nrf2) transcription factor and SOD1 promoter [39]. The dissociation from Keap1 is a prerequisite for Nrf2 translocation to the nucleus. The activated Nrf2 re-localizes into the nucleus where it binds to ARE=adenine/uracil-rich element sequences and activates the expression of different cytoprotective target genes. Moreover, an ARE-binding element, located between −356 and −330 from the transcription start site and targeted by Nrf2, has been identified in SOD1 promoter [40]. By means of a probe harbouring the SOD1 ARE element, we reported the presence of a dynamic protein-DNA complex, which suggested that after H_2O_2 treatment, the cis-acting ARE sequence in SOD1 promoter plays an important role by recruiting multiple TFs and/or cofactors, probably co-operating to modulate SOD1 mRNA induction under oxidative stress. ChIP assay followed by qRT-PCR with primers designed to flank the ARE element in SOD1 promoter showed that Nrf2 occupancy at the ARE elements in SOD1 promoter did not change after H_2O_2 treatment. We also reported a minimal increased association at the ARE element in NQO1 gene, a well-known Nrf2 gene target, thus indicating that Nrf2 cannot gain access to SOD1 5′-flanking region in a native chromatin context. SOD1 mRNA up-regulation in response to H_2O_2 oxidative treatment might indeed be ascribed to the involvement of other transcriptional factors. These data suggested that SOD1 promoter is not a canonical downstream target of the Nrf2 regulatory network and that Nrf2 may act as a 'constitutive' TF, binding to SOD1 ARE sequence even without stimulus, while H_2O_2 treatment could induce changes in the chromatin conformation with consequent changes in the relationship between the different TFs. In regard to SOD1 gene, it has been wrongly considered a housekeeping gene; however, its inducible transcription is finely regulated by *cis*-acting sequences and the corresponding transactive factors [39].

3.2. Post-transcriptional regulation

Until now, post-transcriptional control mechanisms of SOD1 expression are still unexplored; nevertheless, post-transcriptional control represents a specific and punctual regulatory mechanism for gene expression which can easily modify protein levels in response to extracellular stimuli [41, 42]. Variations in gene expression are often the result of synergy between transcriptional and post-transcriptional regulatory mechanisms [28]. Very few data on post-transcriptional regulation of SOD1 have been reported so far. Two species of SOD1 mRNA with different 3′UTR lengths which produce *in vitro* different quantities of SOD1 protein have been identified. Kilk and colleagues [43] reported that the ability of long mRNA to produce more SOD1 enzyme seems to be related to specific sequences located in the 3′UTR; moreover, they identified the presence of AREs in this region (AUUUA, CUUUA, AUUUG, GUUUUA, AUUUU, and AUUUC). In general, AREs represent the docking sites for different RNA-binding proteins (RBPs), which can affect the metabolism of the target transcripts [44]. Among ARE-binding RBPs, ELAV (or Hu) proteins play a critical role [45]; ELAV family comprises the neuron-specific members HuB, HuC, and HuD [46] and the ubiquitously expressed HuR. ELAV proteins act primarily as positive regulators of gene expression; they can increase the stability and/or translation of target mRNAs whose proteins have fundamental cellular functions.

Given the lack of data on this issue in ALS pathogenesis, Cereda's group [26] focused its attention on the modulation of SOD1 mRNA levels by post-transcriptional mechanisms, in particular via ELAV proteins. Considering that oxidative stress plays a critical role in sporadic ALS, and that it is a trigger of ELAV activation, by treating human neuroblastoma SH-SY5Y cells with 1 mM H_2O_2, a significant up-regulation of SOD1 mRNA levels was reported [47].

Milani and collaborators [47] also analysed the 3′UTR region of SOD1 mRNA and, by means a bioinformatics analysis, they identified within SOD1 3′UTR primary sequence the presence of AREs that are putative ELAV-binding sites. These data were consistent with the results reported by Lopez de Silanes and colleagues [48]; REMSA and immunoprecipitation coupled with real-time qPCR experiments demonstrated that the recombinant HuR protein bound specifically and directly to the ARE-bearing probe of SOD1. In parallel, ELAV accumulates in the cytoplasm; this intracellular relocation is in line with the role of ELAV/HuR as a nuclear-cytoplasmic shuttling protein. Indeed, ELAV's influence on target mRNAs depends on its localization in the cytoplasm, where these proteins stabilize target mRNAs and regulate their translation [49]. Taken together, these data seem to indicate that oxidative stress promotes SOD1 induction probably mediated by ELAV-dependent mechanisms. Moreover, the kinase-triggered phosphorylation of ELAV/HuR is crucial for the modulation of its function and allows it to associate extracellular signals to specific post-transcriptional events elicited by this RBP [50, 51]. Finally, Milani and co-authors [47] also reported an enhanced perinuclear and cytoplasmic expression of ELAV in the cerebral motor cortex of SALS patients compared to healthy subjects, suggesting that the up-regulated RBP proteins may be more available and massively enrolled in the positive regulation of target mRNAs, such as SOD1. Remarkably, positivity for cytoplasmic ELAV was paralleled by increased levels of both SOD1 mRNA and protein [47].

SOD1 post-transcriptional regulation may also be mediated by microRNAs (miRNAs). miRNAs are small non-protein-coding RNAs, which act as key post-transcriptional regulators of gene expression by base pairing to the 3′UTR of the target mRNAs, causing translational silencing and mRNA decay [52, 53], as it was reported for miR-377 in human and mouse mesangial cells which diminished SOD1 protein levels [54].

In consideration of all these findings, we can conclude that the increase in SOD1 gene expression is the consequence of an intricate process related both to the activation of a transcriptional mechanism involving Pol II, and also other mechanisms such as chromatin changes and epigenetic variations, mRNA, and protein stabilization

Author details

Diamanti Luca[1*], Zucchi Elisabetta[2], Pansarasa Orietta[3], Ceroni Mauro[1] and Cereda Crisitna[3]

*Address all correspondence to: lukdiamonds@libero.it

1 Department of Brain and Behavioral Sciences, University of Pavia, Pavia, Italy; 'C. Mondino' National Neurological Institute, Pavia, Italy

2 Department of Brain and Behavioral Sciences, University of Pavia, Pavia, Italy

3 Laboratory of Experimental Neurobiology, 'C. Mondino' National Neurological Institute, Pavia, Italy

References

[1] McCord JM, Fridovich I. Superoxide dismutase. An enzymic function for erythrocuprein (hemocuprein), J Biol Chem. 1969; 244(22):6049–55.

[2] Chang LY, Slot JW, Geuze JH, Crapo JD. Molecular immunocytochemistry of the CuZn superoxide dismutase in rat hepatocytes, J Cell Biol. 1988; 107(6, part 1):2169–79.

[3] Rosen DR, Siddique T, Patterson D, Figlewicz DA, Sapp P, Hentati A, Donaldson D, Goto J, O'Regan JP, Deng HX, et al. Mutations in Cu/Zn superoxide dismutase gene are associated with familial amyotrophic lateral sclerosis. Nature. 1993; 362(6415):59–62.

[4] Chiò A, Battistini S, Calvo A, Caponnetto C, Conforti FL, Corbo M, Giannini F, Mandrioli J, Mora G, Sabatelli M; ITALSGEN Consortium, Ajmone C, Mastro E, Pain D, Mandich P, Penco S, Restagno G, Zollino M, Surbone A. Genetic counselling in ALS: facts, uncertainties and clinical suggestions. J Neurol Neurosurg Psychiatr. 2014; 85(5): 478–85.

[5] Ryberg H, Bowser R. Protein biomarkers for amyotrophic lateral sclerosis. Expert Rev Proteom. 2008; 5(2):249–62.

[6] Bowser R, Lacomis D. Applying proteomics to the diagnosis and treatment of ALS and related diseases. Muscle Nerve. 2009; 40(5):753–62.

[7] Otto M, Bowser R, Turner M, Berry J, Brettschneider J, Connor J, Costa J, Cudkowicz M, Glass J, Jahn O, et al. Roadmap and standard operating procedures for biobanking and discovery of neurochemical markers in ALS. Amyotroph Lateral Scler. 2012; 13(1): 1–10.

[8] Wong M, Martin LJ. Skeletal muscle-restricted expression of human SOD1 causes motor neuron degeneration in transgenic mice. Hum Mol Genet. 2010; 19:2284–302.

[9] Winkler EA, Sengillo JD, Sullivan JS, Henkel JS, Appel SH, Zlokovic BV. Blood-spinal cord barrier breakdown and pericyte reductions in amyotrophic lateral sclerosis. Acta Neuropathol. 2013; 125:111.

[10] Krüger T, Lautenschläger J, Grosskreutz J, Rhode H. Proteome analysis of body fluids for amyotrophic lateral sclerosis biomarker discovery. Proteom Clin Appl. 2013; 7(1–2):123–35.

[11] Gibson GE, Huang HM. Oxidative processes in the brain and non-neuronal tissues as biomarkers of Alzheimer's disease. Front Biosci. 2002; 7:d1007–15.

[12] Robberecht W, Sapp P, Viaene MK, Rosen D, McKenna-Yasek D, Haines J, Horvitz R, Theys P, Brown R Jr. Cu/Zn superoxide dismutase activity in familial and sporadic amyotrophic lateral sclerosis. J Neurochem. 1994; 62(1):384–7.

[13] Bowling AC, Barkowski EE, McKenna-Yasek D, Sapp P, Horvitz HR, Beal MF, Brown RH Jr. Superoxide dismutase concentration and activity in familial amyotrophic lateral sclerosis. J Neurochem. 1995; 64(5):2366–9.

[14] Garofalo O, Figlewicz DA, Thomas SM, Butler R, Lebuis L, Rouleau G, Meininger V, Leigh PN. Superoxide dismutase activity in lymphoblastoid cells from motor neuron disease/amyotrophic lateral sclerosis (MND/ALS) patients. J Neurol Sci. 1995; 129(Suppl):90–2.

[15] Curti D, Malaspina A, Facchetti G, Camana C, Mazzini L, Tosca P, Zerbi F, Ceroni M. Amyotrophic lateral sclerosis: oxidative energy metabolism and calcium homeostasis in peripheral blood lymphocytes. Neurology. 1996; 47(4):1060–4.

[16] Cova E, Cereda C, Galli A, Curti D, Finotti C, Di Poto C, Corato M, Mazzini G, Ceroni M. Modified expression of Bcl-2 and SOD1 proteins in lymphocytes from sporadic ALS patients. Neurosci Lett. 2006; 399(3):186–90.

[17] Mantovani S, Garbelli S, Pasini A, Alimonti D, Perotti C, Melazzini M, Bendotti C, Mora G. Immune system alterations in sporadic amyotrophic lateral sclerosis patients suggest an ongoing neuroinflammatory process. J Neuroimmunol. 2009; 210(1–2):73–9.

[18] Gagliardi S, Cova E, Davin A, Guareschi S, Abel K, Alvisi E, Laforenza U, Ghidoni R, Cashman JR, Ceroni M, Cereda C. SOD1 mRNA expression in sporadic amyotrophic lateral sclerosis. Neurobiol Dis. 2010; 39(2):198–203.

[19] Kabashi E, Valdmanis PN, Dion P, Rouleau GA. Oxidized/misfolded superoxide dismutase-1: the cause of all amyotrophic lateral sclerosis? Ann Neurol. 2007; 62(6): 553–9.

[20] Gruzman A, Wood WL, Alpert E, Prasad MD, Miller RG, et al. Common molecular signature in SOD1 for both sporadic and familial amyotrophic lateral sclerosis. Proc Natl Acad Sci U S A. 2007; 104:12524–9.

[21] Bosco DA, Morfini G, Karabacak NM, Song Y, Gros-Louis F, et al. Wildtype and mutant SOD1 share an aberrant conformation and a common pathogenic pathway in ALS. Nat Neurosci. 2010; 13:1396–403.

[22] Forsberg K, Jonsson PA, Andersen PM, Bergemalm D, Graffmo KS, et al. Novel antibodies reveal inclusions containing non-native SOD1 in sporadic ALS patients. PLoS One. 2010; 5:e11552.

[23] Forsberg K, Andersen PM, Marklund SL, Brannstrom T. Glial nuclear aggregates of superoxide dismutase-1 are regularly present in patients with amyotrophic lateral sclerosis. Acta Neuropathol. 2011; 121:623–34.

[24] Pasinelli P, Belford ME, Lennon N, Bacskai BJ, Hyman BT, et al. Amyotrophic lateral sclerosis-associated SOD1 mutant proteins bind and aggregate with Bcl-2 in spinal cord mitochondria. Neuron. 2004; 43:19–30.

[25] Ezzi SA, Urushitani M, Julien JP. Wild-type superoxide dismutase acquires binding and toxic properties of ALS-linked mutant forms through oxidation. J Neurochem. 2007; 102:170–8.

[26] Cereda C, Leoni E, Milani P, Pansarasa O, Mazzini G, Guareschi S, Alvisi E, Ghiroldi A, Diamanti L, Bernuzzi S, Ceroni M, Cova E. Altered intracellular localization of SOD1 in leukocytes from patients with sporadic amyotrophic lateral sclerosis. PLoS One. 2013; 8(10):e75916.

[27] Colombo M, Raposo G, Théry C. Biogenesis, secretion, and intercellular interactions of exosomes and other extracellular vesicles. Annu Rev Cell Dev Biol. 2014; 30:255–89.

[28] Milani P, Gagliardi S, Cova E, Cereda C. SOD1 Transcriptional and posttranscriptional regulation and its potential implications in ALS. Neurol Res Int. 2011; 2011:458427.

[29] Seo SJ, Kang SS, Cho G, Rho HM, Jung G. C/EBPα and C/EBPβ play similar roles in the transcription of the human Cu/Zn SOD gene. Gene. 1997; 203:11–5.

[30] Hour TC, Lai YL, Kuan CI, Chou CK, Wang JM, Tu HY, Hu HT, Lin CS, Wu WJ, Pu YS, Sterneck E, Huang AM. Transcriptional up-regulation of SOD1 by CEBPD: a potential target for cisplatin resistant human urothelial carcinoma cells. Biochem Pharmacol. 2010; 80:325–34.

[31] Afonso V, Santos G, Collin P, Khatib AM, Mitrovic DR, Lomri N, Leitman DC, Lomri A. Tumor necrosis factor-alpha down-regulates human Cu/Zn superoxide dismutase 1 promoter via JNK/AP-1 signaling pathway. Free Radic Biol Med. 2006; 41(5):709–21.

[32] Minc E, de Coppet P, Masson P, Thiery L, Dutertre S, Amor-Guéret M, Jaulin C. The human copper-zinc superoxide dismutase gene (SOD1) proximal promoter is regulated by Sp1, Egr-1, and WT1 via non-canonical binding sites. J Biol Chem. 1999; 274:503–9.

[33] Baldelli S, Aquilano K, Rotilio G, Ciriolo MR. Glutathione and copper, zinc superoxide dismutase are modulated by overexpression of neuronal nitric oxide synthase. Int J Biochem Cell Biol. 2008; 40:2660–70.

[34] Cho JS, Chang MS, Rho HM. Transcriptional activation of the human Cu/Zn superoxide dismutase gene by 2,3,7,8-tetrachlorodibenzo-p-dioxin through the xenobiotic-responsive element. Mol Genet Genom. 2001; 266:133–41.

[35] Santos GM, Afonso V, Barra GB, Togashi M, Webb P, Neves FA, Lomri N, Lomri A. Negative regulation of superoxide dismutase-1 promoter by thyroid hormone. Mol Pharmacol. 2006; 70:793–800.

[36] Vallabhapurapu S, Karin M. Regulation and function of NF-kappaB transcription factors in the immune system. Annu Rev Immunol. 2009; 27:693–733.

[37] Sen CK, Packer L. Antioxidant and redox regulation of gene transcription. FASEB J. 1996; 10:709–20.

[38] Rojo AI, Salinas M, Martín D, Perona R, Cuadrado A. Regulation of Cu/Zn-superoxide dismutase expression via the phosphatidylinositol 3 kinase/Akt pathway and nuclear factor-kappaB. J Neurosci. 2004; 24:7324–34.

[39] Dell'Orco M, Milani P, Arrigoni L, Pansarasa O, Sardone V, Maffioli E, Polveraccio F, Bordoni M, Diamanti L, Ceroni M, Peverali FA, Tedeschi G, Cereda C. Hydrogen peroxide-mediated induction of SOD1 gene transcription is independent from Nrf2 in a cellular model of neurodegeneration. Biochim Biophys Acta. 2016; 1859:315–23.

[40] Park EY, Rho HM. The transcriptional activation of the human copper/zinc superoxide dismutase gene by 2,3,7,8-tetrachlorodibenzo-p-dioxin through two different regulator sites, the antioxidant responsive element and xenobiotic responsive element. Mol Cell Biochem. 2002; 240:47–55.

[41] Keene JD. RNA regulons: coordination of post-transcriptional events. Nat Rev Genet. 2007; 8:533–43.

[42] Abdelmohsen K, Kuwano Y, Kim HH, Gorospe M. Posttranscriptional gene regulation by RNA-binding proteins during oxidative stress: implications for cellular senescence. Biol Chem. 2008; 389:243–55.

[43] Kilk A, Laan M, Torp A. Human CuZn superoxide dismutase enzymatic activity in cells is regulated by the length of the mRNA. FEBS Lett. 1995; 362:323–7.

[44] Chen CY, Shyu AB. AU-rich elements: characterization and importance in mRNA degradation. Trends Biochem Sci. 1995; 20:465–70.

[45] Antic D, Keene JD. Embryonic lethal abnormal visual RNA-binding proteins involved in growth, differentiation, and posttranscriptional gene expression. Am J Hum Genet. 1997; 61:273–8.

[46] Pascale A, Amadio M, Quattrone A. Defining a neuron: neuronal ELAV proteins. Cell Mol Life Sci. 2008; 65:128–40.

[47] Milani P, Amadio M, Laforenza U, Dell'Orco M, Diamanti L, Sardone V, Gagliardi S, Govoni S, Ceroni M, Pascale A, Cereda C. Posttranscriptional regulation of SOD1 gene expression under oxidative stress: potential role of ELAV proteins in sporadic ALS. Neurobiol Dis. 2013; 60:51–60.

[48] López de Silanes I, Zhan M, Lal A, Yang X, Gorospe M. Identification of a target RNA motif for RNA-binding protein HuR. Proc Natl Acad Sci U S A. 2004; 101:2987–92.

[49] Colombrita C, Silani V, Ratti A. ELAV proteins along evolution: back to the nucleus? Mol Cell Neurosci. 2013; 56:447–55.

[50] Doller A, Schlepckow K, Schwalbe H, Pfeilschifter J, Eberhardt W. Tandem phosphorylation of serines 221 and 318 by protein kinase Cdelta coordinates mRNA binding and nucleocytoplasmic shuttling of HuR. Mol Cell Biol. 2010; 30:1397–410.

[51] Amadio M, Bucolo C, Leggio GM, Drago F, Govoni S, Pascale A. The PKCbeta/HuR/VEGF pathway in diabetic retinopathy. Biochem Pharmacol. 2010; 80:1230–7.

[52] Pillai RS, Bhattacharyya SN, Filipowicz W. Repression of protein synthesis by miRNAs: how many mechanisms? Trends Cell Biol. 2007; 17:118–26.

[53] Filipowicz W, Bhattacharyya SN, Sonenberg N. Mechanisms of post-transcriptional regulation by microRNAs: are the answers in sight? Nat Rev Genet. 2008; 9:102–14.

[54] Wang Q, Wang Y, Minto AW, Wang J, Shi Q, Li X, Quigg RJ. MicroRNA-377 is up-regulated and can lead to increased fibronectin production in diabetic nephropathy. FASEB J. 2008; 22:4126–35.

Chapter 5

Role of Cysteine Residue of Mutant Cu, Zn-Superoxide Dismutase (SOD1) in the Pathogenesis of Amyotrophic Lateral Sclerosis (ALS)

Seiichi Nagano and Toshiyuki Araki

Additional information is available at the end of the chapter

http://dx.doi.org/10.5772/63160

Abstract

Mutations of *Cu, Zn-superoxide dismutase (SOD1)* gene have been identified in a subset of familial amyotrophic lateral sclerosis (ALS). Conformational change, that is, misfolding, of mutant SOD1 underlies its toxic gain of function for motor neuronal degeneration. Mutant SOD1 is prone to cause oxidative stress through the copper exposed on the protein by misfolding. The protein structure of SOD1 is critically affected by the redox state of cysteine residues, especially of Cys111. Oxidative modification of Cys111, which is enhanced in mutant SOD1, causes destabilization of the dimer interface to promote misfolding and aggregation of the protein. Substitution of Cys111 to serine alleviated the degeneration of motor neurons as well as the misfolding and aggregate formation of mutant SOD1 in the spinal cord of transgenic mice. It indicates that Cys111 is a crucial residue for the pathogenesis of ALS by mutant SOD1.

Keywords: amyotrophic lateral sclerosis, Cu, Zn-superoxide dismutase, cysteine residues, oxidative stress, monomerized SOD1

1. Introduction

Amyotrophic lateral sclerosis (ALS) is a fatal degenerative disease of motor neurons, which affects skeletal muscle strength of the whole body. About 10% of ALS cases are affected in a familial trait, 25–30% of which are caused by mutations of *Cu, Zn-superoxide dismutase (SOD1)* gene [1]. Although many causative genes of ALS have been identified so far, *SOD1* is still the second frequent responsible gene for ALS next to *C9orf72* [2]. Since the identification of the gene in 1993, research emphasis for ALS has been placed on uncovering the pathogenic

INTECH
open science | open minds

© 2016 The Author(s). Licensee InTech. This chapter is distributed under the terms of the Creative Commons Attribution License (http://creativecommons.org/licenses/by/3.0), which permits unrestricted use, distribution, and reproduction in any medium, provided the original work is properly cited.

mechanism of motor neuronal death by the disease-causing mutant SOD1. We review the recent concept of neuronal toxicity by mutant SOD1 in relation to the posttranslational modification of SOD1 at cysteine residues, especially at Cys111, which is closely related to its conformational change, in ALS pathogenesis.

2. Conformational change and copper-mediated oxidative toxicity of mutant SOD1

SOD1 is a metal-binding antioxidant enzyme expressed ubiquitously in the body, and it functions to convert prooxidant superoxide anions to hydrogen peroxide and oxygen to remove the oxidative stress [3]. SOD1 forms a homodimer to accomplish its full enzymatic activity. Each subunit binds one atom each of copper and zinc. Copper works for the enzymatic activity, whereas zinc has an important role in maintaining the stable structure of SOD1 protein.

More than 150 different mutations of *SOD1* gene have been found in familial ALS patients so far, and they are scattered throughout the entire coding sequence of the gene regardless of specific functional domains. The enzymatic activity of mutant SOD1 is not necessarily reduced compared to that of wild-type SOD1 [4]. Moreover, mice deficient of *Sod1* gene do not cause symptoms of motor neuronal dysfunction, whereas transgenic mice that express mutant SOD1, but not wild-type SOD1, develop progressive motor paralysis and degeneration of motor neurons depending on the expression level of mutant SOD1 in the spinal cord [5, 6]. It means that the pathogenic mechanism of mutant SOD1 for the degeneration of motor neurons is derived from the gain of a specific aberrant function rather than a decrease in the enzyme activity of the protein.

What is the determinant of motor neuronal toxicity by mutant SOD1? Although the nature of mutant SOD1 toxicity has not been fully elucidated, conformational abnormality, that is, misfolding, of mutant SOD1 protein is deeply involved in the pathogenesis of familial ALS [7]. Misfolded SOD1 is subject to dissociate into monomers, which binds together abnormally to form oligomers or further high molecular weight aggregates in cells. Abnormal protein accumulation in neurons can impair their important cellular functions such as axonal transport [8] and degradation machinery of proteins [9]. SOD1-positive inclusion bodies have been actually detected in degenerating motor neurons in the spinal cords of familial ALS patients and mutant SOD1 transgenic mice [10, 11]. Therefore, it is important to understand the common mode of conformational change in mutant SOD1, which will lead to suppress the onset of ALS derived from SOD1 mutations.

Once SOD1 is misfolded, copper or zinc bound to the subunit of SOD1 is also prone to be exposed from the compact dimer structure. Because copper is catalytically redox-active, abnormal chemical reactions can occur to generate reactive oxygen (ROS) or nitrogen (RNS) species apart from the original SOD1 activity. Mutant SOD1, unlike wild-type SOD1, has a potential to generate ROS and RNS such as hydroxyl radicals [12, 13] and peroxynitrite [14] in a copper-dependent manner *in vitro*, which can be inhibited by copper chelators in cultured cells [15].

We first thought that mutant SOD1 is involved in the degeneration of motor neurons by causing oxidative stress through an adverse enzymatic reaction with copper on the protein, and we examined therapeutic effects of G93A mutant SOD1 transgenic mice by removal of the oxidative stress. As a result, a copper-chelating agent trientine and an antioxidant ascorbic acid showed a protective effect either alone, yet a higher beneficial effect was achieved by the combined use of these reagents [16, 17]. Furthermore, to confirm the validity of this hypothesis, the mutant SOD1 mice were bred with metallothionein I/II-deficient mice and the impact of the gene on motor paralysis was analyzed. Metallothionein is an endogenous protein that binds copper to prevent it from being prooxidant in cells. The decrease or halt of metallothionein I/II expression exacerbated the ALS symptoms in a gene dosage-dependent manner [18]. Copper-mediated toxicity in mutant SOD1 was also reinforced with other reports that decreasing intracellular copper, by treatment with copper chelators or by genetic reduction of copper uptake, alleviated ALS phenotype in mutant SOD1 transgenic mice [19–21]. Moreover, the upregulation of metallothionein expression has been shown to attenuate the disease course in mice [22, 23]. These data suggest that copper-mediated oxidative chemistry underlies the pathogenesis of familial ALS linked to mutations of *SOD1* gene, possibly triggered by misfolding of the mutant protein.

3. Conformational change and oxidation of cysteine residues in mutant SOD1

The subunit structure and dimer formation of SOD1 is critically affected by the binding state of copper and zinc, as well as the redox state of cysteine residues in the protein [24]. Human SOD1 has four cysteine residues (Cys6, Cys57, Cys111, and Cys146) in a subunit. Cys57 and Cys146 form an intra-subunit disulfide bond that maintains the rigid structure and enzymatic activity of SOD1 protein, whereas Cys6 and Cys111 are present in a reduced state having free sulfhydryl groups. Cys6 is deeply buried in the core of the subunit and less accessible by other molecules, while Cys111 is located on the protein surface. The intra-subunit Cys57-Cys146 disulfide bond of SOD1 is physiologically formed by copper chaperone for SOD1 (CCS) coupled with copper incorporation into the enzymatic active site, meaning that the metal coordination and disulfide formation are mechanistically related to each other for the conformation of SOD1 protein [25]. Reduction of the Cys57-Cys146 disulfide bond and/or deprivation of metals make human wild-type SOD1 liable to misfold, resulting in monomerization [26].

Modification of amino acid residues, especially by oxidative stress, can be a critical factor to enhance the misfolding of proteins [27]. Cysteine is in particular susceptible to oxidative modification, since its sulfhydryl moiety is readily attacked by redox-active substrates such as glutathione or peroxides to form S-S or S-O covalent modification. Sulfhydryl groups also crosslink each other to form intra- or intermolecular disulfide bond, which have important roles to maintain or disrupt physiological conformation of proteins.

Oxidative reactivity and modification of Cys111, such as glutathionylation [28, 29] and peroxidation [30], is documented with human or chick wild-type SOD1. Because Cys111 is located on the edge of the dimer interface of each subunit, the modification of Cys111 can interrupt the dimer contact at the interface stereochemically and cause the dissociation of SOD1. Molecular dynamic simulations of SOD1 imply that the region including Cys111 is important for the residue interaction network in the protein and is likely to affect the dimer interface through the network and may disrupt their coupled motions [31]. Indeed, it was noted *in vitro* that the Cys111 modification caused wild-type SOD1 liable to monomerize and decrease its enzymatic activity [32]. On the other hand, substitution of Cys111 to serine (C111S) is known to increase the structural stability and resistance to heat inactivation of wild-type SOD1 [33], also implying that the mode of Cys111 may regulate the conformational state of SOD1.

Changes in the redox state of cysteine residues have been reported in ALS-linked mutant SOD1. Mutant SOD1 exhibits aberrant vulnerability to mild reducing conditions, which cleave the intra-subunit Cys57-Cys146 disulfide bond to destabilize the SOD1 dimer [34]. The dimer dissociation results in the exposure of the hydrophobic region of the SOD1 subunit and promotes aggregation of the protein [35]. Alternatively, insoluble mutant SOD1 oligomers can be formed by crosslinking via inter-subunit disulfide bonds at Cys57 and Cys146 [26] or by disulfide scrambling of all four cysteine residues [36]. Such insoluble SOD1 oligomers were also detected in the spinal cord of mutant SOD1 transgenic mice in parallel to the disease onset [37]. These oligomers were mostly reversed by a reducing reagent, supposing that disulfide-mediated crosslinking at cysteine residues is a major factor for mutant SOD1 to form aggregates and ALS phenotype. Conversely, replacement of cysteine residues, especially of Cys6 and Cys111, decreased disulfide-crosslinked mutant SOD1 oligomers and aggregate formation, and improved cell viability in cultured cells [38, 39]. Glutaredoxins, which specifically catalyze the reduction of protein-SSG-mixed disulfides, significantly increased the solubility of mutant SOD1 and protected neuronal cells [39, 40]. On the other hand, the intermolecular disulfide binding at cysteines is shown to have a limited effect on the aggregation of mutant SOD1 [41].

With regard to Cys111, posttranslational modifications of Cys111 per se are also known in mutant SOD1. The change of the protein structure, which would affect the hindrance of Cys111 near the dimer interface, can enhance oxidative modification of Cys111 at the sulfhydryl moiety by substrates in mutant SOD1. Mutant SOD1 is commonly glutathionylated at Cys111 [42], and Cys111-peroxidized SOD1 is detected in the inclusion bodies of spinal motor neurons in G93A mutant SOD1 transgenic mice [30]. Those indicate the pathogenic significance of Cys111-oxidized SOD1 for misfolding and aggregation to acquire neuronal toxicity. Moreover, even in the spinal cord of sporadic ALS patients without SOD1 mutation, misfolded SOD1 deposits have been detected and the SOD1 species are peroxidized at Cys111, indicating that misfolding and aggregation of wild-type SOD1 may also be a factor in the pathogenesis of sporadic ALS [43]. However, in the vast majority of sporadic ALS, an RNA-binding protein TDP-43 is well known to mislocalize from the nucleus and deposit in the cytoplasm [44, 45]. SOD1 does not interact or co-localize with TDP-43 in general in such cases [46], which is

http://dx.doi.org/10.5772/63160

inconsistent with the hypothesis mentioned above. Although the involvement of Cys111-mediated misfolded SOD1 may be limited in sporadic ALS, the theory is attractive and further investigation will be needed.

4. Molecular link between copper-mediated chemistry and cysteine oxidation in mutant SOD1

Then, what is the molecular mechanism by which mutant SOD1 causes the copper-mediated oxidative stress in relation to misfolding of the protein? In case that mutant SOD1 enhances an aberrant side reaction through the discoordinated copper due to the abnormality of the protein structure, we can develop treatment strategies by identifying the responsible site and its conformational state in the protein. To clarify a possible aberrant interaction of mutant SOD1 with copper, we fractionated cell lysates from the spinal cord of SOD1 transgenic mice and SOD1 expressing cultured cells by immobilized metal affinity chromatography (IMAC), a method that separates proteins based on their affinities with an immobilized metal such as copper [47]. Mutant SOD1 was eluted commonly in an aberrant fraction with high affinity for copper, in addition to that with low affinity for copper seen in wild-type SOD1 as well. Considering that mutant SOD1 is separated into two distinct fractions and the interaction of proteins on IMAC is determined by topology of metal-coordinating residues on solvent-facing surfaces [48], conformational transition from the native to non-native state is implicated in the high-affinity fraction for the copper of mutant SOD1.

Therefore, we further analyzed mutant SOD1 in the high-affinity fraction for copper to know its biochemical characteristics compared to that in the low-affinity fraction. Existence of Cys111 was critical to the appearance of the high-affinity fraction species, and mutant SOD1 was in a monomer state and oxidatively modified at Cys111 in this fraction [49]. Peroxidation of wild-type SOD1 forced by oxidants such as hydrogen peroxide made it to monomerize and generate the high-affinity fraction species by copper IMAC. Furthermore, these mutant SOD1 and Cys111-peroxidized wild-type SOD1 showed higher thiol oxidase activity, an adverse side activity reported in SOD1 [50], than untreated wild-type SOD1. These results indicate that mutant SOD1 is labile to be monomerized by peroxidaton of Cys111 near the dimer interface, which will expose the copper of the protein and raise its reactivity to cause oxidative stress, and eventually forms intracellular aggregates or inclusion bodies to cause neurodegeneration (**Figure 1**).

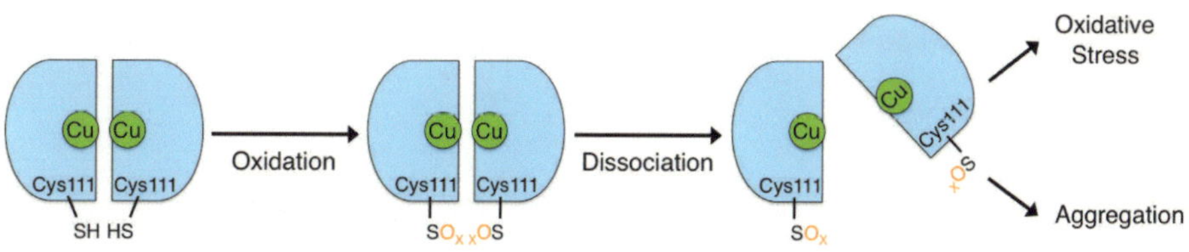

Figure 1. Proposed model of mutant SOD1 toxicity.

Oxidation of Cys111 leads mutant SOD1 dimers to dissociate into monomers, which causes oxidative stress through the copper and aggregate formation of the monomers.

5. Role of cysteine-mediated conformational change of mutant SOD1 in ALS pathogenesis

Although we determined the importance of oxidative modification of Cys111 for conformational change and copper-mediated aberrant chemistry of mutant SOD1, it has not been proved whether the modification of Cys111 is actually relevant to the pathogenesis of ALS by mutant SOD1 *in vivo*. Transgenic mice of mutant SOD1 that has simultaneous substitutions of all metal-coordinating residues and free cysteines (Cys6 and Cys111) were generated and had no pathology or motor symptoms [51]. However, it is difficult to confirm the direct contribution of Cys111 in these mice. To verify the importance of Cys111 solely, we conducted the study of transgenic mice expressing ALS-linked mutant SOD1 (H46R) with or without substitution of Cys111 to serine [52]. Both lines of transgenic mice (H46R and H46R/C111S SOD1 mice) were created, respectively, and were observed whether to obtain motor paralysis and the degeneration of motor neurons.

As a result, H46R SOD1 mice developed motor paralysis most quickly at 5 months of age, and reached the lifetime at 6 months of age. On the other hand, the onset of motor paralysis in H46R/C111S SOD1 mice was late at about 12 months of age, and their lifetime was extended to about 14 months after birth (**Figure 2**). Disease duration from the onset to lifetime was also significantly prolonged in H46R/C111S SOD1 mice than that in H46R SOD1 mice. The number of spinal motor neurons was decreased and the tibialis anterior muscle was atrophic at the time of endpoint in H46R SOD1 mice, while these indexes were preserved at the same age of H46R/C111S SOD1 mice. Activation of astrocytes and microglia, the phenomenon seen in the spinal cord of other mutant SOD1 transgenic mice as a modifying factor of neurodegeneration [53, 54], was also observed at endpoint in the spinal cord of H46R SOD1 mice, whereas it was not apparent in H46R/C111S SOD1 mice at the same time point.

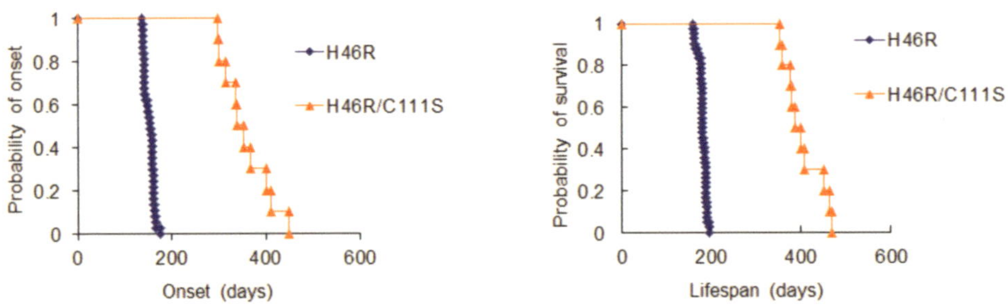

Figure 2. Kaplan-Meier curves of the onset and lifespan of H46R and H46R/C111S SOD1 mice.

Both the time at onset and lifespan were significantly extended in H46R/C111S SOD1 mice compared to those in H46R SOD1 mice.

Next, we examined the redox state of Cys111 in SOD1 and the presence of misfolded/insoluble SOD1 in the liver and spinal cord of these mice as well as of wild-type SOD1 transgenic mice. Cys111-peroxidized SOD1 was detected in H46R SOD1 mice from the early presymptomatic age regardless of organs, although it was trivial in wild-type SOD1 transgenic mice. On the other hand, misfolded and insolubly aggregated SOD1 was found only in the spinal cord in parallel to the disease onset of the mice. The SOD1 species was not seen at the same age of H46R/C111S SOD1 mouse; however, it was observed in the same way as H46R SOD1 mice at endpoint. These results indicate that mutant SOD1 is more prone to be attacked at Cys111 by oxidants than wild-type SOD1 due to a slight structural difference, and peroxidation of Cys111 is important to push the mutant SOD1 into misfolding at the early phase of the disease. However, considering that misfolding and aggregation of Cys111-peroxidized mutant SOD1 are defined to the spinal cord, other factors may exist to enhance or suppress the misfolding of the SOD1 in the spinal cord or liver, respectively. In fact, the expression of an important protective factor, for example, heat shock factor-1, is reported to be relatively low in motor neurons [55]. The difference in clearance efficiency of the SOD1 protein in each organ or cell type may also explain the specificity of mutant SOD1 misfolding and aggregation.

As mentioned before, insoluble high molecular weight species of mutant SOD1 is likely to consist of aggregates crosslinked with inter-subunit disulfide bonds of cysteine residues including Cys111. To verify the significance of this phenomenon in our ALS model, we analyzed the reactivity of the insoluble aggregates to a reducing reagent in the spinal cord of H46R SOD1 mice. The majority of the insoluble aggregates were maintained even in the presence of the reagent. We further examined H46R SOD1 mice by mating with thioredoxin 1 transgenic mice, to see whether the motor symptoms could be alleviated according to inhibition of the disulfide bond-mediated SOD1 crosslinking. Thioredoxin 1 is an antioxidative protein present in the cytoplasm as well as SOD1, and has an effect to revert oxidatively formed protein disulfide bonds to sulfhydryls by reducing reaction. We did not see any change in the course of motor paralysis, decrease of motor neurons, glial activation, or deposition of SOD1 aggregates in H46R SOD1 mice with hemizygous thioredoxin 1 transgenic background. No suppressive effect of the disease was observed even in the SOD1 mice with homozygous thioredoxin 1 transgenic background, excluding the possibility that the expression level of thioredoxin 1 was insufficient to have the effect (Nagano S, unpublished data). It indicates that the involvement of inter-subunit disulfide bonds of cysteine residues may be limited in our H46R mutant SOD1 disease model. More intense study will be needed in other mutant SOD1 mouse models to know the role of inter-subunit disulfide crosslinking in the mutant SOD1 neurotoxicity.

6. Conclusions

We have shown that Cys111 drives the pathogenicity of mutant SOD1 by demonstrating that the substitution of a single residue in mutant SOD1 significantly reduces the disease phenotype of ALS model mice. Cys111 of mutant SOD1 is peroxidized and promotes misfolding of the protein to generate reducing reagent-resistant, high molecular weight insoluble SOD1 species.

It is promising to create a new therapeutic strategy for mutant SOD1-related ALS by developing reagents that inhibit the modification of Cys111 or subsequent monomerization of the mutant SOD1. Dimedone, a trapping reagent of sulfenylated (-SOH) cysteines to block further peroxidation [56], or bis-maleimidoethane, a crosslinker that is shown to crosslink between Cys111 of each SOD1 subunit to inhibit monomerization [49], may be candidates, but the problem is that these reagents have no specificity for SOD1. The reagent that binds specifically to a pocket of SOD1 dimer interface was developed by in silico drug screening approach and had a suppressive effect for monomerization of mutant SOD1 *in vitro* [57]. Clinical application will be achieved by developing a drug having higher effect and permeability into the central nervous system using the reagent as a lead compound. Alternatively, considering that misfolded wild-type or mutant SOD1 is likely to be propagated to the neighboring neurons [58] to cause further misfolding of SOD1 and the spread of the disease, antibody therapy targeting Cys111 or dimer interface of SOD1 may also be effective to inhibit the progress of ALS.

Author details

Seiichi Nagano* and Toshiyuki Araki*

*Address all correspondence to: nagano@ncnp.go.jp and taraki@ncnp.go.jp

Department of Peripheral Nervous System Research, National Institute of Neuroscience, National Center of Neurology and Psychiatry, Tokyo, Japan

References

[1] Rosen DR, Siddique T, Patterson D, Figlewicz DA, Sapp P, Hentati A, Donaldson D, Goto J, O'Regan JP, Deng HX, Rahmani Z, Krizus A, Mckenna-Yasek D, Cayabyab A, Gaston SM, Berger R, Tanzi, RE, Halperin JJ, Herzfeldt B, Van Den Bergh R, Hung WY, Bird T, Deng G, Mulder DW, Smyth C, Laing NG, Soriano E, Pericak–Vance MA, Haines J, Rouleau GA, Gusella JS, Horvitz HR, Brown RHJ. Mutations in Cu/Zn superoxide dismutase gene are associated with familial amyotrophic lateral sclerosis. Nature. 1993;362:59–62.

[2] Scotter EL, Chen HJ, Shaw CE. TDP-43 proteinopathy and ALS: insights into disease mechanisms and therapeutic targets. Neurotherapeutics. 2015;12:352–363.

[3] Valentine JS, Doucette PA, Zittin Potter S. Copper-zinc superoxide dismutase and amyotrophic lateral sclerosis. Annu Rev Biochem. 2005;74:563–593.

[4] Borchelt DR, Lee MK, Slunt HS, Guarnieri M, Xu ZS, Wong PC, Brown RH Jr, Price DL, Sisodia SS, Cleveland DW. Superoxide dismutase 1 with mutations linked to familial

amyotrophic lateral sclerosis possesses significant activity. Proc Natl Acad Sci USA. 1994;91:8292–8296.

[5] Reaume AG, Elliott JL, Hoffman EK, Kowall NW, Ferrante RJ, Siwek DF, Wilcox HM, Flood DG, Beal MF, Brown RH Jr, Scott RW, Snider WD. Motor neurons in Cu/Zn superoxide dismutase-deficient mice develop normally but exhibit enhanced cell death after axonal injury. Nat Genet. 1996;13:43–47.

[6] Gurney ME, Pu H, Chiu AY, Dal Canto MC, Polchow CY, Alexander DD, Caliendo J, Hentati A, Kwon YW, Deng HX, Chen W, Zhai P, Sufit RL, Siddique T. Motor neuron degeneration in mice that express a human Cu, Zn superoxide dismutase mutation. Science. 1994;264:1772–1775.

[7] Chattopadhyay M, Valentine JS. Aggregation of copper-zinc superoxide dismutase in familial and sporadic ALS. Antioxid Redox Signal. 2009;11:1603–1614. doi: 10.1089/ARS.2009.2536.

[8] Tateno M, Kato S, Sakurai T, Nukina N, Takahashi R, Araki T. Mutant SOD1 impairs axonal transport of choline acetyltransferase and acetylcholine release by sequestering KAP3. Hum Mol Genet. 2009;18:942–955. doi: 10.1093/hmg/ddn422.

[9] Yerbury JJ, Ooi L, Dillin A, Saunders DN, Hatters DM, Beart PM, Cashman NR, Wilson MR, Ecroyd H. Walking the tightrope: proteostasis and neurodegenerative disease. J Neurochem. 2016, in press. doi: 10.1111/jnc.13575.

[10] Shibata N, Hirano A, Kobayashi M, Siddique T, Deng HX, Hung WY, Kato T, Asayama K. Intense superoxide dismutase-1 immunoreactivity in intracytoplasmic hyaline inclusions of familial amyotrophic lateral sclerosis with posterior column involvement. J Neuropathol Exp Neurol. 1996;55:481–490.

[11] Bruijn LI, Becher MW, Lee MK, Anderson KL, Jenkins NA, Copeland NG, Sisodia SS, Rothstein JD, Borchelt DR, Price DL, Cleveland DW. ALS-linked SOD1 mutant G85R mediates damage to astrocytes and promotes rapidly progressive disease with SOD1-containing inclusions. Neuron. 1997;18:327–338.

[12] Wiedau-Pazos M, Goto JJ, Rabizadeh S, Gralla EB, Roe JA, Lee MK, Valentine JS, Bredesen DE. Altered reactivity of superoxide dismutase in familial amyotrophic lateral sclerosis. Science. 1996;271:515–518.

[13] Yim MB, Kang JH, Yim HS, Kwak HS, Chock PB, Stadtman ER. A gain-of-function of an amyotrophic lateral sclerosis-associated Cu,Zn-superoxide dismutase mutant: an enhancement of free radical formation due to a decrease in Km for hydrogen peroxide. Proc Natl Acad Sci USA. 1996;93:5709–5714.

[14] Estévez AG, Crow JP, Sampson JB, Reiter C, Zhuang Y, Richardson GJ, Tarpey MM, Barbeito L, Beckman JS. Induction of nitric oxide-dependent apoptosis in motor neurons by zinc-deficient superoxide dismutase. Science. 1999;286:2498–2500.

[15] Ghadge GD, Lee JP, Bindokas VP, Jordan J, Ma L, Miller RJ, Roos RP. Mutant superoxide dismutase-1-linked familial amyotrophic lateral sclerosis: molecular mechanisms of neuronal death and protection. J Neurosci. 1997;17:8756–8766.

[16] Nagano S, Ogawa Y, Yanagihara T, Sakoda S. Benefit of a combined treatment with trientine and ascorbate in familial amyotrophic lateral sclerosis model mice. Neurosci Lett. 1999;265:159–162.

[17] Nagano S, Fujii Y, Yamamoto T, Taniyama M, Fukada K, Yanagihara T, Sakoda S. The efficacy of trientine or ascorbate alone compared to that of the combined treatment with these two agents in familial amyotrophic lateral sclerosis model mice. Exp Neurol. 2003;179:176–180.

[18] Nagano S, Satoh M, Sumi H, Fujimura H, Tohyama C, Yanagihara T, Sakoda S. Reduction of metallothioneins promotes the disease expression of familial amyotrophic lateral sclerosis mice in a dose-dependent manner. Eur J Neurosci. 2001;13:1363–1370.

[19] Hottinger AF, Fine EG, Gurney ME, Zurn AD, Aebischer P. The copper chelator d-penicillamine delays onset of disease and extends survival in a transgenic mouse model of familial amyotrophic lateral sclerosis. Eur J Neurosci. 1997;9:1548–1551.

[20] Kiaei M, Bush AI, Morrison BM, Morrison JH, Cherny RA, Volitakis I, Beal MF, Gordon JW. Genetically decreased spinal cord copper concentration prolongs life in a transgenic mouse model of amyotrophic lateral sclerosis. J Neurosci. 2004;24:7945–7950.

[21] Tokuda E, Ono S, Ishige K, Watanabe S, Okawa E, Ito Y, Suzuki T. Ammonium tetrathiomolybdate delays onset, prolongs survival, and slows progression of disease in a mouse model for amyotrophic lateral sclerosis. Exp Neurol. 2008;213:122–128. doi: 10.1016/j.expneurol.2008.05.011.

[22] Hashimoto K, Hayashi Y, Watabe K, Inuzuka T, Hozumi I. Metallothionein-III prevents neuronal death and prolongs life span in amyotrophic lateral sclerosis model mice. Neuroscience. 2011;189:293–298. doi: 10.1016/j.neuroscience.2011.05.034.

[23] Tokuda E, Okawa E, Watanabe S, Ono S. Overexpression of metallothionein-I, a copper-regulating protein, attenuates intracellular copper dyshomeostasis and extends lifespan in a mouse model of amyotrophic lateral sclerosis caused by mutant superoxide dismutase-1. Hum Mol Genet. 2014;23:1271–1285. doi: 10.1093/hmg/ddt517.

[24] Sheng Y, Chattopadhyay M, Whitelegge J, Valentine JS. SOD1 aggregation and ALS: role of metallation states and disulfide status. Curr Top Med Chem. 2012;12:2560–2572.

[25] Culotta VC, Klomp LW, Strain J, Casareno RL, Krems B, Gitlin JD. The copper chaperone for superoxide dismutase. J Biol Chem. 1997;272:23,469–23,472.

[26] Furukawa Y, O'Halloran TV. Amyotrophic lateral sclerosis mutations have the greatest destabilizing effect on the apo- and reduced form of SOD1, leading to unfolding and oxidative aggregation. J Biol Chem. 2005;280:17,266–17,274.

[27] Parakh S, Spencer DM, Halloran MA, Soo KY, Atkin JD. Redox regulation in amyotrophic lateral sclerosis. Oxid Med Cell Longev. 2013;2013:408681. doi: 10.1155/2013/408681.

[28] Kajihara J, Enomoto M, Seya K, Sukenaga Y, Katoh K. Physicochemical properties of charge isomers of recombinant human superoxide dismutase. J Biochem. 1988;104:638–642.

[29] Schininà ME, Carlini P, Polticelli F, Zappacosta F, Bossa F, Calabrese L. Amino acid sequence of chicken Cu, Zn-containing superoxide dismutase and identification of glutathionyl adducts at exposed cysteine residues. Eur J Biochem. 1996;237:433–439.

[30] Fujiwara N, Nakano M, Kato S, Yoshihara D, Ookawara T, Eguchi H, Taniguchi N, Suzuki K. Oxidative modification to cysteine sulfonic acid of Cys111 in human copper-zinc superoxide dismutase. J Biol Chem. 2007;282:35,933–35,944.

[31] Khare SD, Dokholyan NV. Common dynamical signatures of familial amyotrophic lateral sclerosis-associated structurally diverse Cu, Zn superoxide dismutase mutants. Proc Natl Acad Sci USA. 2006;103:3147–3152.

[32] Wilcox KC, Zhou L, Jordon JK, Huang Y, Yu Y, Redler RL, Chen X, Caplow M, Dokholyan NV. Modifications of superoxide dismutase (SOD1) in human erythrocytes: a possible role in amyotrophic lateral sclerosis. J Biol Chem. 2009;284:13,940–13,947. doi: 10.1074/jbc.M809687200.

[33] Lepock JR, Frey HE, Hallewell RA. Contribution of conformational stability and reversibility of unfolding to the increased thermostability of human and bovine superoxide dismutase mutated at free cysteines. J Biol Chem. 1990;265:21,612–21,618.

[34] Tiwari A, Hayward LJ. Familial amyotrophic lateral sclerosis mutants of copper/zinc superoxide dismutase are susceptible to disulfide reduction. J Biol Chem. 2003;278:5984–5992.

[35] Tiwari A, Xu Z, Hayward LJ. Aberrantly increased hydrophobicity shared by mutants of Cu,Zn-superoxide dismutase in familial amyotrophic lateral sclerosis. J Biol Chem. 2005;280:29,771–29,779.

[36] Toichi K, Yamanaka K, Furukawa Y. Disulfide scrambling describes the oligomer formation of superoxide dismutase (SOD1) proteins in the familial form of amyotrophic lateral sclerosis. J Biol Chem. 2013;288:4970–4980. doi: 10.1074/jbc.M112.414235.

[37] Furukawa Y, Fu R, Deng HX, Siddique T, O'Halloran TV. Disulfide cross-linked protein represents a significant fraction of ALS-associated Cu, Zn-superoxide dismutase aggregates in spinal cords of model mice. Proc Natl Acad Sci USA. 2006;103:7148–7153.

[38] Niwa J, Yamada S, Ishigaki S, Sone J, Takahashi M, Katsuno M, Tanaka F, Doyu M, Sobue G. Disulfide bond mediates aggregation, toxicity, and ubiquitylation of familial amyotrophic lateral sclerosis-linked mutant SOD1. J Biol Chem. 2007;282:28,087–28,095.

[39] Cozzolino M, Amori I, Pesaresi MG, Ferri A, Nencini M, Carrì MT. Cysteine 111 affects aggregation and cytotoxicity of mutant Cu,Zn-superoxide dismutase associated with familial amyotrophic lateral sclerosis. J Biol Chem. 2008;283:866–874.

[40] Ferri A, Fiorenzo P, Nencini M, Cozzolino M, Pesaresi MG, Valle C, Sepe S, Moreno S, Carrì MT. Glutaredoxin 2 prevents aggregation of mutant SOD1 in mitochondria and abolishes its toxicity. Hum Mol Genet. 2010;19:4529–4542. doi: 10.1093/hmg/ddq383.

[41] Karch CM, Borchelt DR. A limited role for disulfide cross-linking in the aggregation of mutant SOD1 linked to familial amyotrophic lateral sclerosis. J Biol Chem. 2008;283:13,528–13,537. doi: 10.1074/jbc.M800564200.

[42] McAlary L, Yerbury JJ, Aquilina JA. Glutathionylation potentiates benign superoxide dismutase 1 variants to the toxic forms associated with amyotrophic lateral sclerosis. Sci Rep. 2013;3:3275. doi: 10.1038/srep03275.

[43] Bosco DA, Morfini G, Karabacak NM, Song Y, Gros-Louis F, Pasinelli P, Goolsby H, Fontaine BA, Lemay N, McKenna-Yasek D, Frosch MP, Agar JN, Julien JP, Brady ST, Brown RH Jr. Wild-type and mutant SOD1 share an aberrant conformation and a common pathogenic pathway in ALS. Nat Neurosci. 2010;13:1396–1403. doi: 10.1038/nn.2660.

[44] Neumann M, Sampathu DM, Kwong LK, Truax AC, Micsenyi MC, Chou TT, Bruce J, Schuck T, Grossman M, Clark CM, McCluskey LF, Miller BL, Masliah E, Mackenzie IR, Feldman H, Feiden W, Kretzschmar HA, Trojanowski JQ, Lee VM. Ubiquitinated TDP-43 in frontotemporal lobar degeneration and amyotrophic lateral sclerosis. Science. 2006;314:130–133.

[45] Arai T, Hasegawa M, Akiyama H, Ikeda K, Nonaka T, Mori H, Mann D, Tsuchiya K, Yoshida M, Hashizume Y, Oda T. TDP-43 is a component of ubiquitin-positive tau-negative inclusions in frontotemporal lobar degeneration and amyotrophic lateral sclerosis. Biochem Biophys Res Commun. 2006;351:602–611.

[46] Mackenzie IR, Bigio EH, Ince PG, Geser F, Neumann M, Cairns NJ, Kwong LK, Forman MS, Ravits J, Stewart H, Eisen A, McClusky L, Kretzschmar HA, Monoranu CM, Highley JR, Kirby J, Siddique T, Shaw PJ, Lee VM, Trojanowski JQ. Pathological TDP-43 distinguishes sporadic amyotrophic lateral sclerosis from amyotrophic lateral sclerosis with SOD1 mutations. Ann Neurol. 2007;61:427–434.

[47] Watanabe S, Nagano S, Duce J, Kiaei M, Li QX, Tucker SM, Tiwari A, Brown RH Jr, Beal MF, Hayward LJ, Culotta VC, Yoshihara S, Sakoda S, Bush AI. Increased affinity for copper mediated by cysteine 111 in forms of mutant superoxide dismutase 1 linked to amyotrophic lateral sclerosis. Free Radic Biol Med. 2007;42:1534–1542.

[48] Porath J, Carlsson J, Olsson I, Belfrage G. Metal chelate affinity chromatography, a new approach to protein fractionation. Nature. 1975;258:598–599.

[49] Kishigami H, Nagano S, Bush AI, Sakoda S. Monomerized Cu, Zn-superoxide dismutase induces oxidative stress through aberrant Cu binding. Free Radic Biol Med. 2010;48:945–952. doi: 10.1016/j.freeradbiomed.2010.01.008.

[50] Winterbourn CC, Peskin AV, Parsons-Mair HN. Thiol oxidase activity of copper, zinc superoxide dismutase. J Biol Chem. 2002;277:1906–1911.

[51] Prudencio M, Lelie H, Brown HH, Whitelegge JP, Valentine JS, Borchelt DR. A novel variant of human superoxide dismutase 1 harboring amyotrophic lateral sclerosis-associated and experimental mutations in metal-binding residues and free cysteines lacks toxicity *in vivo*. J Neurochem. 2012;121:475–485. doi: 10.1111/j.1471-4159.2012.07690.x.

[52] Nagano S, Takahashi Y, Yamamoto K, Masutani H, Fujiwara N, Urushitani M, Araki T. A cysteine residue affects the conformational state and neuronal toxicity of mutant SOD1 in mice: relevance to the pathogenesis of ALS. Hum Mol Genet. 2015;24:3427–3439. doi: 10.1093/hmg/ddv093.

[53] Yamanaka K, Chun SJ, Boillee S, Fujimori-Tonou N, Yamashita H, Gutmann DH, Takahashi R, Misawa H, Cleveland DW. Astrocytes as determinants of disease progression in inherited amyotrophic lateral sclerosis. Nat Neurosci. 2008;11:251–253. doi: 10.1038/nn2047.

[54] Boillée S, Yamanaka K, Lobsiger CS, Copeland NG, Jenkins NA, Kassiotis G, Kollias G, Cleveland DW. Onset and progression in inherited ALS determined by motor neurons and microglia. Science. 2006;312:1389–1392.

[55] Kondo N, Katsuno M, Adachi H, Minamiyama M, Doi H, Matsumoto S, Miyazaki Y, Iida M, Tohnai G, Nakatsuji H, Ishigaki S, Fujioka Y, Watanabe H, Tanaka F, Nakai A, Sobue G. Heat shock factor-1 influences pathological lesion distribution of polyglutamine-induced neurodegeneration. Nat Commun. 2013;4:1405. doi: 10.1038/ncomms2417.

[56] Lo Conte M, Carroll KS. The redox biochemistry of protein sulfenylation and sulfinylation. J Biol Chem. 2013;288:26,480–26,488. doi: 10.1074/jbc.R113.467738.

[57] Ray SS, Nowak RJ, Brown RH Jr, Lansbury PT Jr. Small-molecule-mediated stabilization of familial amyotrophic lateral sclerosis-linked superoxide dismutase mutants against unfolding and aggregation. Proc Natl Acad Sci USA. 2005;102:3639–3644.

[58] Münch C, O'Brien J, Bertolotti A. Prion-like propagation of mutant superoxide dismutase-1 misfolding in neuronal cells. Proc Natl Acad Sci USA. 2011;108:3548–3553. doi: 10.1073/pnas.1017275108.

Chapter 6

Influence of Repeats in the Protein Chain on its Aggregation Capacity for ALS-Associated Proteins

Oxana V. Galzitskaya

Additional information is available at the end of the chapter

http://dx.doi.org/10.5772/63104

Abstract

Studies of diseases associated with pathological irreversible aggregation of proteins have become of special relevance and attracted the attention of researchers throughout the world because of the appearance of a new conceptual model based on the capacity of some proteins to self-assemble by the prion mechanism. Along with direct prion diseases, such as bovine rabies and Creutzfeldt-Jakob disease in humans, a great number of neurodegenerative disorders associated with the formation of aggregates through the prion mechanism are revealed. These disorders include Alzheimer's and Parkinson's diseases, amyotrophic lateral sclerosis, Huntington disease, and mucoviscidosis, some types of diabetes and hereditary cataracts. The listed diseases are caused by transition of a "healthy" protein or peptide molecule from the native conformation to a very stable "pathological" form. In this case, molecules in the "pathological" conformation aggregate specifically, forming amyloid fibrils that can multiply infinitely. An important result of studying the molecular mechanisms of prion diseases and different proteinopathies, associated with the formation of pathological aggregations by the prion mechanism, is the discovery of protein chain regions responsible for their aggregation. The ability to regulate aggregation (fibrillation) of proteins can be the focal tool for the drug development. Herein by the example of 29 RNA-binding proteins with prion-like domains, we demonstrate what role the amino acid repeats in prion-like domains can play. For these proteins, quite different repeats are revealed in the disordered part of the protein chain predicted with bioinformatics methods. Ten proteins of the 29 RNA-binding proteins are involved in the development of some diseases. The prion-like domains of FUS, TAF15, and EWS are critical for the aggregation of proteins associated with human neurodegenerative diseases. Proteins of this family are involved not only in neurodegenerative diseases, such as amyotrophic lateral sclerosis (ALS), Huntington disease, spinocerebral ataxy, and dentatorubral pallidoluysian atrophy, but also in the formation of human mixoid liposarcoma. It can be suggested that the presence of a great number of repeats in prion-like domains of RNA-binding proteins can accelerate the formation of a dynamic beta-structure and

INTECH
open science | open minds

© 2016 The Author(s). Licensee InTech. This chapter is distributed under the terms of the Creative Commons Attribution License (http://creativecommons.org/licenses/by/3.0), which permits unrestricted use, distribution, and reproduction in any medium, provided the original work is properly cited.

pathological aggregates, which are crucibles of amyotrophic lateral sclerosis (ALS) pathogenesis.

Keywords: disordered regions, repeats, motifs of low complexity, Alzheimer's disease, amyotrophic lateral sclerosis (ALS)

1. Introduction

Misfolded proteins leading to formation of protein aggregations are a reason for many diseases. There is no definite answer to the question what causes death of cells where such aggregations have been found: is this the cell defence mechanism or plain death? In a normal state, cells that accumulate such aggregations are usually programmed to death or apoptosis. Cell fragments subjected to apoptosis are removed by phagocytic cells. However, aggregations like amyloid fibrils are known to be resistant to the action of different proteases [1] that can impede the effective termination of efferocytosis and, as a result, accumulate in tissues. In any case, there is undoubtedly close association of the formation of aggregations and the development of many fatal diseases. There are several models describing the process of fibril formation. For example, in order to begin aggregation, proteins should be preliminarily unfolded or partially folded [2]. As known, the generation of fibrils is facilitated by denaturing conditions. At the same time, aggregation of peptides and proteins involved in pathogenesis of such types of amyloidosis as type II diabetes, Alzheimer's, and Parkinson's diseases does not necessitate preliminary unfolding of a protein molecule. But these data sooner support the general rule, because under physiological conditions most of these proteins have no definite structure, i.e., are natively unstructured [3]. However, most natively unfolded protein in vivo does not aggregate [4]. Moreover, unstructured proteins are resistant to denaturing conditions, i.e., to the factors bringing about stress, and, in the first place, high temperatures [5]. It was demonstrated that the absence of structure does not correlate with the aggregation capacity [6]. Therefore to avoid spontaneous self-assembly of a protein molecule, the evolutionary selection has led to an increased content of such amino acids as proline and glycine that inhibit protein aggregation [7] and to an increased content of charged amino acids [8]. On the contrary, due to a large number of amyloidogenic regions, globular proteins have developed capacity to avoid aggregation because of rapid folding into a globular structure. This shows that protein unfolding is necessary but not sufficient for activation of amyloid fibrils. It is most likely that there should be special motifs of amino acid sequences exposed to the solvent, which are more liable to aggregation than other regions of the amino acid sequences. Experimental data corroborate the hypothesis that there are small regions of a protein molecule responsible to the amyloidogenic behavior [9–11].

2. Role of repeats in protein aggregation

It has remained unclear what the mechanism of the earliest stage of initiation of the pathologic irreversible aggregation of proteins is and how this process is triggered in healthy organisms. It is supposed that the key role in the development of systematic amyloidosis belongs to the so-called primes or factors accelerating pathologic aggregation. Such primes can be infectious agents as well protein molecule regions containing motifs of low complexity, especially when these motifs are recurrent. It was shown that the more frequently the repeats occur in a protein sequence, the less structured the protein is. Generally, most homo-repeats are not structured [12–15]. Nevertheless, this is not characteristic of fibrillar proteins [16], the capacity of which to aggregation depends strongly on the amino acid sequence of the protein [17–19]. For example, if the identity of the amino acid sequence of immunoglobulin domains is lower than 30–40%, the proteins lose their capacity to co-aggregation [18]. Using the bioinformatics analysis, it has been established that in a large number of multidomain proteins the identity of amino acid sequences of their domains is below 40%. It suggests a conclusion that in this way the domains avoid mutual aggregation.

The existence of repeats in proteins and the clarification of their special roles are in the focus of attention of researchers. The role of different repeats is studied actively, including repeats such as PGMG (GPGM) and PNN upon biomineralization of PM27 proteins [20], NPNA (NANP) repeats in circumsporozoite protein of *Plasmodium falciparum*, YSPTSPS repeats in RNA-polymerase II, PHGGGWGQ repeats in prion protein, YGHGGG(N) and YNHGGG(G) repeats in plant proteins rich in glycine, PGQGQQ, PGQGQQGQQ, and GYYPTSOQQ repeats in wheat gluten, and FGGMGGGKGG repeat in bivalves (*Aequipecten abductin*). As a rule, conformational loops formed by these repeats are stabilized upon interaction with different cations; they are characterized by noncovalent interactions, particularly, interactions of aromatic groups. It was demonstrated that many tandem repeats add plasticity and mobility to the protein [21]. A leader on the occurrence of repeats in proteins is *P. falciparum* where 35% proteins of 5300 have repeats. Moreover, *P. falciparum* contains 24% proteins with prion-like domains rich in asparagine, whereas flies have only 3.4% of such proteins [22]. The occurrence frequency of asparagine repeats in our HRaP database (http://bioinfo.protres.ru/hrap/) [14] shows that *P. falciparum* is the leader. Of interest is the fact that one of the functions of these homorepeats is connected with the parasitic life [14]. For example, the sequence of the protein from *P. falciparum* (ID Q8IKW2_PLAF7 1304 aa 493.P_falciparum) has asparagine homorepeats of different lengths, the maximal length reaching 41 amino acids. The basic functions of this protein are associated with processes such as deacylation of proteins and "silence" of chromatin [14].

3. Cell stress and generation of stress granules

Cell stress can also be an important factor of initiation of aggregation even though each cell has developed an intricate defence system, because it is subjected to destructive stress action at regular intervals. A striking example of waiting till stress is over in the formation of stress granules (SG), when the nontranslated mRNA and RNA-binding proteins are assembled in ribonucleoprotein (RNP) complexes in order to terminate protein synthesis and thereby maintain cell energy. In this case, only those proteins that are synthesized are required for cell survival [23]. This means that after termination of the stress action, SGs disintegrate rapidly and the "released" mRNA resumes its functioning. However, if due to some reasons, the residence time of such proteins in SGs increases or their concentration in SGs exceeds the norm, disintegration of SGs can be impeded, creating favorable conditions for generation of the "center of aggregation initiation" that may induce transition to irreversible pathologic protein aggregation [24]. A detailed analysis of the mechanism of assembly and disassembly of SGs can provide a new insight into the development of diseases associated with this process and suggest novel therapeutic approaches. Since the main function of SGs is protection of cells from stress, many investigations are conducted to reveal factors shifting the balance of reversible aggregation towards pathology after stress termination (**Figure 1**).

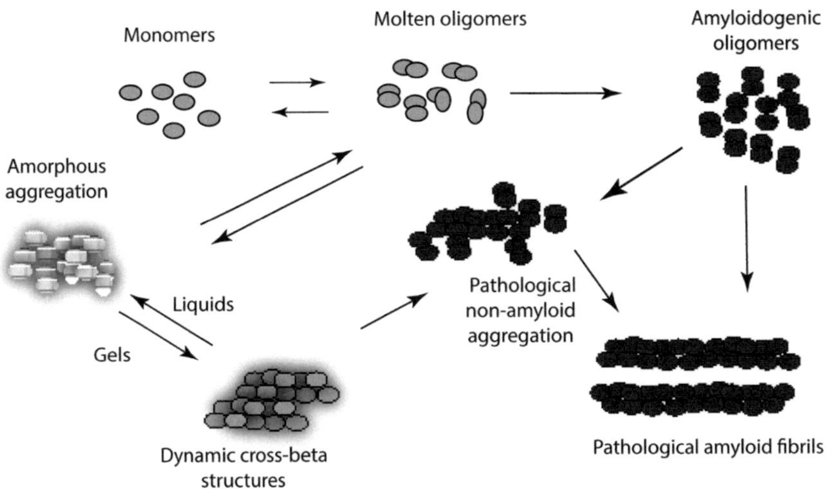

Figure 1. Schematic representation of different conformational states of self-assembly and disintegration of prion-like domains and a possible transition to irreversible pathologic aggregation. Modified and adapted from Li et al. [25].

It is assumed that due to self-assembly, RNA-binding proteins can facilitate formation of SGs using prion-like domains [26–28]. At any rate, it has been established that namely the structured part of RNA-binding proteins is responsible for the formation of hydrogel and binding to it [29]. Thus, protein FUS maintained its capacity to form gel even without the removal of the C-terminal region that corresponds to the RNA-binding domain and lost this capacity upon removal of the N-terminal unstructured region corresponding to the prion-like domain. The capacity to bind to hydrogel has been established for proteins such as hnRNPA2, RBM3 RNA-binding proteins, hnRNPA1, TIA1, CPEB2, FMRP, CIRBP, TDP43, and yeast Sup35. The formation of hydrogel was also demonstrated for the hnRNPA2 protein, and it was shown that proteins are retained to a different degree by hydrogel formed of different proteins [29].

http://dx.doi.org/10.5772/63104

4. The role of RNA-binding proteins with prion-like domains in diseases

Studies of the human genome have allowed isolating a set of RNA-binding proteins with a canonical RNA-binding motif. For example, prion-like domains were predicted for 29 of the 210 RNA-binding proteins for human diseases [30]. Ten of these 29 proteins are associated with neurodegenerative diseases, i.e., proteinopathies [31]. In this chapter, we focus our attention on isolation of repeats in well-studied proteins of the FET/TET family that are included in this group of 10. To elucidate the mechanism of pathologic aggregation of proteins, we have set ourselves the task to determine what repeats of amino acid residues in RNA-binding proteins can be responsible for reversible and irreversible aggregation.

The prion-like domains predicted for TDP-43 and FUS overlap with the region containing a large number of glycine residues. The prion-like domains are critical for aggregation of these proteins associated with human neurodegenerative diseases [32]. It was found that protein TAF15 is also involved in the development of disorder such as amyotrophic lateral sclerosis (ALS) or Lou Gering's disease [33]. At first, this protein was discovered using a bioinformatics analysis as a possible candidate and later it was revealed in ALS patients. It turned out that this protein has very similar properties to those of TDP-43 and FUS proteins involved in this disease. The only difference is that mutations of the protein associated with this disease are capable of higher aggregation in vitro than the wild-type protein, exert a stronger effect on the lifetime, and lead to incorrect localization of proteins in the spinal cord of mammals [33].

Among 29 candidates of RNA-binding proteins with predicted prion-like domains, the first and second places belong to FUS and TAF15, whereas TDP-43 is the 10th in this list [34]. Probably, it is expedient to pay attention to the first 10 proteins because the third place belongs to protein EWS [35]. They should also be detected in ALS patients.

5. Members of the FET family: FUS, EWS, TAF15

Members of the FET family are very similar RNA-binding proteins containing the following main domains in their structure: a SYGQ-rich N-terminal prion-like domain enriched with uncharged polar amino acids (asparagine, glutamine, serine, and tyrosine) and glycine [36], an RNA-binding motif (RNA-recognition motif, RRM), a "zinc finger" motif, and several RGG domains rich in glycine [37–39]. Three proteins (FUS, EWS, and TAF15) also have a nuclear location signal (NLS) that is recognized by the nuclear receptor transportin and is responsible for protein transport from the cytoplasm into the nucleus and back [27, 40–43]. Genes of the FET family are expressed practically everywhere. Proteins of this family are involved in regulation of different stages of gene expression, including transcription, pre-mRNA splicing, mRNA transport, and also take part in DNA repair [44–46]. The family name stems from three capital letters of its three members: proteins FUS/TLS (fused in sarcoma or translocated in liposarcoma), EWS (Ewing's sarcoma), and TAF15 (TATA-binding protein-associated factor 2N) [47]. These RNA-binding proteins participate in many cell processes, including transcription, pre-mRNA splicing, DNA repair, and mRNA transport in neurons [44–46]. As a rule, under stress conditions such RNA-binding proteins shift from the nucleus into the cytoplasm and take part in the formation of SGs, after which they return to the nucleus. This cycle is multiply repeated during the cell lifetime, and it is not excluded that under such conditions errors may occur in its functioning. The mechanism of activity of FET proteins, their cellular localization, and determination of domains involved in different processes are to be clarified.

Prion-like domains of these proteins associated with human neurodegenerative diseases are critical for their aggregation [32]. Proteins of this family are involved not only in neurodegenerative diseases, such as ALS [33], Huntington's disease, spinocerebellar ataxia, and dentatorubral cerebellar atrophy [48], but also in the development of human mixoid liposarcoma [49–51].

5.1. FUS: Its functions, structural peculiarities of a prion-like domain, mutations associated with diseases

A member of the FET family is the RNA-binding protein FUS, for which a number of mutations associated with ALS have been revealed [27, 40–43, 52]. Under normal conditions, this protein is localized mostly in the nucleus, whereas under pathologic conditions its aggregations are accumulated in the cytoplasm. It was demonstrated on several cell models that FUS delocalized in the cytoplasm was accumulated in SGs. This permitted a conclusion that a high concentration of the protein facilitates generation of protein aggregations under FUS pathology [53, 54]. Nonetheless an exact mechanism by which this transformation occurs remains unclear. It is not excluded that prion-like domains affect aggregation-like prions or fibril formation analogous to amyloidogenesis. It is also possible that FUS, accumulated in large amounts, aggregates in the cytoplasm independently of its capacity to sequestration in SGs. The protein accumulation can also facilitate dysfunction of the protein intracellular degradation systems that frequently occurs parallel to neurodegenerative disorders [55]. It should be noted that under sporadic ALS diseases, the control of splicing of a large amount of genes is violated [56]. The FUS protein also regulates alternative splicing, as a rule binding to transcripts containing large introns. Therefore, accumulation of FUS in the cytoplasm can result in the loss of its function in the nucleus and consequently violation of the alternative splicing of a number of genes, e.g., coding proteins associated with the growth and development of axons and the cell cytoskeleton [57]. This version is in agreement with the results obtained on a drosophila model, when an increased FUS concentration in the cell was extremely toxic for organisms that can also cause dysfunction during splicing. In addition, enhanced expression of the gaz gene of the fus ortholog caused death at the pupal stage [58].

In transgenic *Caenorhabditis elegans* worms, in which serine 57 was removed in protein FUS, paralysis occurred much earlier when compared to transgenic species with a full-sized FUS protein [59]. Therewith, the sequence of the FUS protein itself corresponded to that of the FUS protein from the human proteome. This mutation (removal of serine 57) is associated with the sporadic form of ALS [60]. It has been shown that for aggregation and toxicity of yeasts a prion-like (1–239) and an RGG2 (374–422) domains are required, though FUS (1–359) is sufficient for aggregation in models of neuroblastoma cells [54]. Domain RGG3 does not affect aggregation, and mutations in (502–526) lead only to the protein accumulation in the cytoplasm and its insertion in SGs. In yeasts, FUS was accumulated only in the cytoplasm [61]. Some components of SGs, such as translation initiation factors and poly-A-binding proteins, suppress toxicity of FUS aggregations. It is important that many proteins associated with RNA metabolism can affect the toxicity of FUS aggregations.

To verify the hypothesis that dislocation of FUS from the nucleus into the cytoplasm leads to the loss of its function in the nucleus, Murakami et al. created transgenic animals with double gene expression. One of these genes (fus) having the N-terminus, labeled with red fluorescent protein RFP, could not move into the cytoplasm under the action of stress, and the other gene (mutant GFP-fus-P525L) was uniformly distributed both over the nucleus and the cytoplasm. After heat shock, most of GFP-FUS-P525L moved into the SGs, whereas GFP-RUS remained in the cytoplasm. Therewith, the damaging effect was the same as in the experiment with expression of only GFP-fus-P525L. Therefore, the authors concluded that accumulation and aggregation of FUS in the cytoplasm are more neurotoxic than that when FUS lost its function in the nucleus [62].

In any case, formation of such aggregations is the reason for apoptosis, i.e., the process of programmed cell death. Apoptosis is characterized by retaining fragmentation of intracellular components with retention of the integrity of the plasmatic membrane that facilitates fast phagocytosis.

5.2. Role of FET proteins in the formation of stress granules

To understand the mechanism of assembly and disassembly of SGs, it is necessary to know what regions of the chain of RNA-binding proteins can perform the function of a prime and what the role of unstructured regions of simple complexity is. It is worth noting that in many respects protein FUS is a perfect model for studying processes involved in the formation of protein aggregations by the prion mechanism. To search for and reveal properties of prion-like domains, we have chosen three proteins from the FET/TET family of 29 RNA-binding proteins of the human proteome, the structures of which included prion-like domains [31]. The prediction was made using the algorithm developed by Alberti et al. [63], which is based on the choice of protein regions of 60 amino acid residues, similar in the amino acid content to the prion domains of yeast proteins, such as Sup35, Ure2p, and Rnq1p [64]. As a rule, these regions are rich in hydrophilic amino acid residues such as glutamine, asparagine, and tyrosine. In the range of proteins used in the prediction of prion-like domains, the first and second places belonged to FUS and TAF15 among 29 candidates of RNA-binding proteins, and the third was protein EWS [35].

The experiments, devoted to disclosing the capacity of protein FUS to aggregate, demonstrated that upon deletion of the most part of the predicted prion-like domain the protein lost its capacity to self-assemble; however, the formed aggregations did not reveal toxicity (**Figure 2**) [67]. Some components of SGs, such as translation initiation factors and poly-A-binding proteins, suppress toxicity of FUS aggregation [67]. It is important that proteins associated with RNA metabolism can affect the toxicity of FUS aggregations. Prion-like (1–239) and RGG2

(374–422) domains are also required for aggregation and toxicity of yeasts, although FUS (1–359) is sufficient for simulations on the neuroblastoma cell culture [68]. Domain RGG3 does not affect aggregation, and mutations at (502–526) result only in accumulation of the protein in the cytoplasm and its insertion in SGs [24, 69]. It should be mentioned that in contrast to mammalian cells, in yeast cells protein FUS is accumulated largely in the cytoplasm [61]. This may be connected with the fact that NLS FUS is not recognized by nuclear receptors of yeasts [65]. In mammalian cells, protein FUS is accumulated in the cytoplasm only when it has mutations distorting the reverse transport into the nucleus [69].

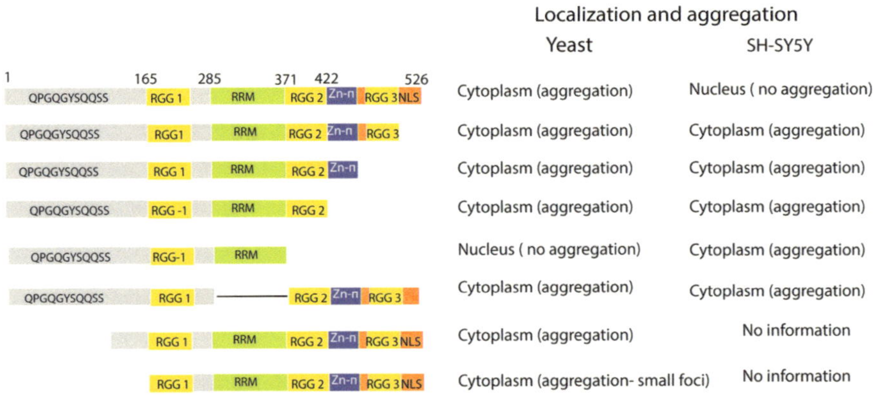

Figure 2. Effect of different constructions of FUS on aggregation and toxicity in yeasts and aggregation and localization in SGs in cell culture of the SH-SY5Y neuroblastoma [65, 66].

The N-terminal domain of FUS has 27 different variants of GYG, GYS, SYG, and SYS triplets (that can be designated as [G/S]Y[G/S] repeats) [70]. Four mutants were obtained with a different number of substituted tyrosine residues for serine ones to demonstrate that namely tyrosine residues are responsible for the formation of hydrogel. There were 5, 9, 15 substitutions and all 27. Neither of the mutants could form hydrogel, however, all of them could equally well bind to it. Mutants with substituted residues 5 and 9 could bind to hydrogel, but the remaining mutants could not [70].

5.3. Disordered regions in proteins of the FET family and search for partners for interactions with these proteins

For all three proteins, the IsUnstruct program [15] predicts the presence of unstructured domains, as a rule, at the N and C termini of the polypeptide chain. Unstructured proteins often play the role of hubs, i.e., have a capacity to concentrate a large number of partners around them (it is accepted that when there are more than five partners, it is a hub) [71]. To what extent is this role validated? To answer this question, it is necessary to determine the presence of functional sites in the protein considered. The search for the number of partners in the STRING database revealed that it exceeds 5 [72] (see **Figure 3**). Usually upon binding to a partner, natively unfolded proteins can acquire a structure that imparts a certain function to

http://dx.doi.org/10.5772/63104

them. In other words, the conformation of unstructured proteins is "dictated" by the interaction partners. This explains their capacity to perform different functions both in the cell and in the extracellular space. For example, the analyzed RNA-binding proteins have regions with large amounts of glycine in addition to large amounts of asparagine, glutamine, and tyrosine, which also facilitates their unfolded state and performance of various functions in the cell because these proteins are involved in the formation of RNP complexes, control of DNA transcription, pre-mRNA splicing, protein posttranslational modification, and many other vital functions [73]. According to the STRING database (version 10), the number of partners is 44 for TAF15, 132 for EWS (**Figure 3**), and 218 for FUS.

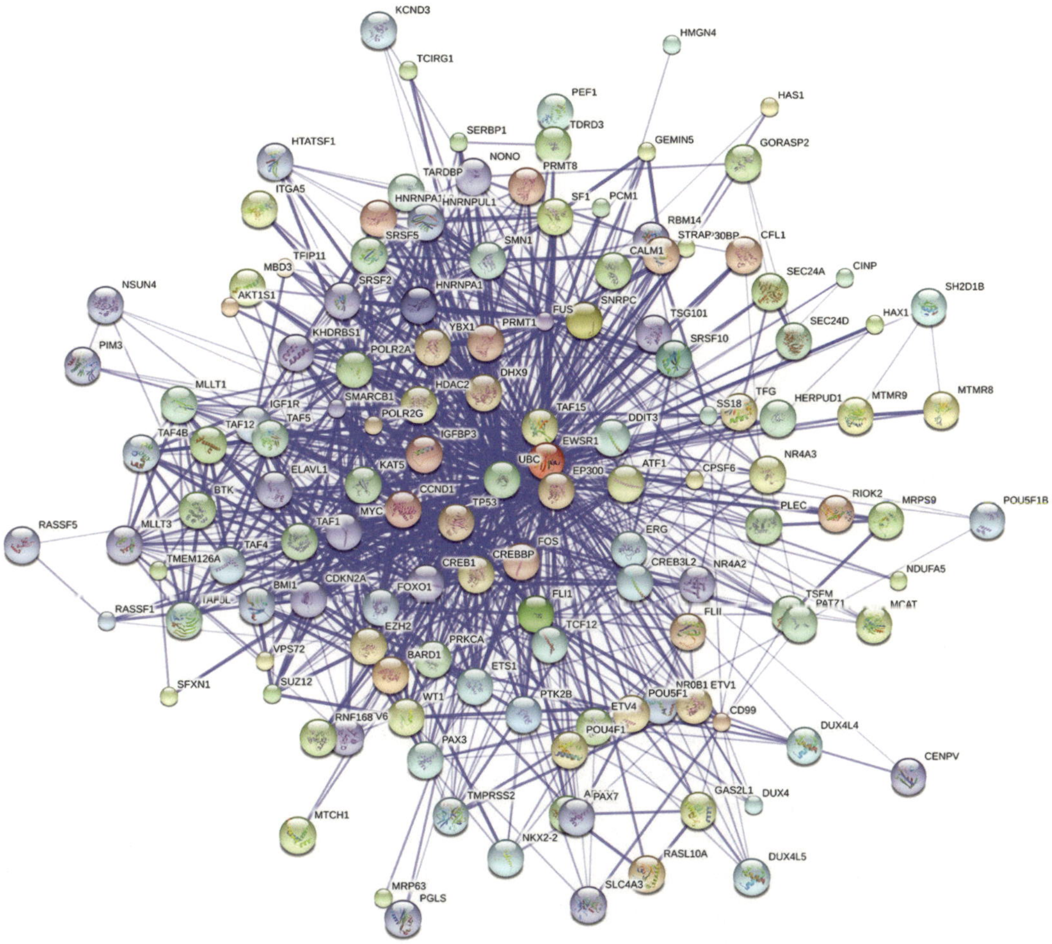

Figure 3. The list of partners for EWS has been obtained from the STRING database using the information from the data bases, data about homologies, possible co-expression, experimental confirmation about interactions, etc. The boundary condition for entry in the list of partners is probability of interactions equal to 0.4. Transparency of edges connecting vertices in the graph designates probability of interaction. The more transparent of edge, the less probability of interaction.

These proteins contain many motifs of simple complexity. As shown, the portion of proteins, included in periodic fragments or homorepeats, is an order of magnitude lower in eukaryotic proteomes than in bacterial ones [74, 75]. The proteins with periodic fragments are extremely nonuniformly distributed both over the kingdoms and over organisms within each kingdom [74, 75]. It is worth underlining that these repeated motifs can be located in the region not predicted as prion-like. It is known that protein Ure2 has regions in the carboxy-terminal domain affecting the capacity of the amino-terminal domain to become prion-like [76]. The available data for FUS allow us to conclude that the presence of both a prion-like domain and a C-terminal region corresponding to the RGG2 region (see **Figure 2**) is important for pathologic aggregation. It is most likely that the RNA-binding domain also contributes to the pathologic aggregation. The RNA-binding motif (RRM) in proteins RUS and TAF15 is highly identical and is retained from species to species. On the contrary, the RNA-binding motif (RRM) in protein EWS differs remarkably from other members of the family and does not preserve 100% identity in different species. For example, for FET proteins, the following amyloidogenic regions, revealed using program FoldAmyloid [77], can be indicated in the RNA-binding domain (RRM): AIYVQ/ADFFK/MIHIYL/VEWFD for EWS; TIFVQ/INLYT/IDWFD for TAF15; and TIFVQ/INLYT/IDWFD for FUS.

The prediction of unstructured regions in proteins of the FET/TET family using program IsUnstruct allowed us to isolate two unstructured domains at the N and C termini and one structured region, corresponding to the RNA-binding domain. **Figure 4** shows probability profiles for amino acid residues of the FET/TET proteins, which make it possible to determine whether they are structured or unstructured. Motifs in the amino acid sequence are shown by different colors. These proteins are characterized by the presence of a large number of homorepeats when one amino acid is recurrent many times. Generally, the longer are the repeats, the higher is the probability that the aggregated protein containing and it is associated with the development of a disease. For example, protein FUS is characterized by five unstructured patterns from the pattern library obtained by us from the Protein Data Bank: GSHM, GGGGSGG, GGGGG, GGSGGGGSGGG, and RGGGGSG. The occurrence of these patterns in the given protein in different organisms (human, monkey, pig, mouse, quicken and fish) can be found in our HRaP database, containing data on the occurrence of unstructured patterns and homorepeats in 122 proteomes [14]. For protein TAF15, the glycine-rich recurrent motif is well isolated at the C-terminus: DRGGGYGG/DRSSGGGYSG/DRGSRGGYGG, which is characteristic of many animals and fish [78]. We isolated 22 repeats, and the Uniprot program finds 21 repeats at the C terminus: GRGGRGG/DRGGYGG (**Figure 4**). As concerns EWS, we can observe 14 repeats as SYSQAPS in the prion-like domain (the N-terminal part) and 6 repeats (DRGRGGPGG) in the C-terminal part (**Figure 4**). It should be noted that 15 imperfect repeated motifs (QPGQGYSQQSS) are positioned in a prion-like region (the N-terminal part) and four repeats (DDRRGGRGGY) in the C-terminal one for FUS (**Figure 4**).

As known, protein regions enriched in glycine residues cannot have a rigid spatial structure; therefore, the main function characterizing this protein region is determined by a number of adjacent amino acid residues. It should be noted that in the mentioned proteins with high toxic aggregation, the glycine repeats adjoin arginine, serine, and tyrosine. Domains rich in glycine

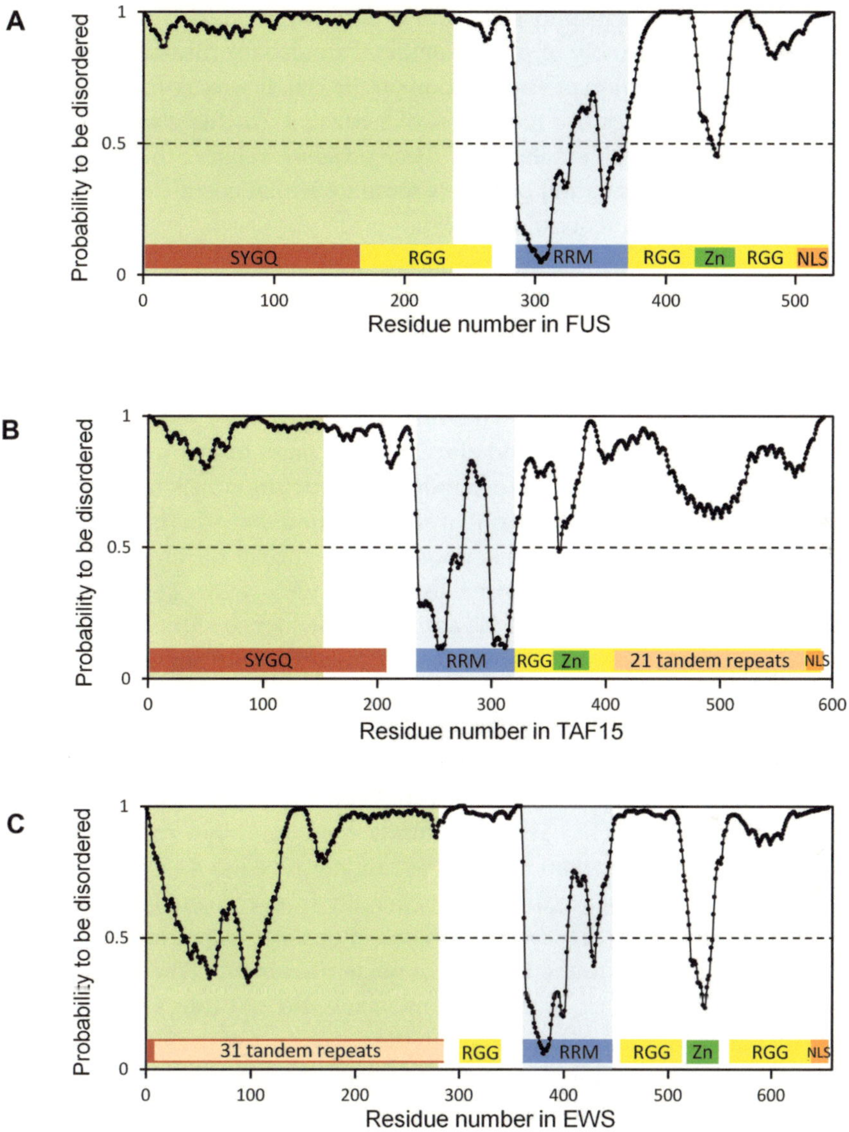

Figure 4. Probability profiles of amino acid residues in proteins of the FET/TET family (A for FUS, B for TAF15, and C for EWS) according to which it is possible to predict possible formation of the structure or its absence by the IsUnstruct program [15].

and arginine (RGG) are known to be responsible for the interaction of proteins with each other and with RNA. As a rule, these interactions are controlled by methylation of arginine [79], whereas phosphorylation of serine residues affects the direct mutual interaction of prion-like domains [45, 80]. Of interest is the fact that deletion of serine (S57), the mutation associated with sporadic form of ALS [81], induced paralysis in transgenic *C. elegans* species, that took place much faster than in transgenic species with a full-sized human FUS [82]. These data make it possible to suggest that phosphorylation and dephosphorylation of serine residues are critical not only for self-assembly of prion domains but also for disassembly by aggregation when required, e.g., termination of stress action on the cell. It was assumed that the presence of tyrosine residues facilitates the formation of hydrogel. In this connection, it should be mentioned that in spite of high similarity of these proteins, relative to other members of the family, the cytoplasmic aggregation of FUS is more toxic that correlates with longer glycine repeats in the amino acid sequence of FUS [33].

5.4. Zinc-finger motif in proteins of the FET family

All proteins of the FET/TET family are characterized by the presence of a zinc-finger motif. The exclusion is the EWS protein in chickens, because here the zinc-finger motif has not been determined [78]. As known, a classic zinc-finger motif forms a loop, where two cysteine residues and two histidine residues bind zinc ions. The main function of a classic zinc-finger motif is the binding of DNA, which corresponds to its structure consisting of two to three beta-sheets in the N-terminal region of the protein and one alpha-helix in its C-terminal region. As for the FET/TET family of proteins, the amino acid sequence of the zinc-finger motif in them differs significantly from the classic consensus motif (Cys-X_{2-4}-Cys-X_3-Phe-X_5-Leu-X_2-His-X_3-His) [83]. It should be noticed here that the amino acid sequence of this motif in proteins FUS and EWS is highly similar, which is preserved in all organisms studied by us. Our plots on the prediction of the structure demonstrated quite well the correspondence of this motif and the predicted structure (**Figure 4**: proteins FUS and EWS, second peak from the bottom, blue). On the contrary, in TAF15, this motif differs somewhat not only from FUS and EWS but also in the organisms studied by us; according to our prediction, it forms no structure (**Figure 4**). It is important that in proteins of the FET/TET family the zinc-finger motif occurs only once, contrary to the classic variant when it occurs as tandem repeats. As a rule, if the zinc-finger motif occurs once and its sequence differs considerably from the canonical one, the functions of this motif can differ remarkably from the classic motif. For example, it can both be bound to RNA and have no relation to the binding of nucleic acids [83]. The removal of this motif together with the terminal part of the FUS molecule did not affect the protein ability to aggregate and have toxicity either in yeasts or in the cell culture of the SH-SY5Y neuroblastoma [67]. Additional studies should be conducted to reveal the functions of the zinc-finger motif in proteins of the FET/TET family.

6. Conclusion: Repeats are a general characteristics of prion-like domains

In this study, we have analyzed RNA-binding proteins with prion-like domains, such as TAF15, FUS, and EWS. Using the FoldAmyloid program [77], we revealed the existence of amyloidogenic regions in the RRM domain in all three proteins of the FET family. This allows us to suggest that when the binding to RNA is violated, the proteins can aggregate spontaneously forming amyloid fibrils. In this case, protein FUS can aggregate both upon the removal of RRM and at point mutations in this domain [65, 66]. Further studies should be conducted to clarify whether aggregation of protein FUS in the presence of RRM does not lead to the formation of irreversible pathologic aggregations and functions only by the mechanism of assembly and possible disassembly under favorable conditions analogous to the functioning of SGs. We have also found that in all members of the FET/TET family the zinc-finger motif does not correspond to the classical one because it concerns both the location of tandem repeats and the amino acid sequence. Moreover, according to our prediction, in the FUS and TAF15 proteins, it does not even form any structure. Based on this, we can propose that in proteins of the FET/TET family the zinc-finger motif is not responsible for the DNA binding, but performs other functions determination of which requires further investigations.

We have also predicted unstructured regions corresponding both to prion-like domains and to additional regions, where we have revealed several recurrent amino acid motifs—tandem repeats. In addition, these proteins are characterized by the occurrence of homorepeats when one amino acid is multiply recurrent. The length of homorepeats can affect not only the capacity to aggregate but also the toxicity in an aggregated state. Correspondingly, the larger is the number of repeats, the higher is the probability that the aggregated protein containing them is associated with the development of the disease. We have established that protein FUS contains five disordered patterns from the pattern library obtained from the protein data bank: GSHM, GGGGSGG, GGGGG, GGSGGGGSGGG, and RGGGGSG, which are not located in the prion-like domain predicted for FUS. For other members of this family, these patterns are not characteristic and, as known, are less toxic when compared to FUS. When a larger part of the prion-like domain in protein FUS was removed (100 residues of the 165), it retained its capacity to aggregate [65], but lost completely the ability to form gel and display toxicity. These results allow us to suggest that the presence of short repeats in the unstructured prion-like domain of RNA-binding proteins is required for fast formation of a dynamic cross-beta structure of SGs [84].

Acknowledgements

I thank T.B. Kuvshinkina, E.I. Leonova, I.V. Sokolovsky, and N.V. Dovidchenko for assistance in the chapter preparation. This study was supported by the Russian Science Foundation No. 14-14-00536.

Author details

Oxana V. Galzitskaya

Address all correspondence to: ogalzit@vega.protres.ru

Institute of Protein Research, Russian Academy of Sciences, Pushchino, Russia

References

[1] Söderberg L, Dahlqvist C, Kakuyama H, Thyberg J, Ito A, Winblad B, et al. Collagenous Alzheimer amyloid plaque component assembles amyloid fibrils into protease resistant aggregates. FEBS J. 2005;272:2231–6.

[2] Dobson CM. Protein misfolding, evolution and disease. Trends Biochem. Sci. 1999;24:329–32.

[3] Rochet JC, Lansbury PT. Amyloid fibrillogenesis: themes and variations. Curr. Opin. Struct. Biol. 2000;10:60–8.

[4] Uversky VN, Gillespie JR, Fink AL. Why are "natively unfolded" proteins unstructured under physiologic conditions? Proteins. 2000;41:415–27.

[5] Tompa P. Intrinsically unstructured proteins. Trends Biochem. Sci. 2002;27:527–33.

[6] Linding R, Schymkowitz J, Rousseau F, Diella F, Serrano L. A comparative study of the relationship between protein structure and beta-aggregation in globular and intrinsically disordered proteins. J. Mol. Biol. 2004;342:345–53.

[7] Rauscher S, Baud S, Miao M, Keeley FW, Pomès R. Proline and glycine control protein self-organization into elastomeric or amyloid fibrils. Structure 2006. 14:1667–76.

[8] Kovacs E, Tompa P, Liliom K, Kalmar L. Dual coding in alternative reading frames correlates with intrinsic protein disorder. Proc. Natl. Acad. Sci. U. S. A. 2010;107:5429–34.

[9] Tenidis K, Waldner M, Bernhagen J, Fischle W, Bergmann M, Weber M, et al. Identification of a penta- and hexapeptide of islet amyloid polypeptide (IAPP) with amyloidogenic and cytotoxic properties. J. Mol. Biol. 2000;295:1055–71.

[10] von Bergen M, Friedhoff P, Biernat J, Heberle J, Mandelkow EM, Mandelkow E. Assembly of tau protein into Alzheimer paired helical filaments depends on a local sequence motif ((306)VQIVYK(311)) forming beta structure. Proc. Natl. Acad. Sci. U. S. A. 2000;97:5129–34.

[11] Ivanova MI, Sawaya MR, Gingery M, Attinger A, Eisenberg D. An amyloid-forming segment of beta2-microglobulin suggests a molecular model for the fibril. Proc. Natl. Acad. Sci. U. S. A. 2004;101:10584–9.

[12] Huntley MA, Golding GB. Simple sequences are rare in the Protein Data Bank. Proteins. 2002;48:134–40.

[13] Lobanov MY, Galzitskaya OV. Disordered patterns in clustered Protein Data Bank and in eukaryotic and bacterial proteomes. PLoS One. 2011;6:e27142.

[14] Lobanov MY, Sokolovskiy IV, Galzitskaya OV. HRaP: database of occurrence of HomoRepeats and patterns in proteomes. Nucleic Acids Res. 2014;42:D273–8.

[15] Lobanov MY, Sokolovskiy IV, Galzitskaya OV. IsUnstruct: prediction of the residue status to be ordered or disordered in the protein chain by a method based on the Ising model. J. Biomol. Struct. Dyn. 2013;31:1034–43.

[16] Jorda J, Xue B, Uversky VN, Kajava AV. Protein tandem repeats - the more perfect, the less structured. FEBS J. 2010;277:2673–82.

[17] Tanaka M, Chien P, Yonekura K, Weissman JS. Mechanism of cross-species prion transmission: an infectious conformation compatible with two highly divergent yeast prion proteins. Cell. 2005;121:49–62.

[18] Wright CF, Teichmann SA, Clarke J, Dobson CM. The importance of sequence diversity in the aggregation and evolution of proteins. Nature. 2005;438:878–81.

[19] Krebs MRH, Morozova-Roche LA, Daniel K, Robinson CV, Dobson CM. Observation of sequence specificity in the seeding of protein amyloid fibrils. Protein Sci. Publ. Protein Soc. 2004;13:1933–8.

[20] Harkey MA, Klueg K, Sheppard P, Raff RA. Structure, expression, and extracellular targeting of PM27, a skeletal protein associated specifically with growth of the sea urchin larval spicule. Dev. Biol. 1995;168:549–66.

[21] Matsushima N, Yoshida H, Kumaki Y, Kamiya M, Tanaka T, Izumi Y, et al. Flexible structures and ligand interactions of tandem repeats consisting of proline, glycine, asparagine, serine, and/or threonine rich oligopeptides in proteins. Curr. Protein Pept. Sci. 2008;9:591–610.

[22] Singh GP, Chandra BR, Bhattacharya A, Akhouri RR, Singh SK, Sharma A. Hyper-expansion of asparagines correlates with an abundance of proteins with prion-like domains in Plasmodium falciparum. Mol. Biochem. Parasitol. 2004;137:307–19.

[23] Lindquist S. Regulation of protein synthesis during heat shock. Nature. 1981;293:311–4.

[24] Bosco DA, Lemay N, Ko HK, Zhou H, Burke C, Kwiatkowski TJ, et al. Mutant FUS proteins that cause amyotrophic lateral sclerosis incorporate into stress granules. Hum. Mol. Genet. 2010;19:4160–75.

[25] Li YR, King OD, Shorter J, Gitler AD. Stress granules as crucibles of ALS pathogenesis. J. Cell Biol. 2013;201:361–72.

[26] Bosco DA, Lemay N, Ko HK, Zhou H, Burke C, Kwiatkowski TJ, et al. Mutant FUS proteins that cause amyotrophic lateral sclerosis incorporate into stress granules. Hum. Mol. Genet. 2010;19:4160–75.

[27] Dormann D, Rodde R, Edbauer D, Bentmann E, Fischer I, Hruscha A, et al. ALS-associated fused in sarcoma (FUS) mutations disrupt Transportin-mediated nuclear import. EMBO J. 2010;29:2841–57.

[28] Liu-Yesucevitz L, Bassell GJ, Gitler AD, Hart AC, Klann E, Richter JD, et al. Local RNA translation at the synapse and in disease. J. Neurosci. Off. J. Soc. Neurosci. 2011;31:16086–93.

[29] Kato M, Han TW, Xie S, Shi K, Du X, Wu LC, et al. Cell-free formation of RNA granules: low complexity sequence domains form dynamic fibers within hydrogels. Cell. 2012;149:753–67.

[30] Alberti S, Halfmann R, King O, Kapila A, Lindquist S. A systematic survey identifies prions and illuminates sequence features of prionogenic proteins. Cell. 2009;137:146–58.

[31] King OD, Gitler AD, Shorter J. The tip of the iceberg: RNA-binding proteins with prion-like domains in neurodegenerative disease. Brain Res. 2012;1462:61–80.

[32] Aguzzi A, Rajendran L. The transcellular spread of cytosolic amyloids, prions, and prionoids. Neuron. 2009;64:783–90.

[33] Couthouis J, Hart MP, Shorter J, DeJesus-Hernandez M, Erion R, Oristano R, et al. A yeast functional screen predicts new candidate ALS disease genes. Proc. Natl. Acad. Sci. 2011;108:20881–90.

[34] King OD, Gitler AD, Shorter J. The tip of the iceberg: RNA-binding proteins with prion-like domains in neurodegenerative disease. Brain Res. 2012;1462:61–80.

[35] Tan AY, Manley JL. The TET family of proteins: functions and roles in disease. J. Mol. Cell Biol. 2009;1:82–92.

[36] Zinszner H, Albalat R, Ron D. A novel effector domain from the RNA-binding protein TLS or EWS is required for oncogenic transformation by CHOP. Genes Dev. 1994;8:2513–26.

[37] Bentmann E, Neumann M, Tahirovic S, Rodde R, Dormann D, Haass C. Requirements for stress granule recruitment of fused in sarcoma (FUS) and TAR DNA-binding protein of 43 kDa (TDP-43). J. Biol. Chem. 2012;287:23079–94.

[38] Lerga A, Hallier M, Delva L, Orvain C, Gallais I, Marie J, et al. Identification of an RNA binding specificity for the potential splicing factor TLS. J. Biol. Chem. 2001;276:6807–16.

[39] Iko Y, Kodama TS, Kasai N, Oyama T, Morita EH, Muto T, et al. Domain architectures and characterization of an RNA-binding protein, TLS. J. Biol. Chem. 2004;279:44834–40.

[40] Gal J, Zhang J, Kwinter DM, Zhai J, Jia H, Jia J, et al. Nuclear localization sequence of FUS and induction of stress granules by ALS mutants. Neurobiol. Aging. 2011;32:27–40.

[41] Ito D, Seki M, Tsunoda Y, Uchiyama H, Suzuki N. Nuclear transport impairment of amyotrophic lateral sclerosis-linked mutations in FUS/TLS. Ann. Neurol. 2011;69:152–62.

[42] Kino Y, Washizu C, Aquilanti E, Okuno M, Kurosawa M, Yamada M, et al. Intracellular localization and splicing regulation of FUS/TLS are variably affected by amyotrophic lateral sclerosis-linked mutations. Nucleic Acids Res. 2011;39:2781–98.

[43] Niu C, Zhang J, Gao F, Yang L, Jia M, Zhu H, et al. FUS-NLS/Transportin 1 complex structure provides insights into the nuclear targeting mechanism of FUS and the implications in ALS. PLoS One. 2012;7:e47056.

[44] Ishigaki S, Masuda A, Fujioka Y, Iguchi Y, Katsuno M, Shibata A, et al. Position-dependent FUS-RNA interactions regulate alternative splicing events and transcriptions. Sci. Rep. 2012;2:529.

[45] Rogelj B, Easton LE, Bogu GK, Stanton LW, Rot G, Curk T, et al. Widespread binding of FUS along nascent RNA regulates alternative splicing in the brain. Sci. Rep. 2012;2:603.

[46] Fujii R, Okabe S, Urushido T, Inoue K, Yoshimura A, Tachibana T, et al. The RNA binding protein TLS is translocated to dendritic spines by mGluR5 activation and regulates spine morphology. Curr. Biol. 2005;15:587–93.

[47] Anderson P, Kedersha N. Stress granules: the Tao of RNA triage. Trends Biochem. Sci. 2008;33:141–50.

[48] Doi H, Koyano S, Suzuki Y, Nukina N, Kuroiwa Y. The RNA-binding protein FUS/TLS is a common aggregate-interacting protein in polyglutamine diseases. Neurosci. Res. 2010;66:131–3.

[49] Kwiatkowski TJ Jr, Bosco DA, Leclerc AL, Tamrazian E, Vanderburg CR, Russ C, et al. Mutations in the FUS/TLS gene on chromosome 16 cause familial amyotrophic lateral sclerosis. Science. 2009;323:1205–8.

[50] Vance C, Rogelj B, Hortobágyi T, De Vos KJ, Nishimura AL, Sreedharan J, et al. Mutations in FUS, an RNA processing protein, cause familial amyotrophic lateral sclerosis type 6. Science. 2009;323:1208–11.

[51] Crozat A, Aman P, Mandahl N, Ron D. Fusion of CHOP to a novel RNA-binding protein in human myxoid liposarcoma. Nature. 1993;363:640–4.

[52] Zhang ZC, Chook YM. Structural and energetic basis of ALS-causing mutations in the atypical proline-tyrosine nuclear localization signal of the Fused in Sarcoma protein (FUS). Proc. Natl. Acad. Sci. U. S. A. 2012;109:12017–21.

[53] Mitchell JC, McGoldrick P, Vance C, Hortobagyi T, Sreedharan J, Rogelj B, et al. Overexpression of human wild-type FUS causes progressive motor neuron degeneration in an age- and dose-dependent fashion. Acta Neuropathol. (Berl.). 2013;125:273–88.

[54] Shelkovnikova TA, Robinson HK, Connor-Robson N, Buchman VL. Recruitment into stress granules prevents irreversible aggregation of FUS protein mislocalized to the cytoplasm. Cell Cycle Georget. Tex. 2013;12:3194–202.

[55] Bossy-Wetzel E, Schwarzenbacher R, Lipton SA. Molecular pathways to neurodegeneration. Nat. Med. 2004;10 Suppl:S2–9.

[56] Rabin SJ, Kim JMH, Baughn M, Libby RT, Kim YJ, Fan Y, et al. Sporadic ALS has compartment-specific aberrant exon splicing and altered cell-matrix adhesion biology. Hum. Mol. Genet. 2010;19:313–28.

[57] Orozco D, Edbauer D. FUS-mediated alternative splicing in the nervous system: consequences for ALS and FTLD. J. Mol. Med (Berl.) 2013;91:1343–54.

[58] Xia R, Liu Y, Yang L, Gal J, Zhu H, Jia J. Motor neuron apoptosis and neuromuscular junction perturbation are prominent features in a Drosophila model of Fus-mediated ALS. Mol. Neurodegener. 2012;7:10.

[59] Vaccaro A, Tauffenberger A, Aggad D, Rouleau G, Drapeau P, Parker JA. Mutant TDP-43 and FUS cause age-dependent paralysis and neurodegeneration in *C. elegans*. PLoS One. 2012;7:e31321.

[60] Belzil VV, Valdmanis PN, Dion PA, Daoud H, Kabashi E, Noreau A, et al. Mutations in FUS cause FALS and SALS in French and French Canadian populations. Neurology. 2009;73:1176–9.

[61] Ju S, Tardiff DF, Han H, Divya K, Zhong Q, Maquat LE, et al. A yeast model of FUS/TLS-dependent cytotoxicity. PLoS Biol. 2011;9:e1001052.

[62] Murakami T, Yang S-P, Xie L, Kawano T, Fu D, Mukai A, et al. ALS mutations in FUS cause neuronal dysfunction and death in *Caenorhabditis elegans* by a dominant gain-of-function mechanism. Hum. Mol. Genet. 2012;21:1–9.

[63] Alberti S, Halfmann R, King O, Kapila A, Lindquist S. A systematic survey identifies prions and illuminates sequence features of prionogenic proteins. Cell. 2009;137:146–58.

[64] Shorter J, Lindquist S. Hsp104 catalyzes formation and elimination of self-replicating Sup35 prion conformers. Science. 2004;304:1793–7.

[65] Sun Z, Diaz Z, Fang X, Hart MP, Chesi A, Shorter J, et al. Molecular determinants and genetic modifiers of aggregation and toxicity for the ALS disease protein FUS/TLS. PLoS Biol. 2011;9:e1000614.

[66] Shelkovnikova TA, Robinson HK, Connor-Robson N, Buchman VL. Recruitment into stress granules prevents irreversible aggregation of FUS protein mislocalized to the cytoplasm. Cell Cycle Georget. Tex. 2013;12:3194–202.

[67] Sun Z, Diaz Z, Fang X, Hart MP, Chesi A, Shorter J, et al. Molecular determinants and genetic modifiers of aggregation and toxicity for the ALS disease protein FUS/TLS. PLoS Biol. 2011;9:e1000614.

[68] Shelkovnikova TA, Robinson HK, Connor-Robson N, Buchman VL. Recruitment into stress granules prevents irreversible aggregation of FUS protein mislocalized to the cytoplasm. Cell Cycle Georget. Tex. 2013;12:3194–202.

[69] Dormann D, Rodde R, Edbauer D, Bentmann E, Fischer I, Hruscha A, et al. ALS-associated fused in sarcoma (FUS) mutations disrupt Transportin-mediated nuclear import. EMBO J. 2010;29:2841–57.

[70] Kato M, Han TW, Xie S, Shi K, Du X, Wu LC, et al. Cell-free formation of RNA granules: low complexity sequence domains form dynamic fibers within hydrogels. Cell. 2012;149:753–67.

[71] Kim PM, Sboner A, Xia Y, Gerstein M. The role of disorder in interaction networks: a structural analysis. Mol. Syst. Biol. 2008;4:179.

[72] Jensen LJ, Kuhn M, Stark M, Chaffron S, Creevey C, Muller J, et al. STRING 8--a global view on proteins and their functional interactions in 630 organisms. Nucleic Acids Res. 2009;37:D412–6.

[73] Fisette J-F, Montagna DR, Mihailescu M-R, Wolfe MS. A G-rich element forms a G-quadruplex and regulates BACE1 mRNA alternative splicing. J. Neurochem. 2012;121:763–73.

[74] Jorda J, Kajava AV. Protein homorepeats sequences, structures, evolution, and functions. Adv. Protein Chem. Struct. Biol. 2010;79:59–88.

[75] Lobanov MY, Galzitskaya OV. Occurrence of disordered patterns and homorepeats in eukaryotic and bacterial proteomes. Mol. Biosyst. 2012;8:327–37.

[76] Maddelein ML, Wickner RB. Two prion-inducing regions of Ure2p are nonoverlapping. Mol. Cell. Biol. 1999;19:4516–24.

[77] Garbuzynskiy SO, Lobanov MY, Galzitskaya OV. FoldAmyloid: a method of prediction of amyloidogenic regions from protein sequence. Bioinformatics. 2010;26:326–32.

[78] Galzitskaya OV. Reversible and irreversible aggregation of proteins from the FET family: influence of repeats in protein chain on its aggregation capacity. Curr. Protein Pept Sci. 2016;17:319-331.

[79] Bedford MT. Arginine methylation at a glance. J. Cell Sci. 2007;120:4243–6.

[80] Han TW, Kato M, Xie S, Wu LC, Mirzaei H, Pei J, et al. Cell-free formation of RNA granules: bound RNAs identify features and components of cellular assemblies. Cell. 2012;149:768–79.

[81] Belzil VV, Valdmanis PN, Dion PA, Daoud H, Kabashi E, Noreau A, et al. Mutations in FUS cause FALS and SALS in French and French Canadian populations. Neurology. 2009;73:1176–9.

[82] Vaccaro A, Tauffenberger A, Aggad D, Rouleau G, Drapeau P, Parker JA. Mutant TDP-43 and FUS cause age-dependent paralysis and neurodegeneration in C. elegans. PLoS One. 2012;7:e31321.

[83] Lewin B. Genes IX. 9th ed. Sudbury, Mass: Jones and Bartlett Publishers; 2008.

[84] Galzitskaya OV. Repeats are one of the main characteristics of RNA-binding proteins with prion-like domains. Mol. Biosyst. 2015;11:2210–8.

Chapter 7

MicroRNAs in Amyotrophic Lateral Sclerosis

Maria Teresa Gonzalez Garza

Additional information is available at the end of the chapter

http://dx.doi.org/10.5772/62989

Abstract

miRNAs are sequences of 20–22 nucleotides that participate in the development, growth, and cell differentiation by the regulation of the mRNAs.Their possible participation in the development of degenerative diseases has been extensively investigated. Results show quantitative changes in miRNA transcription, to the pathogenesis of various neurodegenerative diseases. In this chapter, the dysregulation of microRNAs reported in the samples taken from amyotrophic lateral sclerosis (ALS) animal model or ALS patients is analyzed. Moreover,their probable participation in the pathogenesis of the disease is also analyzed.

Keywords: ALS, microRNA, miR-206, miR-338-3, miR-9a

1. Introduction

miRNAs are small RNA molecules that do not encode proteins. They are sequences of 20–22 nucleotides that regulate gene expression. miRNAs were identified in 1993 by Lee et al. [1]. Since then numerous studies have been carried out in order to have a better understanding of their functioning as regulators and, in turn, regulating transcription. These molecules are transcribed as a longer RNA between 500 and 3000 nucleotides [2, 3]. Then, a serial enzymatic activity inside the nucleus allows the reduction in the number of nucleotides. These pri-miRNAs are then exposed to an enzymatic process by using Drosha-associated Pasha (also known as DGCR8), resulting in a precursor of 65–75 nucleotides in a loop called pre-miRNA, which is transported to the cytoplasm. Finally, the Dicer enzyme breaks for mature single-stranded fragments comprise 19–25 nucleotides. The last enzymatic activity into cytoplasm provides an miRNA of 20–22 nucleotides with a complementary sequence of seven base pairs that enable an miRNA to bind to the target mRNA [3–6].

INTECH
open science | open minds

© 2016 The Author(s). Licensee InTech. This chapter is distributed under the terms of the Creative Commons Attribution License (http://creativecommons.org/licenses/by/3.0), which permits unrestricted use, distribution, and reproduction in any medium, provided the original work is properly cited.

The consequence of that complementary interaction could provide the inhibition of translation or the reduction in the stability of the mRNA resulting in the decrease of the target protein expression [7]. The importance of these small molecules in gene expression has led to numerous studies, which aimed at better understanding of its functioning as regulators and, in turn, the regulation of transcription. Another characteristic is its possibility to target several mRNAs given a major potential to regulate gene expression or a specific mRNA that can be regulated by multiple miRNAs [8–10]. Although most authors observed a downregulation by miRNAs, there are examples of upregulation by miRNAs as well. The ability of a single miRNA to act both in repression and activation depends on the number of nucleotides that can mate or phase of the cell cycle in which it is generated [11–16].

In order to homogenize the nomenclature of miRNAs for the pre-miRNA and the pri-miRNA, they are referred to as uncapitalized "mir," for the mature form of the miRNA as miR and MIR for the gene that encodes them [17].

Considering the complexity of the capacity and functions of these small molecules, they have been linked to several diseases such as cancer [18, 19], autoimmune diseases [20, 21], cardiovascular diseases [22–26], and, of particular interest to our group, are those related to neurological diseases.

General reviews on the participation of miRNAs in neurodegenerative diseases have been emerging, and the research on specific neurological diseases confirms a dysregulation biogenesis of these small molecules [27–31]. Impaired concentration of blood miRNAs has been reported in patients with stroke, Alzheimer disease, Huntington disease, Parkinson Disease, and Amyotrophic Lateral Sclerosis (ALS) [30–46]. In this chapter, ALS disease will be analyzed in more detail.

The dysregulation of miRNAs in the samples from ALS patients has been reported by several authors. Until now, it is not clear that which one is the most important dysregulation. This chapter aims at analyzing those reports that shed light on the enrolled miRNAs and their participation in ALS pathology.

2. miR-b2403 and miR-b1336 downregulation

During neuron degeneration in ALS diseases, many alterations on neurofilament have been observed such as the aggregate formation of the perikaryon and proximal axons. In addition, mRNA of low molecular weight neurofilament (NEFL) decreases [47–49]. A number of reports agree that an alteration of NEFL synthesis could contribute to the possible cause of neuron death in ALS patients. Recent reports on the expression analysis of miRNAs, performed on neurons recovered from sporadic ALS patients' spinal cord, confirm the downregulation of miR-b2403 and miR-b1336. These miRNAs modulate NEFL mRNA stability [50]. Consequently, it could be the cause of the decreased mRNA, as previously reported in patients with spinal cord ALS.

http://dx.doi.org/10.5772/62989

3. miR-338-3 upregulation

The overexpression of miR-338-3 was reported in leucocytes of ALS patients. This miRNA regulates gene cytochrome *c* oxidase IV [51]. *In vitro* experiments report that the transfection of miR-338 into the axons of primary sympathetic neurons results in a decrease in mitochondrial COXIV mRNAs and consequently a decrease in enzyme protein levels [52]. This protein belongs to the cytochrome *c* oxidase complex, the ending step in the mitochondrial electron transfer chain. Its downregulation results in a decrease in the ATP level and sensitizes the cells to apoptosis [53, 54]. miR-338 also regulates ATP synthase expression, which is another mitochondrial enzyme. The postmortem samples from the frontal cortex of patients with ALS also report on the upregulation of miR-338-3 [55]. The overexpression of miR-338-3 could induce an axonal respiration functionality and viability damage.

4. miR-29a and miR-29b upregulation

Microarray analysis of miRNAs on samples from three brains of patients with ALS reports the upregulation of miR-29a. This affects the stability and translation of mRNAs of NAV3, a nuclear membrane protein-related neuronal regeneration [55]. Unfortunately, there was a noticeable change in values of the miRNAs for the samples analyzed. In addition, the number of samples was very small so the analysis does not conclude. However, recently Nolan et al. [56] have reported an interesting result. The downregulation of the antiapoptotic Mcl-1 was associated with an upregulation of miR-29a, which enhances the sensitivity of neurons to endoplasmic reticulum stress-induced apoptosis. In previous research, Nolan et al. found a high expression for miR-29a in the brain and spinal cord of a family of ALS mouse model. The intracerebroventricular injection of an miR-29a-specific antagomir does not change disease manifestation, but the change in the life span was observed [57].

5. miR-9a downregulation

TAR DNA-binding protein 43 (TDP-43) is a nuclear protein related to binding the single-stranded DNA, RNA, and proteins [58]. In the nucleus, TDP-43 plays a critical role in regulating RNA splicing as well as modulating microRNA biogenesis. Nevertheless, TDP-43 is a nuclear factor. A mutant form of the TDP-43 protein can be found in the cytoplasm of affected neuron in neurological diseases. TDP-43 is considered a major component of the tau-negative and ubiquitin-positive inclusions in ALS and frontal dementia [59–62]. High levels of TDP-43 are detected in CSF samples from ALS patients [63]. Recently, it was found that miR-9a expression significantly reduced on ALS with the TDP43 A90V mutation [64]. It has been proposed that the genetic interaction studies support the notion that dTDP-43 acts through miR-9a to control the precision of SOP specification [65]. The *in vitro* experiment on mice genetic model tissue, miR-9, demonstrates an upstream regulation of NF mRNAs [66]. In *Drosophila* TDP43 mutants, the miR-9a expression was significantly inhibited [65]. These findings reveal a novel role for endogenous TDP-43 in neuronal specification and suggest that the functions of the FTD/ALS-associated RNA-binding protein TDP-43 ensure the robustness of control genetic programs [65]. Moreover, there is a possibility that TDP-43 may play an important role in miRNA processing, given an miR-9 downregulation reported on *in vitro* experiments [64].

6. miR-206 downregulation

Though the main feature is the death of motor neurons, other cells contribute to disease like muscle cells. In fact, in ALS animal models it was observed that motor neuron death starts with neuromuscular junction destruction and distal axonal degeneration [67]. The direct partners of the injured motor axons may respectively be the recipients or initiators of the initial damage. The bidirectional signaling between motor neurons and skeletal muscle fibers at neuromuscular synapses has been studied in an animal model. miR-206 is specifically expressed in skeletal muscle and linked to many disorders in skeletal muscle [68]. The expression of miR-206 is regulated by myostatin, TGFβ, and IGF [69, 70]. Moreover, the histone deacetylase 4 and fibroblast growth factor signaling pathways are involved. It was proved that a response to muscle denervation was activated, which promotes skeletal muscle regeneration in response to injury [71–74]. *In vivo* research performed on the ALS model shows the down-regulation of miR-206s. This deficiency was correlated with the acceleration of the disease progression [73]. In patients, miR-206 functions like a key factor for muscle reinnervation and disease progression [75]. However, sera from ALS patients showed an increase in the circulation of miR-206 as well as in SOD1-G93A mouse. Samples from biopsies of Biceps brachii muscle patients with ALS show that miR-206s are overexpressed in the skeletal muscle and plasma of ALS patients [76, 77]. Nevertheless, this miRNA has no enough data about its relation with disease status; it has been proposed as a marker [78].

7. miR-146a downregulation

Quantitative PCR performed on ALS spinal motor neuron samples showed dysregulation of a large number of miRNAs, such as miR-146a and miR-582-3p. An algorithmic program revealed that these miRNAs are able to interact with NFL mRNA 3′UTR and suggested that the main role of these miRNAs is to suppress NFL mRNA [79]. Additional reports on miR-146 function dysregulation are related to the inflammation process by inflammatory factors such as interleukin 1 and tumor necrosis factor-alpha and another process that functions in the innate immune system by regulating Toll-like receptor signaling [80, 81]. On the other hand, *in vitro* experiments performed with mouse neural stem cells showed their relation with proliferation and differentiation, where miR-146 overexpression promoted spontaneous differentiation of neural stem cells by downstream Notch 1 gene [82].

8. miR-524-5p downregulation

Nevertheless, miR-524-5p was inversely associated with the activity of the MAPK/ERK pathway by suppressing the expression of BRAF and ERK2 proteins on melanoma [83], as a tumor suppressor in glioblastoma by Jagged-1 and Hes-1 downregulation [84] and in gastric cancer cells [85]. The results obtained by the application of miRNA recognition element program, on samples obtained from spinal cord neurons of sporadic ALS patients, showed that this miRNA is able to directly regulate the NFL by downregulating its synthesis in neuron cells. However, in ALS patients, it is decreasing and by consequence there is an overproduction of NFL which is a deleterious effect. On the other hand, the overexpression of miR-524-5p inhibits the MAPK/ERK pathway; apparently these cells could demonstrate a high activity on the MAPK/ERK pathway and cytoplasm NS accumulation.

9. miR-124 downregulation

miR-124 has been found to be the most abundant microRNA expressed in neuronal cells. Its targets are laminin $\gamma1$ and integrin $\beta1$. Nevertheless, experiments to alter expression of miR-124 in neural cells did not appear to affect differentiation [86]. However, later research reports described the role of miR-124 during neuronal differentiation by the overexpression of miR-9* and miR-124 in neural progenitors [87]. In a recent work, it was demonstrated that exosomes containing miR-124a releasing from neurons that can be directly internalized into astrocytes, with a concomitant increase in miR-124a, induce an increase in the levels of GLT1 protein [88]. miR-124a was found downregulated in the spinal cord of mutant SOD1 mouse models. *In vivo* injection of miR-124a into oligonucleotides in the spinal cord of ALS mice significantly prevents further pathological loss of GLT1 protein.

10. Other dysregulate miR

De Felice et al. [51] analyzed 911 mRNA expression by microarray in leukocytes of 14 patients with sporadic ALS. In addition to miR-338-3p, they identified eight miRNAs with changes in expression, e.g., hsa-miR-451, hsa-miR-1275, hsa-miR-328, hsamiR-638, has-miR-149, and the expression decreased for miR583 and miR-665 [51]. Campos-Melo et al. [79] also reported a decrease in most miRNAs, such as miR-146a, miR-524-5, and miR-582-3, from neurons of the spinal cord in the lower back. In addition, miR-b2403 and miR-b1336 are underregulated in the spinal cord samples; both are related to the stabilization of mRNA NEFL as well as miR-338-3 as previously reported [50, 51]. The consequence of the accumulation effects on the NEFL mRNA could be the cause for the decrease in mRNA previously reported in patients with spinal cord ELA [47]. Reports of miRNAs expression analysis performed on the samples of neurons recovered from the brain or spinal cord of ALS patients have been able to confirm a reduction in miRNAs that modulate gene NEFL stability (for the synthesis of light neurofilament), the cytochrome *c* oxidase gene, and protein of the nuclear membrane NAV3 and related neuronal regeneration.

Other cells that contribute to the disease are microglia cells, lymphocytes, and Schwann cells [89–91]. A recent hypothesis is that Schwann and muscle cells are also direct partners of the injured motor axons and may respectively be the recipients or initiators of the initial damage [67, 92].

In a mice ALS model, it has been proved that miR-365 and miR-125b suppress the IL-6/STAT3 pathway in microglia cells with an increase in the levels of TNFα mRNA [93]. This agrees with the fact that TNFα is upregulated in G93A mice and ALS patients [94, 95], which indicates that miR-365 and miR-125b dysregulations might develop the pathological cytokine profile on ALS.

11. Conclusion

Until now, there is no consensus on which miRNA could be the best target for therapy. To alter the cell homeostasis of miRNAs, more than one change is needed for their biogenesis. Similar to previous reports, miRNA can have several target mRNAs and one mRNA can be regulated by different microRNAs. ALS research provides an example of NEFL synthesis alteration, which can be regulated by miR-b2403, miR-b1336, miR-146a, miR-524-5p, and miR-582-3p. Probably, for the development of diseases, the coincidence of more than one dysregulation is necessary, or the accumulative alteration of various changes in the transcriptome, to induce neuron cell death. On the other hand, the dysregulation of miRNAs on neighbor cells participates in ALS pathology, where microglia cells, lymphocytes, Schwann cells, and muscle cells show a dysregulation in the miRNA transcript. Further, miRNAs also participate in neuron death. Nevertheless, research on miRNAs involves looking at miRNAs from the perspective of biomarkers. Moreover, the systematic comparative analysis of their profile between healthy people and ALS patients provides information on which pathways can be suggested as possible targets for directed therapy. In addition, the analysis also provides an opportunity to know more about the development of this disease, metabolic pathways altered, and cells involved in ALS pathology.

Author details

Maria Teresa Gonzalez Garza

Address all correspondence to: mtgonzalezgarza@itesm.mx

School of Medicine, Tecnologico de Monterrey, Monterrey, Mexico

References

[1] Lee RC, Feinbaum RL, Ambros V. The C. elegans heterochronic gene lin-4 encodes small RNAs with antisense complementarity to lin-14. Cell. 1993;75:843–854.

[2] Lee RC, Ambros V. An extensive class of small RNAs in *Caenorhabditis elegans*. Science. 2001;294(5543):862–964.

[3] Lee Y, Ahn C, Han J, Choi H, Kim J, Yim J, Lee J, Provost P, Rådmark O, Kim S, Kim VN. The nuclear RNase III Drosha initiates microRNA processing. Nature. 2003;425(6956):415–419.

[4] Lee Y, Kim M, Han J, Yeom KH, Lee S, Baek SH, Kim VN. MicroRNA genes are transcribed by RNA polymerase II. EMBO J. 2004;23:4051–4605.

[5] Landthaler M, Yalcin A, Tuschl T. The human DiGeorge syndrome critical region gene 8 and its *D. melanogaster* homolog are required for miRNA biogenesis. Curr. Biol. 2004;14:2162–2167.

[6] Schwarz DS, Hutvágner G, Du T, Xu Z, Aronin N, Zamore PD. Asymmetry in the assembly of the RNAi enzyme complex. Cell. 2003;115:199–208.

[7] Bartel DP. MicroRNAs: target recognition and regulatory functions. Cell. 2009;136;215–233. DOI: 10.1016/j.cell.2009.01.002.

[8] Lagos-Quintana M, Rauhut R, Meyer J, Borkhardt A, Tuschl T. New microRNAs from mouse and human. RNA. 2003;9:175–179.

[9] Lim LP, Lau NC, Garrett-Engele P, Grimson A, Schelter JM, Castle J, Bartel DP, Linsley PS, Johnson JM. Microarray analysis shows that some microRNAs downregulate large numbers of target mRNAs. Nature. 2005;433(7027):769–773.

[10] Kamanu TK, Radovanovic A, Archer JA, Bajic VB. Exploration of miRNA families for hypotheses generation. Sci. Rep. 2013;3:2940. DOI: 10.1038/srep02940.

[11] Ørom UA, Nielsen FC, Lund AH. Microrna-10a binds the 5′UTR of ribosomal protein mRNAs and enhances their translation. Mol. Cell. 2008;30:460–471. DOI: 10.1016/j.molcel.2008.05.001.

[12] Buchan JR, Parker R. Molecular biology. The two faces of miRNA. Science. 2007;318:1877–1878.

[13] Ghosh T, Soni K, Scaria V, Halimani M, Bhattacharjee C, Pillai B. MicroRNA-mediated up-regulation of an alternatively polyadenylated variant of the mouse cytoplasmic {beta}-actin gene. Nucl. Acids Res. 2008;36:6318–6332. DOI: 10.1093/nar/gkn624.

[14] Iwasaki S, Tomari Y. Argonaute-mediated translational repression (and activation). Fly (Austin). 2009;3:204–206.

[15] Saraiya AA, Li W, Wang CC. Transition of a microRNA from repressing to activating translation depending on the extent of base pairing with the target. PLoS One. 2013;8(2):e55672. DOI:10.1371/annotation/cb23f7bd-0d8c-4fa2-8ce8-1d641c03f561.

[16] Vasudevan S, Tong Y, Steitz JA. Switching from repression to activation: microRNAs can upregulate translation. Science. 2007;318(5858):1931–1934.

[17] Griffiths-Jones S, Grocock RJ, van Dongen S, Bateman A, Enright AJ. miRBase: microRNA sequences, targets and gene nomenclature. Nucl. Acids Res. 2006;34(Database issue):D140–D144.

[18] Fang Z, Tang J, Bai Y, Lin H, You H, Jin H, Lin L, You P, Li J, Dai Z, Liang X, Su Y, Hu Q, Wang F, Zhang ZY. Plasma levels of microRNA-24, microRNA-320a, and microRNA-423-5p are potential biomarkers for colorectal carcinoma. J. Exp. Clin. Cancer Res. 2015;34:86. DOI: 10.1186/s13046-015-0198-6.

[19] Zhu MY, Zhang W, Yang T. Diverse microRNAs with convergent functions regulate tumorigenesis. Oncol. Lett. 2016;11:915–920.

[20] Singh RP, Massachi I, Manickavel S, Singh S, Rao NP, Hasan S, Mc Curdy DK, Sharma S, Wong D, Hahn BH, Rehimi H. The role of miRNA in inflammation and autoimmunity. Autoimmun. Rev. 2013;12:1160–1165. DOI: 10.1016/j.autrev.2013.07.003.

[21] Jimenez SA, Piera-Velazquez S. Potential role of human-specific genes, human-specific microRNAs and human-specific non-coding regulatory RNAs in the pathogenesis of systemic sclerosis and Sjogren's syndrome[J]. Autoimmun. Rev. 2013;12:1046–1051. DOI: 10.1016/j.autrev.2013.04.004.

[22] Yang B, Lin H, Xiao J, Lu Y, Luo X, Li B, Zhang Y, Xu C, Bai Y, Wang H, Chen G, Wang Z. The muscle-specific microRNA miR-1 regulates cardiac arrhythmogenic potential by targeting GJA1 and KCNJ2. Nat. Med. 2007;13:486–491.

[23] Luo X, Lin H, Pan Z, Xiao J, Zhang Y, Lu Y, Yang B, Wang Z. Down-regulation of miR-1/miR-133 contributes to re-expression of pacemaker channel genes HCN2 and HCN4 in hypertrophic heart. J. Biol. Chem. 2008;283:20045–20052. DOI: 10.1074/jbc.M801035200.

[24] Callis TE, Pandya K, Seok HY, Tang RH, Tatsuguchi M, Huang ZP, Chen JF, Deng Z, Gunn B, Shumate J, Willis MS, Selzman CH, Wang DZ. MicroRNA-208a is a regulator of cardiachypertrophy and conduction in mice. J. Clin. Invest. 2009;119:2772–2786. DOI: 10.1172/JCI36154.

[25] Shan H, Zhang Y, Lu Y, Pan Z, Cai B, Wang N, Li X, Feng T, Hong Y, Yang B. Downregulation of miR-133 and miR-590 contributes to nicotine-induced atrial remodelling in canines. Cardiovasc. Res. 2009;83:465–472. DOI: 10.1093/cvr/cvp130.

[26] Matkovich SJ, Wang W, Tu Y, Eschenbacher WH, Dorn LE, Condorelli G, Diwan A, Nerbonne JM, Dorn GW II. MicroRNA-133a protects against myocardial fibrosis and modulates electrical repolarization without affecting hypertrophy in pressure-over-

loaded adult hearts. Circ. Res. 2010;106:166–175. DOI: 10.1161/CIRCRESAHA.109.202176.

[27] Nelson PT, Wang WX, Rajeev BW. MicroRNAs (miRNAs) in neurodegenerative diseases. Brain Pathol. 2008;18:130–138. DOI: 10.1111/j.1750-3639.2007.00120.x.

[28] Abe M, Bonini NM. MicroRNAs and neurodegeneration: role and impact. Trends Cell Biol. 2013;23:30–36. DOI: 10.1016/j.tcb.2012.08.013.

[29] Maciotta S, Meregalli M, Torrente Y. The involvement of microRNAs in neurodegenerative diseases. Front. Cell Neurosci. 2013;7:265. DOI: 10.3389/fncel.2013.00265.

[30] Gascon E, Gao F-B. The emerging roles of microRNAs in the pathogenesis of frontotemporal dementia–amyotrophic lateral sclerosis (FTD-ALS) spectrum disorders. J. Neurogenet. 2014;28:30–40. DOI: 10.3109/01677063.2013.876021.

[31] Volonte C, Apolloni S, Parisi C. MicroRNAs: newcomers into the ALS picture. CNS Neurol. Disord. Drug Targets. 2015;14:194–207.

[32] Zeng L, Liu J, Wang Y, Wang L, Weng S, Tang Y, Zheng C, Cheng Q, Chen S, Yang GY. MicroRNA-210 as a novel blood biomarker in acute cerebral ischemia. Front. Biosci. (Elite Ed.). 2011;3:1265–1272.

[33] Gan CS, Wang CW, Tan KS. Circulatory microRNA-145 expression is increased in cerebral ischemia. Genet. Mol. Res. 2012;11:147–152. DOI: 10.4238/2012.January.27.1.

[34] Ouyang YB, Stary CM, Yang GY, Giffard R. microRNAs: innovative targets for cerebral ischemia and stroke. Curr. Drug. Targets. 2013;14:90–101.

[35] Sepramaniam S, Tan JR, Tan KS, DeSilva DA, Tavintharan S, Woon FP, Wang CW, Yong FL, Karolina DS, Kaur P, Liu FJ, Lim KY, Armugam A, Jeyaseelan K. Circulating microRNAs as biomarkers of acute stroke. Int. J. Mol. Sci. 2014;15:1418–1432. DOI: 10.3390/ijms15011418.

[36] Hébert SS, Horré K, Nicolaï L, Papadopoulou AS, Mandemakers W, Silahtaroglu AN, Kauppinen S, Delacourte A, De Strooper B. Loss of microRNA cluster miR-29a/b-1 in sporadic Alzheimer's disease correlates with increased BACE1/beta-secretase expression. Proc. Natl. Acad. Sci. U. S. A. 2008;105:6415–6420. DOI: 10.1073/pnas.0710263105.

[37] Smith P, Al Hashimi A, Girard J, Delay C, Hébert SS. In vivo regulation of amyloid precursor protein neuronal splicing by microRNAs. J. Neurochem. 2011;116:240–247. DOI: 10.1111/j.1471-4159.2010.07097.x.

[38] Absalon S, Kochanek DM, Raghavan V, Krichevsky AM. MiR-26b, upregulated in Alzheimer's disease, activates cell cycle entry, tau-phosphorylation, and apoptosis in postmitotic neurons. J. Neurosci. 2013;33:14645–14659. DOI: 10.1523/JNEUROSCI.1327-13.2013.

[39] Banzhaf-Strathmann J, Benito E, May S, Arzberger T, Tahirovic S, Kretzschmar H, Fischer A, Edbauer D. MicroRNA-125b induces tau hyperphosphorylation and

cognitive deficits in Alzheimer's disease. EMBO J. 2014;33:1667–1680. DOI: 10.15252/embj.201387576.

[40] Gaughwin PM, Ciesla M, Lahiri N, Tabrizi SJ, Brundin P, Björkqvist M. Hsa-miR-34b is a plasma-stable microRNA that is elevated in pre-manifest Huntington's disease. Hum. Mol. Genet. 2011;20:2225–2237. DOI: 10.1093/hmg/ddr111.

[41] Hoss AG, Labadorf A, Latourelle JC, Kartha VK, Hadzi TC, Gusella JF, MacDonald ME, Chen JF, Akbarian S, Weng Z, Vonsattel JP, Myers RH. miR-10b-5p expression in Huntington's disease brain relates to age of onset and the extent of striatal involvement. BMC Med. Genom. 2015;8:10. DOI: 10.1186/s12920-015-0083-3.

[42] Müller S. In silico analysis of regulatory networks underlines the role of miR-10b-5p and its target BDNF in Huntington's disease. Transl. Neurodegener. 2014;3:17. DOI: 10.1186/2047-9158-3-17. eCollection 2014.

[43] Junn E, Lee KW, Jeong BS, Chan TW, Im JY, Mouradian MM. Repression of alpha-synuclein expression and toxicity by microRNA-7. Proc. Natl. Acad. Sci. U. S. A. 2009;106:13052–13057. DOI: 10.1073/pnas.0906277106.

[44] Doxakis E. Post-transcriptional regulation of alpha-synuclein expression by mir-7 and mir-153. J. Biol. Chem. 2010;285:12726–12734. DOI: 10.1074/jbc.M109.086827.

[45] Margis R, Margis R, Rieder CR. Identification of blood microRNAs associated to Parkinsonĭs disease. J. Biotechnol. 2011;152(3):96–101. DOI: 10.1016/j.jbiotec.2011.01.023.

[46] Bergeron C, Beric-Maskarel K, Muntasser S, Weyer L, Somerville MJ, Percy ME. Neurofilament light and polyadenylated mRNA levels are decreased in amyotrophic lateral sclerosis motor neurons. J. Neuropathol. Exp. Neurol. 1994;53:221–230.

[47] Wong NK, He BP, Strong MJ. Characterization of neuronal intermediate filament protein expression in cervical spinal motor neurons in sporadic amyotrophic lateral sclerosis (ALS). J. Neuropathol. Exp. Neurol. 2000;59:972–982.

[48] Ge WW, Leystra-Lantz C, Wen W, Strong MJ. Selective loss of trans-acting instability determinants of neurofilament mRNA in amyotrophic lateral sclerosis spinal cord. J. Biol. Chem. 2003;278:26558–26563.

[49] Ishtiaq M, Campos-Melo D, Volkening K, Strong MJ. Analysis of novel NEFL mRNA targeting microRNAs in amyotrophic lateral sclerosis. PLoS One. 2014;9(1):e85653. DOI: 10.1371/journal.pone.0085653. eCollection 2014

[50] De Felice B, Guida M, Coppola C, De Mieri G, Cotrufo R. A miRNA signature in leukocytes from sporadic amyotrophic lateral sclerosis. Gene. 2012;508:35–40. DOI: 10.1016/j.gene.2012.07.058.

[51] Aschraf A, Schwechter AD, Mameza, MG, Natera-Naranjo O, Gioio AE, Kaplan BB. MicroRNA-338 regulates local cytochrome oxidase IV mRNA levels and oxidative

phosphorylation in the axons of sympathetic neurons. J. Neurosci. 2008;28:12581–12590, DOI: 10.1523/JNEUROSCI.3338-08.2008.

[52] Li Y, Park JS, Deng JH, Bai Y. Cytochrome c oxidase subunit IV is essential for assembly and respiratory function of the enzyme complex. J. Bioenerg. Biomembr. 2006;38:283–291.

[53] Kar AN, Sun CY, Reichard K, Gervasi NM, Pickel J, Nakazawa K, Gioio AE, Kaplan BB. Dysregulation of the axonal trafficking of nuclear-encoded mitochondrial mRNA alters neuronal mitochondrial activity and mouse behavior. Dev. Neurobiol. 2014;74:333–350. DOI: 10.1002/dneu.22141.

[54] Shioya M, Obayashi S, Tabunoki H, Arima K, Saito Y, Ishida T, Satoh J. Aberrant microRNA expression in the brains of neurodegenerative diseases: miR-29a decreased in Alzheimer disease brains targets neurone navigator 3. Neuropathol. Appl. Neurobiol. 2010;36:320–330. DOI: 10.1111/j.1365-2990.2010.01076.x.

[55] Nolan K, Walter F, Tuffy LP, Poeschel S, Gallagher R, Haunsberger S, Bray I, Stallings RL, Concannon CG, Prehn JH. ER stress-mediated upregulation of miR-29a enhances sensitivity to neuronal apoptosis. Eur. J. Neurosci. 2016;43(5):640–652. doi:10.1111/ejn.13160.

[56] Nolan K, Mitchem MR, Jimenez-Mateos EM, Henshall DC, Concannon CG, Prehn JH. Increased expression of microRNA-29a in ALS mice: functional analysis of its inhibition. J. Mol. Neurosci. 2014;53:231–241. DOI: 10.1007/s12031-014-0290-y.

[57] Buratti E. Functional significance of TDP-43 mutations in disease. Adv. Genet. 2015;91:1–53. DOI: 10.1016/bs.adgen.2015.07.001.

[58] Arai T, Hasegawa M, Akiyama H, Ikeda K, Nonaka T, Mori H, Mann D, Tsuchiya K, Yoshida M, Hashizume Y, Oda T. TDP-43 is a component of ubiquitin-positive tau-negative inclusions in frontotemporal lobar degeneration and amyotrophic lateral sclerosis. Biochem. Biophys. Res. Commun. 2006;351(3):602–611.

[59] Arai T, Hasegawa M, Nonoka T, Kametani F, Yamashita M, Hosokawa M, Niizato K, Tsuchiya K, Kobayashi Z, Ikeda K, Yoshida M, Onaya M, Fujishiro H, Akiyama H. Phosphorylated and cleaved TDP-43 in ALS, FTLD and other neurodegenerative disorders and in cellular models of TDP-43 proteinopathy. Neuropathology. 2010;30(2):170–181.

[60] Hasegawa M, Nonaka T, Tsuji H, Tamaoka A, Yamashita M, Kametani F, Yoshida M, Arai T, Akiyama H. Molecular dissection of TDP-43 proteinopathies. J. Mol. Neurosci. 2011;45(3):480–485.

[61] Neumann M, Kwong LK, Sampathu DM, Trojanowski JQ, Lee VM. TDP-43 proteinopathy in frontotemporal lobar degeneration and amyotrophic lateral sclerosis: protein misfolding diseases without amyloidosis. Arch. Neurol. 2007;64(10):1388–1394

[62] Kasai T, Tokuda T, Ishigami N, Sasayama H, Foulds P, Mitchell DJ, Mann DM, Allsop D, Nakagawa M. Increased TDP-43 protein in cerebrospinal fluid of patients with amyotrophic lateral sclerosis. Acta Neuropathol. 2009;117(1):55–62.

[63] Zhang Z, Almeida S, Lu Y, Nishimura AL, Peng L, Sun D, Wu B, Karydas AM, Tartaglia MC, Fong JC, Miller BL, Farese RV Jr, Moore MJ, Shaw CE, Gao FB. Downregulation of microRNA-9 in iPSC-derived neurons of FTD/ALS patients with TDP-43 mutations. PLoS One. 2013;8(10):e76055.

[64] Li Z, Lu Y, Xu XL, Gao FB. The FTD/ALS-associated RNA-binding protein TDP-43 regulates the robustness of neuronal specification through microRNA-9a in *Drosophila*. Hum. Mol. Genet. 2013;22(2):218–225.

[65] Haramati S, Chapnik E, Sztainberg Y, Eilam R, Zwang R, Gershoni N, McGlinn E, Heiser PW, Wills AM, Wirguin I, Rubin LL, Misawa H, Tabin CJ, Brown R Jr, Chen A, Hornstein E. miRNA malfunction causes spinal motor neuron disease. Proc. Natl. Acad. Sci. U. S. A. 2010;107(29):13111–13116.

[66] Dupuis L, Loeffler JP. Neuromuscular junction destruction during amyotrophic lateral sclerosis: insights from transgenic models. Curr. Opin. Pharmacol. 2009;9(3):341–346.

[67] Ma G, Wang Y, Li Y, Cui L, Zhao Y, Zhao B, Li K. MiR-206, a key modulator of skeletal muscle development and disease. Int. J. Biol. Sci. 2015;11(3):345–352.

[68] Rachagani S, Cheng Y, Reecy JM. Myostatin genotype regulates muscle-specific miRNA expression in mouse pectoralis muscle. BMC Res. Notes. 2010;3:297.

[69] Winbanks CE, Wang B, Beyer C, Koh P, White L, Kantharidis P, Gregorevic P. TGF-beta regulates miR-206 and miR-29 to control myogenic differentiation through regulation of HDAC4. J. Biol. Chem. 2011;286(16):13805–13814.

[70] van Rooij E, Liu N, Olson EN. MicroRNAs flex their muscles. Trends Genet. 2008;24(4): 159–166.

[71] Williams AH, Liu N, van Rooij E, Olson EN. MicroRNA control of muscle development and disease. Curr. Opin. Cell Biol. 2009;21(3):461–469

[72] Williams AH, Valdez G, Moresi V, Qi X, McAnally J, Elliott JL, Bassel-Duby R, Sanes JR, Olson EN. MicroRNA-206 delays ALS progression and promotes regeneration of neuromuscular synapses in mice. Science. 2009;326(5959):1549–1554.

[73] Liu N, Williams AH, Maxeiner JM, Bezprozvannaya S, Shelton JM, Richardson JA, Bassel-Duby R, Olson EN. microRNA-206 promotes skeletal muscle regeneration and delays progression of Duchenne muscular dystrophy in mice. J. Clin. Invest. 2012;122(6):2054–2065.

[74] Bruneteau G, Simonet T, Bauché S, Mandjee N, Malfatti E, Girard E, Tanguy ML, Behin A, Khiami F, Sariali E, Hell-Remy C, Salachas F, Pradat PF, Fournier E, Lacomblez L, Koenig J, Romero NB, Fontaine B, Meininger V, Schaeffer L, Hantaï D. Muscle histone

deacetylase 4 upregulation in amyotrophic lateral sclerosis: potential role in reinnervation ability and disease progression. Brain. 2013;136(Pt 8):2359–2368.

[75] Russell AP, Wada S, Vergani L, Hock MB, Lamon S, Léger B, et al. Disruption of skeletal muscle mitochondrial network genes and miRNAs in amyotrophic lateral sclerosis. Neurobiol Dis. 2012;49C:107–117.

[76] Andrade H, Albuquerque M, Peluzzo T, Dogni D, Nucci A, Lopes-Cendes I, Franca M, Avansini S. Hsa-miR-424 and has-miR-206 are overexpressed in the skeletal muscle and plasma of patients with amyotrophic lateral sclerosis (ALS). Neurology. 2015;84(14 Suppl):P2.054

[77] Toivonen JM, Manzano R, Oliván S, Zaragoza P, García-Redondo A, Osta R. MicroRNA-206: a potential circulating biomarker candidate for amyotrophic lateral sclerosis. PLoS One. 2014;9(2):e89065.

[78] Campos-Melo D, Droppelmann CA, He Z, Volkening K, Strong MJ. Altered microRNA expression profile in amyotrophic lateral sclerosis: a role in the regulation of NFL mRNA levels. Mol. Brain. 2013;6:26.

[79] Sonkoly E, Ståhle M, Pivarcsi A. MicroRNAs and immunity: novel players in the regulation of normal immune function and inflammation. Semin. Cancer Biol. 2008;18(2):131–140.

[80] Sheedy FJ, O'Neill LA. Adding fuel to fire: microRNAs as a new class of mediators of inflammation. Ann. Rheum. Dis. 2008;67(Suppl 3):iii50–iii55.

[81] Xiao WZ, Lu AQ, Liu XW, Li Z, Zi Y, Wang ZW. Role of miRNA-146 in proliferation and differentiation of mouse neural stem cells. Biosci. Rep. 2015;35(5):e00245.

[82] Liu SM, Lu J, Lee HC, Chung FH, Ma N. miR-524-5p suppresses the growth of oncogenic BRAF melanoma by targeting BRAF and ERK2. Oncotarget. 2014;5(19):9444–9459.

[83] Chen L, Zhang W, Yan W, Han L, Zhang K, Shi Z, Zhang J, Wang Y, Li Y, Yu S, Pu P, Jiang C, Jiang T, Kang C. The putative tumor suppressor miR-524-5p directly targets Jagged-1 and Hes-1 in glioma. Carcinogenesis. 2012;33(11):2276–2282.

[84] Li FQ, Xu B, Wu YJ, Yang ZL, Qian JJ. Differential microRNA expression in signet-ring cell carcinoma compared with tubular adenocarcinoma of human gastric cancer. Genet. Mol. Res. 2015;14(1):739–747.

[85] Cao X, Pfaff SL, Gage FH. A functional study of miR-124 in the developing neural tube. Genes Dev. 2007;21(5):531–536.

[86] Yoo AS, Staahl BT, Chen L, Crabtree GR. MicroRNA-mediated switching of chromatin-remodelling complexes in neural development. Nature. 2009;460(7255):642–646.

[87] Morel L, Regan M, Higashimori H, Ng SK, Esau C, Vidensky S, Rothstein J, Yang Y. Neuronal exosomal miRNA-dependent translational regulation of astroglial glutamate transporter GLT1. J. Biol. Chem. 2013;288(10):7105–7116.

[88] Ilieva H, Polymenidou M, Cleveland DW. Non-cell autonomous toxicity in neurodegenerative disorders: ALS and beyond. J. Cell Biol. 2009;187(6):761–772

[89] Boillee S, Vande Velde C, Cleveland DW. ALS: a disease of motor neurons and their nonneuronal neighbors. Neuron. 2006;52(1):39–59.

[90] Lobsiger CS, Boillee S, McAlonis-Downes M, Khan AM, Feltri ML, Yamanaka K, Cleveland DW. Schwann cells expressing dismutase active mutant SOD1 unexpectedly slow disease progression in ALS mice. Proc. Natl. Acad. Sci. U. S. A. 2009;106(11):4465–4470.

[91] Chen K, Northington FJ, Martin LJ. Inducible nitric oxide synthase is present in motor neuron mitochondria and Schwann cells and contributes to disease mechanisms in ALS mice. Brain Struct. Funct. 2010;214(2–3):219–234.

[92] Parisi C, Arisi I, D'Ambrosi N, Storti AE, Brandi R, D'Onofrio M, Volonté C. Dysregulated microRNAs in amyotrophic lateral sclerosis microglia modulate genes linked to neuroinflammation. Cell Death Dis. 2013;4:e959.

[93] Poloni M, Facchetti D, Mai R, Micheli A, Agnoletti L, Francolini G, Mora G, Camana C, Mazzini L, Bachetti T. Circulating levels of tumour necrosis factor-alpha and its soluble receptors are increased in the blood of patients with amyotrophic lateral sclerosis. Neurosci. Lett. 2000;287(3):211–214.

[94] Hensley K, Fedynyshyn J, Ferrell S, Floyd RA, Gordon B, Grammas P, Hamdheydari L, Mhatre M, Mou S, Pye QN, Stewart C, West M, West S, Williamson KS. Message and protein-level elevation of tumor necrosis factor alpha (TNF alpha) and TNF alpha-modulating cytokines in spinal cords of the G93A-SOD1 mouse model for amyotrophic lateral sclerosis. Neurobiol. Dis. 2003;14(1):74–80.

[95] D'Ambrosi N, Finocchi P, Apolloni S, Cozzolino M, Ferri A, Padovano V, Pietrini G, Carrì MT, Volonté C. The proinflammatory action of microglial P2 receptors is enhanced in SOD1 models for amyotrophic lateral sclerosis. J. Immunol. 2009;183(7):4648–4656.

Chapter 8

Tiny microRNAs Fine-Tune Amyotrophic Lateral Sclerosis Regulation

Utpal Bhadra, Anisha Pal, Jagamohan Chhatai and
Manika Pal Bhadra

Additional information is available at the end of the chapter

http://dx.doi.org/10.5772/63528

Abstract

Progressing muscle wasting and dramatic neurodegeneration of upper and lower motor neurons are the initial symptoms of amyotrophic lateral sclerosis (ALS) that eventually cause aetiology or death in quick succession. The functional mechanism of ALS is non-cell autonomous but it strongly influences on non-neural cells including microglia, astrocyte muscles and T cell. In ALS, neurodegeneration is triggered by at least four gene mutations that are not related to any classical signalling pathways, molecular mechanism or known cellular ingredients. MicroRNA is endogenous tiny non-coding RNA, which is required for fine-tuning or micromanaging protein expression post transcriptionally. In this review, we identified numerous microRNAs and their possible targets in ALS-related genes. These microRNAs misprocess ALS-related protein-coding genes via microRNA-gene circuits. This result sheds a strong link between microRNA and ALS genes. The mechanistic insight of multiple microRNAs related to ALS is required to treat neuro-inflammation and neuro-degradation. It is proposed that the micro-regulation of multiple microRNAs is involved in generation of unique neuroprotective agent against ALS. Therefore, a classical and novel microRNA-mediated therapy might unravel an alternative strategy for ALS-related neurodegeneration. This strategy indeed implicates real promises to illustrate a unique impact for ALS cure.

Keywords: amyotrophic lateral sclerosis (ALS), small microRNA, hotspot, microRNA-mediated therapy, neurodegeneration

INTECH
open science | open minds

© 2016 The Author(s). Licensee InTech. This chapter is distributed under the terms of the Creative Commons Attribution License (http://creativecommons.org/licenses/by/3.0), which permits unrestricted use, distribution, and reproduction in any medium, provided the original work is properly cited.

1. Overview and introduction

Amyotrophic lateral sclerosis (ALS) is an important neuromuscular disease [1]. ALS was recognized back in 1850 by the English neurophysiologist Augustus Waller for the appearance of shrivelled nerve fibres. In 1869, in a scientific literature it was described and named ALS by the French neurologist Jean-Martin Charcot [2]. ALS, otherwise known as Lou Gehrig's disease, caused a baseball player, Lou Gehrig, to retire from his peak season. This New York Yankees player was called the iron horse for his contribution in the field (adapted from http://www.hopkinsmedicine.org/neurology_neurosurgery/centers_clinics/als/conditions/als_amyotrophic_lateral_sclerosis.html, http://www.biography.com/people/lou-gehrig-9308266).

Gradual degeneration of motor neurons in the brain and spinal cord is sought after to characterize this disease [1]. After the disease contracts, the motor neurons can no longer deliver impulses to the muscles, resulting in atrophy of muscles and muscle weakness (**Figure 1**). ALS does not disrupt a person's intellectual reasoning, vision, hearing or sense of taste, smell and touch. Mostly, ALS does not affect a person's bowel, sexual or bladder functions. ALS is often referred to as a neurodegenerative syndrome because the disease becomes evident in various

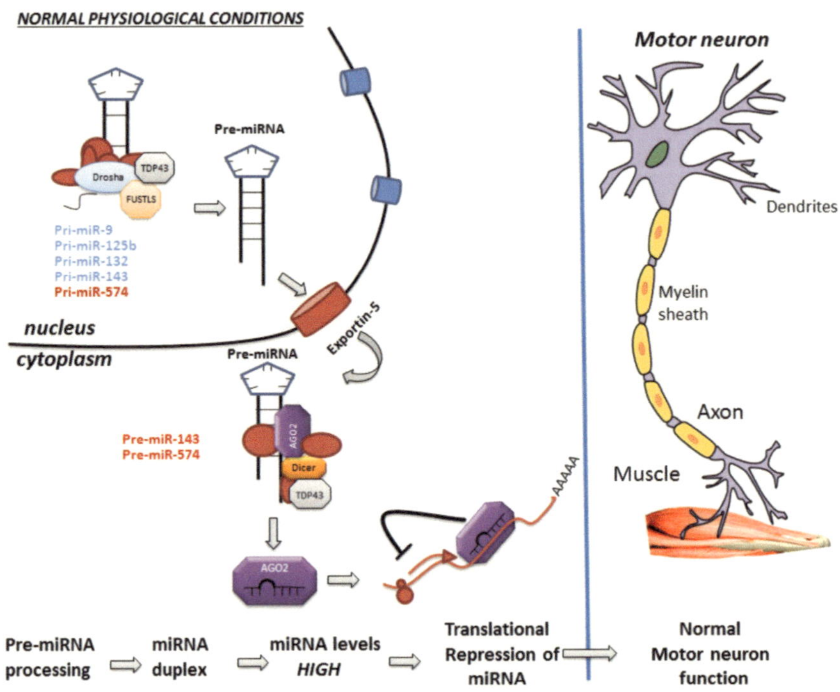

Figure 1. Under normal physiological condition, pri-miRNAs are processed in nucleus by Drosha along with its partner DGCR8. Recently it has been revealed that interactions with TDP-43 and FUS–TLS enhance miRNA biogenesis. In this diagram the pri-miRNAs, regulated by TDP-43, have been shown in blue colour, and the pri-miRNAs, regulated by FUS–TLS, have been shown in red colour. It has also been demonstrated that TDP43 associates with Dicer complex and helps in the processing of pre-miR-143 and pre-miR-574 into mature miRNAs in cytoplasm (adapted from Bicker S, Schratt G. MicroRNAs in ALS: small pieces to the puzzle. EMBO J. 2015;34[3]:2601–3 and Ref. [21]).

http://dx.doi.org/10.5772/63528

patterns. ALS occurs scarcely and spontaneously. Currently, there is no straightforward and classical cure for ALS (adapted from http://www.hopkinsmedicine.org/neurology_neurosurgery/centers_clinics/als/conditions/als_amyotrophic_lateral_sclerosis.html, http://emedicine.medscape.com/article/1170097-clinical).

MicroRNAs are the tiny endogenous non-coding RNA that represses protein synthesis post-transcriptionally by coupling at the 3′ untranslated leader sequences of target mRNAs [4]. MicroRNA micro-manages a broad range of biological process including developmental decisions, cellular differentiation, programmed cell death for pattern formation, and many pivotal roles in different human diseases [5]. At least 500–1000 microRNAs are found in vertebrate [6]. However, each microRNA can target numerous mRNAs [7]. It is suggested that 30–40% of human transcriptome is under control of different miRNA-gene circuits.

Biogenesis, processing and functional mechanism of microRNA are unique. Four different functional processes are involved in microRNA-mediated gene expression where (1) co-translational protein synthesis is disrupted, (2) translation elongation is inhibited, (3) translation product is terminated prematurely and finally (4) translation initiation is disrupted. MicroRNA inhibits their functional targets by sequestering to target mRNAs [8].

Basically, microRNA can be used as a fine-tuner for different gene regulatory networks. Especially numerous microRNAs are expressed in different sites of the brains [9]. They participate in the functional mechanism of brain development. They have important roles in brain morphogenesis, neuronal differentiation, dendrite and spine developments, synaptic structure formation and neuronal plasticity, etc. [10]. Multiple clusters of microRNA play important parts in different acute and chronic pathological disorders in the brain. In this review we have mentioned a set of microRNA that produce a distinct cluster in different ALS-related genes. The dysregulation of these microRNAs collectively misregulates multiple mRNAs related to ALS and other neurological diseases. Multiple microRNAs can simultaneously control several endogenous mRNAs because 3′ UTR of an mRNA can have complementary sites for a cluster of microRNAs; conversely a single microRNA can regulate multiple mRNAs [11]. In protein homeostasis, different cellular events participate with different microRNAs. However, different microRNAs may involve various mediators to control gene expression [12].

2. Symptoms of ALS

"ALS is like a lit candle: it melts your nerves and leaves your body a pile of wax. Often, it begins with the legs and works its way up. You lose control of your thigh muscles, so that you cannot support yourself standing. You lose control of your trunk muscles, so that you cannot sit up straight. By the end, if you are still alive, you are breathing through a tube in a hole in your throat, while your soul, perfectly awake, is imprisoned inside a limp husk, perhaps able to blink, or cluck a tongue, like something from a science fiction movie, the man frozen inside his own flesh. This takes no more than 5 years from the day you contract the disease". Courtesy from "Tuesdays with Morrie" by Mitch Albom.

Each individual patient may experience symptoms differently. Symptoms may include:

- Twitching and cramping of muscles, especially those in the hands and feet
- Loss of motor control in the hands and arms
- Impaired use of the arms and legs
- Weakness and fatigue
- Tripping and falling
- Dropping things
- Uncontrollable periods of laughing or crying
- Slurred or thick speech and difficulty in projecting the voice

As the disease progresses, symptoms may comprise:

- Shortness of breath
- Difficulty in breathing
- Difficulty in swallowing
- Paralysis (adapted from http://www.hopkinsmedicine.org/neurology_neurosurgery/centers_clinics/als/conditions/als_amyotrophic_lateral_sclerosis.html)

3. Symptom statistics

ALS occurs between the ages of 40 years and 70 years, but the disease can occur at a younger age also. It affects throughout the world without any ethnic, racial or socioeconomic boundaries. ALS is responsible for almost five of every 100,000 deaths in people aged 20 or older. The frequent age for ALS is after 60 years age. The incidence of ALS is five times higher than Huntington's disease and almost equal to multiple sclerosis. Fifty percent of affected patients live at least three or more years after diagnosis, 20 percent live 5 years or more and up to 10 percent will survive more than 10 years (adapted from http://www.hopkinsmedicine.org/neurology_neurosurgery/centers_clinics/als/conditions/als_amyotrophic_lateral_sclerosis.html).

4. Medical classification of ALS

Making a proper diagnosis in ALS is complicated because symptoms can vary in each patient. Based on the symptom, ALS can be classified in five broad ranges based on the disease symbol:

Classical ALS – characterized by the deterioration of upper and lower motor neurons [nerve cells]. This symptom generally affects more than two-thirds of patients with the disease.

http://dx.doi.org/10.5772/63528

Primary lateral sclerosis [PLS] – in which case the upper motor neurons deteriorate. If the lower motor neurons are not affected within 2 years, the disease usually remains a pure upper motor neuron disease. It is the rarest form of ALS.

Progressive bulbar palsy [PBP] – this condition starts with difficulties in speaking, chewing and swallowing due to lower motor neuron [nerve cell] deterioration. It affects about 25% of those with ALS.

Progressive muscular atrophy [PMA] – in which the lower motor neurons deteriorate. If the upper motor neurons are unaffected within 2 years of contracting the disease, the disease usually remains a pure lower motor neuron disease.

Familial – that affects more than one member of the same family (adapted from http://www.hopkinsmedicine.org/neurology_neurosurgery/centers_clinics/als/conditions/als_amyotrophic_lateral_sclerosis.html).

5. Tiny small RNA or microRNA

It seems the world of non-coding RNAs is expanding like the universe, with the progress of science. After the discovery of miRNA in 1993, our knowledge about miRNA is increasing exponentially. *Lin-4* was the first miRNA to be discovered, in 1993, by the joint efforts of Victor Ambros's and Gary Ruvkun's laboratories [13]. After that, *let-7* is a heterochronic gene of *Caenorhabditis elegans* and was the second miRNA to be discovered, in 2000, 7 years after the finding of the first miRNA [14]. MicroRNAs [mi-RNAs] are 18–25 nt RNAs produced from a cellular RNA with a stem-loop structure. These evolutionarily conserved, naturally abundant, small, regulatory non-coding RNAs can inhibit gene expression at the post-transcriptional level in a sequence-specific manner [8]. It can be (i) intronic and (ii) intergenic [15].

All miRNAs undergo 5′ capping and 3′ polyadenylation, which are common events in case of mRNA processing also [16]. Intronic miRNAs are produced under host gene promoter [15]. Intergenic miRNAs have own promoter [15]. In the nucleus, genes encoding miRNA are generally transcribed by RNA polymerase II (Pol II) into large primary miRNA transcripts (pri-miRNA) (sized >1 kb) [15–17]. The pri-miRNA is maximally 2.2 kb long [15, 17]. Processing of pri-miRNA:pri-miRNA > pre-miRNA > miRNA [15]. miRNAs bind to the 3′ UTR region of target mRNAs [8]. Once the miRNA binds to a completely complementary region of target mRNA, mRNA gets degraded [18]. miRNA-mediated regulation does not require to have a perfect match with its target-binding region [19]. Only seven-base sequence between second and eighth nucleotides from the 5′ end is called "seed region (sequence)" and a complete match of these sequence is required for degradation of target mRNA[s] [20]. It is believed that the strength of the inhibition varies depending on the sequences [20]. A single miRNA may directly affect the expression of hundreds of proteins at one time and several miRNAs can also target the same mRNA and result in enhanced translational inhibition. It causes post-transcriptional gene control [8].

6. Link between miRNA and ALS

In last few decades, neuroscience has made a remarkable progress. This has led to accumulation of humongous information including neuronal signalling and neuronal circuits. Neuroscience itself is complex and RNA interference (RNAi) molecules have made it much more intricate. The finer details are being searched to cope up with the neurodegenerative disorders. In the postgenomic era, we are still searching mysteries related to non-coding RNA. These small RNA molecules are the controller of our genome.

The microRNA molecules are acting as nodes and links of gene expression. These experts work in various biological functions. Using complementarity against cognate mRNA, this 21–22 nt stretch plays havoc. A miRNA can target several mRNAs, and in combination with other regulatory molecules, it can alter a cell's expression and activity. Neurology includes networking between the cells of nervous system and other cells of the organism. Direct and indirect targets of one miRNA make a cell's system much more complex. ALS is a motor neuron disorder and it has been proved in various reports that ALS can be caused due to dysregulation of miRNAs and thus misexpression of proteins in the cells (**Figure 2**). This chapter deals with the miRNAs which are culprits behind ALS [21].

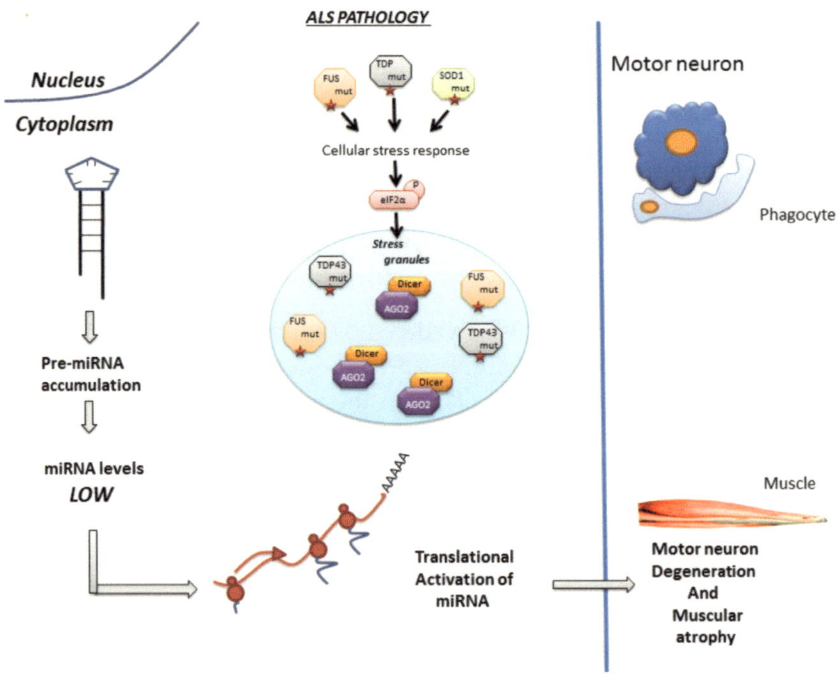

Figure 2. In ALS, there are mutations in multiple genes like TDP-43, FUS–TLS and SOD1 and these results in activation of stress response involving phosphorylation of eIF2α and stress granule formation. In ALS, reduced pre-miRNA processing and decreased levels of different miRNAs are caused by remodelling of Dicer complex in cytoplasm. Thus, the translation of target mRNAs is relieved, resulting in degeneration of motor neurons (adapted from Bicker S, Schratt G. MicroRNAs in ALS: small pieces to the puzzle. EMBO J. 2015;34[3]:2601–3).

7. MicroRNA and its biogenesis pathway

miRNAs, after being discovered in 1993 [13], has come a long way and established itself as one of key regulators at the post-transcriptional level. It gets expressed in wide varieties of organism from plants to humans. Many miRNAs are conserved across several species. These regulatory molecules are of 21–25 nt in length. Many components of miRNA-processing machinery can be found in Archaea and Eukarya, which supports its ancient presence [3]. Databases of different miRNAs are increasing day by day because of its association with several biological processes and diseases. miRNAs account for >3% of all human genes [22, 23]. At first it gained its initial importance because of its involvement in developmental biology. Now it has been noticed that normal miRNA population can be dysregulated in different diseases, and thus, they are being used as biomarker to detect diseases. Sequence-specific regulation by miRNA makes it more specific but it can diversify its function by binding to 3′ UTR sites of several mRNAs.

The miRNA genes can be operated from their own promoter or promoter of another gene [15]. Primary miRNA transcripts are transcribed by RNA pol II in nucleus [16, 17]. Primary transcripts are of multiple hairpin loops. In nucleus Drosha along with DGCR8 cleaves at 3′ end to form pre-miRNAs. Pre-miRNAs have a hanging 3′-OH end [24]. 70 nt structure pre-miRNAs get transported to cytoplasm from nucleus by Ran-GTP and Exportin-5 [24]. In the cytoplasm, RNase-III Dicer enzyme cut at the loop structure of the pre-miRNA to produce passenger strand and guide strand [24]. The thermodynamically unstable strand, i.e. guide strand, works as a mature miRNA [25]. These mature miRNAs get loaded into RISC complex [RNA-induced silencing complex]. RISC complex contains several proteins which are needed for ribonucleotide binding and cleaving the target mRNA. Argonaute protein, GW182 are some of the factors of RISC [8]. Once RISC factor is assembled, the miRNA guides the complex to its target on the basis of complementary base pairing. The complementarity is generally restricted to the second to eighth base from 5′ end of miRNA, which is called "seed" region [25]. This seed region binds to 3′ UTR of target mRNA [19, 20]. The fate of target mRNA depends upon the extent of base pairing to the cognate miRNA [19, 20]. The miRNA will direct the destruction of the target mRNA, who has the perfect or near-perfect pairing [19, 20]. If there is multiple partially complementary site, the accumulation of protein from target mRNAs will be inhibited.

8. miRNA in mammals

miRNAs can inhibit translation in many ways like co-translational protein degradation, inhibition of translation elongation, premature termination of translation, inhibition of translation initiation, deposition of mRNAs in cytoplasmic P-bodies and premature ribosome drop-off [8].

9. Post-initiation mechanisms

Studies in the worm *C. elegans* and in mammalian cell cultures present evidences that miRNAs repress protein synthesis after translation is initiated. The contradictory observation that the targets of miRNAs appear to be actively translated while the corresponding protein product remains undetectable prompted the proposal that the nascent polypeptide chain might get degraded co-translationally. The identity of protease is unknown. Proteasome was excluded as a possibility because proteasome inhibitor does not restore the protein. Several other evidences lead to the suggestion that premature ribosome dissociation is caused by miRNAs [8].

10. Inhibition of translation initiation

There was an observation by a group, where it was observed that the central domain of Argonaute proteins has sequence similarities to the cytoplasmic cap-binding protein *eIF4E* [eukaryotic translation initiation factor 4E], which is necessary for the cap-dependent translation initiation in the cell. *eIF4E* binds to the m7Gppp-cap structure of mRNAs by stacking the methylated base of the cap between two tryptophans. At the equivalent position of the tryptophans in eIF4E, Argonaute proteins have phenylalanines that could mediate a similar interaction between the molecules. Consistently, Kiriakidou et al. [26] showed that human Argonaute 2 (AGO2) binds to m7GTP present on Sepharose beads. It was shown that substituting one or both AGO2 phenylalanines with valine residues suspended the silencing activity. Using human cells it was shown that AGO2 associates with both *eIF6* and large ribosomal subunits. By binding to the large ribosomal subunit, *eIF6* prevents this subunit from joining with the small ribosomal subunit prematurely. *AGO2* recruits *eIF6*, thus stopping the association of the large and small ribosomal subunits, causing translation repression [8, 27].

11. miRNA-mediated mRNA decay

Argonaute proteins prevent the formation of the closed-loop mRNA configuration by a murky mechanism that includes de-adenylation. MicroRNAs trigger de-adenylation and de-capping of the target mRNA. Proteins required for this process are components of the major de-adenylase complex [CAF1, CCR4 and the NOT complex], the de-capping enzyme DCP2 and several de-capping activators. Thus, signal for translation is lost.

P-bodies or cytoplasmic processing bodies are nothing but ribosome-depleted areas inside a cell. Recent studies support the evidence that the mRNAs silenced by miRNAs are localized to P-bodies for storage or degradation. Induced by miRISC and RNA helicase activity, remodelled mRNPs may modify the translation initiation complex at the 5′ end of target mRNAs, which may cause translation repression and localization of mRNAs in P-bodies. P-bodies may facilitate the access of the de-capping factors to the cap structure, thus facilitating mRNA degradation. However, with the help of appropriate signals, stored mRNAs residing in P-bodies could be released and returned to the translational machinery of the cell [8, 28].

12. miRNAs in different parts of the human brain

One of the important processes is microRNA-mediated gene regulation, which is fine-tuning the expression of genes essential for the pathway. Using bioinformatics approach, one can easily understand that the cells of human brain are finely tuned by miRNAs. Prediction of miRNA target sites using bioinformatics approach can give us a whole bunch of gene names. But a major weakness of in silico analysis is the lack of experimental validation. For circumventing such problem, a combinative approach can be implemented where target sites are predicted using multiple programmes. Out of miRNAs, which get expressed in the midbrain, cerebellum, hippocampus and frontal cortex, majority of them are from midbrain while almost equal proportions of microRNAs are expressed in the hippocampus and frontal cortex. The microRNAs in the cerebellum are less in number compared to miRNAs expressed in other regions considered. The target sites of the microRNA expressed in different parts of the brain had been predicted on the 35 genes related to ALS initially. The result obtained from miRanda [version 1.0] indicates that 477 target sites were predicted for mRNAs expressed in midbrain as compared to the target sites [411] predicted for miRNAs expressed in the hippocampus (**Figure 3**). However, total target sites predicted for miRNAs expressed in the cerebellum and frontal cortexes were 175 and 395, respectively (**Figure 3**). The number of targets for miRNAs expressed in cerebellum is considerably less comparing to binding sites for miRNAs expressed in other areas of the brain. Surprisingly, microRNA targets were distributed in the different regions of the genes and are not limited to only in 3′ UTR. Total 1456 target sites were predicted using miRanda for miRNAs considered in the study. Target sites in the 3′ untranslated region are comparatively less. A significant number of targets were also found in the 5′ UTR of the genes. Earlier, there was occurrence of miRNA target sites in coding region and 5′ UTR of genes was considered as exception in animals. But numerous recent evidences have established that microRNAs can target different regions of a gene and microRNA-based regulation is not confined only to 3′ UTR [9, 29]. Experiments aimed at identification of specific parameter or factor for effective targeting of 3′ UTR by miRNAs have failed considerably. Conversely, the existence of miRNA target sites in ORF of Nanog, *OCT4* and *SOX1*, during induction of stem cell pluripotency, reinforces the existence of miRNA-binding sites in other sites of the genes in animals. These results established the notion that microRNA-target sites are not only restricted to 3′ UTR in animals. Such variability in regions also adds cues for anticipating the mode of action especially their role in transcriptional, post-transcriptional and translation inhibition. As the majority of the algorithms developed for miRNA target site prediction consider only 3′ UTR, confirmation of 3′ UTR target site prediction using a combinatorial approach will be helpful. Target sites on ALS-related genes were classified according to the microRNAs expressed in four different regions of the brain (**Figure 3**). As there were less miRNAs expressed in cerebellum, this can explain small number of target sites predicted on genes associated to ALS. Analysis of miRNA targets in each gene associated with ALS showed that there are no target sites that could be detected in 3′ UTR for mRNAs expressed in midbrain for *CASP1, GRIA1, GPX1, DAXX, CAT, SOD1, NEFM, NEFL* and *NEFH* genes. Furthermore 5′ UTR lack any target sites of same miRNAs in *CASP1, GRIA1, GPX1, DAXX, CAT, SOD1, NEFM, NEFL, NEFH, RAC1* and *TNF* genes. The miRNAs expressed in midbrain showed the least number of target sites in *RAC1* and *CASP1* genes, whereas 29 target sites were predicted in *NOS1*. Similar results were there for the miRNAs expressed in the cerebellum for the same genes. For instance, *RAC1* has on one target site whereas *NOS1* has 11 target sites. For miRNAs expressed in the hippocampus, *CASP1* and *GRIA1* genes have a few numbers of predicted sites [4] and *MAP3K5* was predicted to possess maximum target sites [30]. Similarly, *CASP1* and *SOD1* have two target sites each, while 23 target sites had been predicted for *TNFRSF1A* gene for miRNAs, expressed in the frontal cortex. On the other hand, target sites could not be predicted for six genes, namely, *GPX1, CYCS, CHP, CASP3, SOD1* and *RAB5A*, for miRNAs expressed in the cerebellum. No target sites could be predicted in 3′ UTR of *ALS2, BID, CASP1, GRIA1, DAXX, CCS, CAT, CASP9, TOMM40, TNF, SOD1, RAC1, NEFM* and *NEFL* genes. No target site could be predicted in *BCL2, CASP1, GRIA1, DAXX, CYCS, CASP3, TNF, RAC1, NEFM* and *NEFH* genes for miRNAs expressed in the cerebellum. These results demonstrate that the majority of the ALS genes lack any target site for miRNAs expressed in the cerebellum. miRNA targets were found in most of the genes, but surprisingly few genes, *CASP1, GRIA1, DAXX, CAT, SOD1* and *NEFM*, lack any miRNA target site in their 3′ UTR. This shows that complexity of regulations and numerous members of this play give the brain another level of entanglement [9] (**Figure 4**).

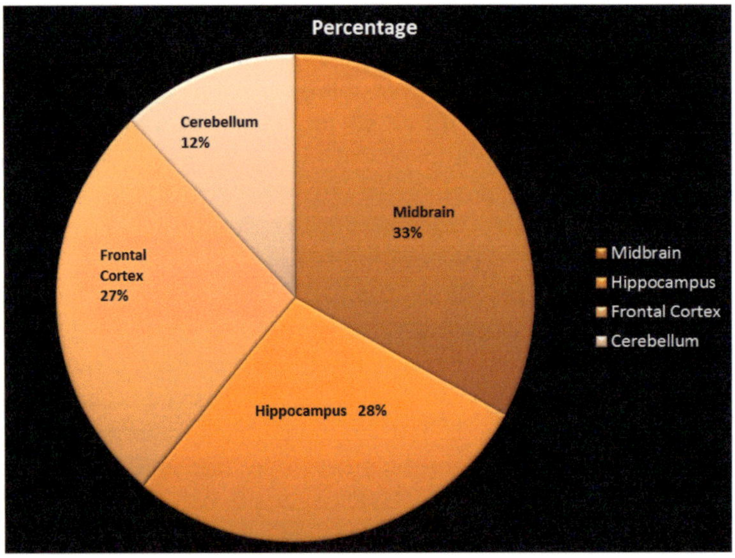

Figure 3. Percentage of miRNAs, expressed in the brain. From this diagram we can have an idea that the regulation of genes by miRNAs is widespread in various parts of the human brain (adapted from Ref. [9]).

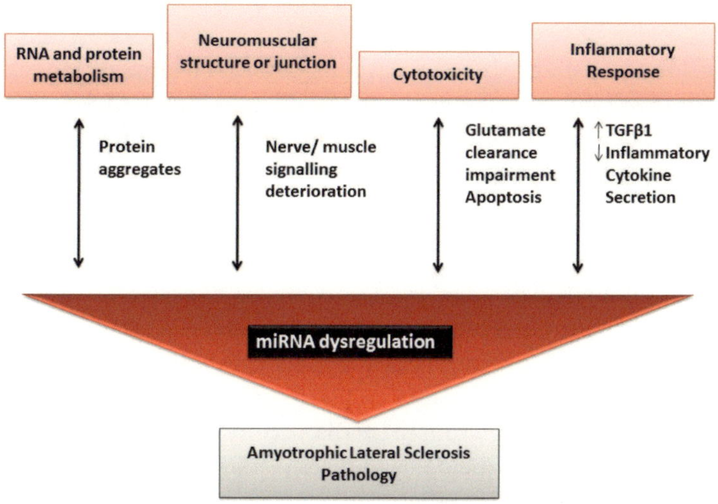

Figure 4. Either dysregulation of miRNA biogenesis and function might result into ALS pathogenesis or ALS pathogenesis can cause dysregulation of miRNA biogenesis and function. Disrupted signalling at the neuromuscular junction, caused by cytotoxicity associated with the faulty glutamate clearance or an overactive inflammatory response, results in neuromuscular degeneration. Dysregulation of key miRNAs triggers the altercations in cell physiology, resulting in ALS pathology (adapted from Ref. [84]).

13. Causative factors in ALS

Most of the cases are sporadic ALS [sALS]. Only 10–15% are usually inherited as an autosomal dominant trait and defined as familial [fALS]. They show comparable etiopathology and they affect same neuronal population [31]. Several ALS genes (*SOD1, Alsin, SETX, SPG11, FUS/TLS, VAPB, ANG, TARDBP, FIG4, OPTN, ATXN2, VCP, UBQLN2, SIGMAR1, CHMP2B, PFN1, SQSTM1, C9ORF72*) and additional chromosomal loci have been identified [32, 33]. Almost two-thirds of the familial cases are due to mutations of *C9ORF72, SOD1, TARDBP* and *FUS* genes. Twenty percent of fALS is because of the mutation of *SOD1* gene, coding for the superoxide dismutase one mitochondrial and cytoplasmic copper/zinc enzyme, responsible for metabolizing naturally occurring, but harmful, superoxide radicals to molecular oxygen and hydrogen peroxide. A massive hexanucleotide-repeat expansion (GGGGCC)n in the first intron of *C9ORF72* gene on the chromosome 9p21is the most frequent cause of ALS identified to date [30, 33]. After identifying several causal genes, it has been hard to find the clear evidence of the pathogenic role of some mutations. The most extensively studied gene, SOD1, still lacks pathogenic feature of the reported missense, nonsense and deletion mutations. Studies suggest that there are multiple genetic factors which contribute to develop ALS ultimately or show phenotypical features. Though the contributions of environmental factors have not been proved, ALS is a combination of genetic and environmental factors. It has been clearly noted that with increasing age, one develops higher risk of ALS. Some reports tell that heavy metals, pesticides and exposure to electromagnetic field might cause ALS [34]. The use of neurotrophic factors like IGF-I, GDNF, VEGF, ADNF-9, colivelin and angiogenin showed potential in therapy of ALS. Talampanel (AMPA antagonist), ceftriaxone (antibiotic), pramipexole/dexpramipexole (dopamine agonists) and arimoclomol (activator of molecular chaperons' protein repair pathway) are amongst the existing drugs to treat ALS. Lately stem cell and immune therapies have been suggested [35]. A comprehensive listing of trials in the USA can be found at ClinicalTrials.gov.

A wealth of evidence supports that ALS is a multifactorial and multisystemic disease, characterized by overlapping different mechanisms, transduction pathways and multicellular crosstalk. Transgenic animals expressing human mutant SOD1 (mSOD1) have helped to reveal that perishing of motor neurons is not the only reason behind ALS but there is active contribution of non-neuronal cells like microglia, astrocytes and muscle and T cells, which differently participate to the different phases of the disease [36, 37]. Expression of mSOD1 within the most vulnerable motor neurons primarily causes for disease onset; synthesis of the mutant protein by interneurons also positively participates to disease initiation [38, 39]. Speeding of disease progression is caused by moSOD-1-mediated injury and neighbouring astrocytes and microglia. Schwann [40] and muscle cells play as direct partners of the injured motor axons, either working as recipients or initiators of the initial damage. These characteristics thus properly earned to ALS the definition of non-cell-autonomous disease [41]. Chimeric mice formed by expressing both mutated and non-mutated SOD1 proved that wild-type nonneuronal cells prolong the survival of motor neurons carrying mSOD1 protein. Neighbouring astrocytes, microglia, oligodendrocytes and Schwann cells can cause the degeneration of motor neurons [42, 43]. Compelling evidence indicates that primary mSOD1-expressing astrocytes from mouse, rat and humans cause motor neurons death by releasing toxic factors into the media while sparing interneurons [44–46]. Astrocytes deriving from neuronal progenitor cells, gathered from fALS and sALS cases, exhibit features of non-cell-autonomous toxicity [47]. There are very few studies of non-cell-autonomous toxicity. Astrocytes expressing mutant TDP43 [TDP43-M337V] participate in ALS pathology only through cell-autonomous processes. It has been studied that conditioned medium from astrocytes that express SOD1-G93A, or SOD1-G86R, or TDP43-A315T leads to extensive motor neuron death via non-cell-autonomous mechanisms. Still, there is a long way left to travel and to unravel mystifying stories behind ALS [21] (**Figures 1** and **3**).

14. The miRNAs involved in ALS regulation

14.1. Effects of miRNA biogenesis related but mutated factors in ALS

Several factors are there, which can affect CNS homeostasis and thereby facilitate neurodegenerative and neuroinflammatory diseases. Perturbation in intricate miRNA network can disrupt neuronal function in cell-autonomous or non-cell-autonomous manner [48–50]. It has been shown that there is cell-type-specific deletion of miRNA-processing enzyme, Dicer in cerebellar Purkinje, or striatal, retinal, spinal and cortical neurons, which leads to degeneration and ataxia [51–54]. Neurodegeneration also occurs after targeted deletion of Dicer in astrocytes, oligodendrocytes and Schwann cells, perhaps because the glial cells have some effects on neuronal survival [55–58] (**Table 1**). Experimental results show that deletion of Dicer directly in spinal motor neurons mimics most of the clinical (e.g. progressive paralysis) and pathological (e.g. astrocytosis and signs of axonopathy) traits of ALS [54]. Several groups have proved that TDP43 and FUS/TLS are involved in multilayered steps of RNA processing and miRNA biogenesis pathway. It has been investigated recently they have role in miRNA-related ALS [59–62]. FUS, nuclear factor complexes with Drosha along with DGCR8. This association is indispensible in miRNA processing in nucleus. Cytoplasmic TDP-43 associates with Dicer, containing TRBP. This interaction facilitates the processing of the specific pre-miRNAs by Dicer, generally a subset of the pre-miRNAs whose yield in the nucleus is regulated by TDP-43, by direct binding to their terminal loops. It was proved that TDP-43 promotes neuronal outgrowth by facilitating miRNA production. Further studies show that TDP-43 has its role in both nucleus and cytoplasm. It associates with DGCR8 containing nuclear Drosha complex in RNA-dependent and RNA-independent fashion. In nucleus, TDP-43 binds to a selected pri-miRNAs, and in cytoplasm, it binds to terminal loops of pre-miRNAs. TDP-43 facilitates neuronal outgrowth through the regulation of miRNA processing [60].

Tissue/cells	**miRNAs**	**Changes**	**Biological function**	**Model**
Skeletal muscle	miR-1/206 family	↓	Myogenic differentiation	TDP-43 mice
CNS	miR-29a	↑	ER stress-induced cell death	SOD1-G93A mice
Skeletal muscle	miR-206, miR-133b	↑	Maintenance and repair of NMJ	SOD1-G93A mice
Human blood serum	miR-206, miR-106b	↑	*Ni*	ALS patients
Lumbar spinal cord	miR-b1336, miR-b2403, miR-sb659	↓	NFL stability	sALS patients
Lumbar spinal cord	miR-b1123, miRb2948, miR-b3265, miR-b5539, miR-sb1217*, miR-sb3998	↑	NFL stability	
epSPCs	miR-124a	↑	epSPC fate	SOD1-G93A mice
epSPC fate	miR-9, miR-19a, miR-19b	↓	epSPC fate	
Brain microglia	miR-155, miR-146b , miR-22, miR-365, miR-125b, miR-214	↑	Microglia activation	SOD1-G93A mice

Tissue/cells	miRNAs	Changes	Biological function	Model
CSF	miR-132-5p, miR-132-3p, miR-143-3p	↓	*Ni*	sALS patients
CSF	miR-143-5p, miR-574-5p	↑	*Ni*	
Neurons	miR-9	↓	*Ni*	*TARDBP* A90V, *TARDBP* M337V patients
Spinal cord	miR-9	↑	Neuronal differentiation	SOD1-G93A mice
Spinal cord	miR-124a	↓	Glutamate transport	SOD1-G93A mice
Spinal cord	miR-558, miR-16-2*, miR-146a*, miR-508-5p, miR-373*, miR-551a, miR-506, miR-518a-5p, miR-518e*, miR-890	↑	NFL stability	sALS human patients
Spinal cord	miR-624, miR-520, miR-524-5p, miR-548a-5p, miR-606, miR-612, miR-647 miR-155, miR-17, miR-19b, miR-20a, miR-24-2*, miR-106a, miR-142-3p, miR-142-5p, miR-146a, miR-146b, miR-223	↓	NFL stability	
Spinal cord	miR-155, miR-17, miR-19b, miR-20a, miR-24-2*, miR-106a, miR-142-3p, miR-142-5p, miR-146a, miR-146b		*Ni*	SOD1-G93A mice
Spinal cord	miR-24-2*, miR-142-3p, miR-142-5p, miR-146a, miR-146b, miR-155		*Ni*	Human patients
Blood leukocytes	miR-338-3p	↑	*Ni*	sALS human patients
	miR-451, miR-1275, miR-328-5P, miR-638, miR-149, miR-665	↓	*Ni*	
Skeletal muscle	miR-23a, miR-29b, miR-206 miR-455	↑	Mitochondrial function	Human patients

Tissue/cells	miRNAs	Changes	Biological function	Model
Spinal cord microglia	miR-544, miR-23, miR-203, miR-340 miR-146. miR-130/miR-301, miR-155, miR-27, miR-16/miR-497/miR-195*, miR-20a/miR-106b/miR-17-5p	↑	*Ni*	SOD1-G93A mice
Spleen monocytes	let-7, miR-15b, miR-16, miR-27a, miR-34a, miR-132, miR-146a, miR-155, miR-223, miR-451	↑	*Ni*	SOD1-G93A mice
CD14+CD16– monocytes	miR-27a, miR-155, miR-146a, miR-32-3p	↑	*Ni*	Human ALS patients
Skeletal muscle	miR-206	↑	Maintenance and repair of NMJ	SOD1-G93A mice

Ni, not investigated in the study (adapted from Ref. [21] with the permission from Bentham Science Publishers).

Table 1. Summarization of dysregulated miRNA in ALS.

One group has reported the changes that occur in the miRNA population followed by TDP-43 knockdown in cultured cells. It was observed that *let-7b* and *miR-663* expression levels are down- and upregulated, respectively (**Table 1**). It was found that both miRNAs can bind to TDP-43 directly in different positions: within the miRNA sequence itself (i.e. let-7b) or in the hairpin precursor (miR-663). Using microarray data and q-PCR, candidate transcripts are identified, whose expression levels are discriminately affected by these TDP-43–miRNA interactions. TDP-43 gets increased in ALS [61] leading to neurotoxicity from both gain and loss of functions. Neurodegeneration and ALS phenotypes are caused by a partial loss of TDP-43 function. TDP-43 toxicity in neighbouring cells has effects on motor neurons. Both dysregulation and dysfunction of TDP-43 are relevant to ALS [53]. Researchers have reported that TDP43 depletion could affect the levels of specific miRNAs in human hepatocarcinoma cells, by potentially binding to their sequence and/or precursor elements [61]. Regulation of miRNA by TDP43 is conserved amongst mammals. TDP43 associating with both nuclear and cytoplasmic microprocessor complexes actively participates in the production of miRNAs indispensable for neuronal outgrowth. Finally, it was noted that the carboxyl-terminal of TDP43, where most ALS mutations reside, is crucial for the interaction with the miRNA-processing complexes [60]. Recent discovery of mutations in the genes, encoding for the RNA-binding proteins TDP43 and FUS/TLS, has proved the key role of regulatory RNA in the pathogenesis of ALS. Both proteins are generally localized within the nucleus, but their mutated forms delocalize and form neuronal inclusions and dystrophic neurites, as well as glial cytoplasmic inclusions. The sensory organ precursor cells of peripheral nervous system of *Drosophila melanogaster* were used as a model to demonstrate that hTDP43 clinical ALS mutations influence early neurogenesis and neuronal specification, through the regulation of miR-9a biogenesis. Further studies in human cells show that TDP43 is an essential element in miRNA biogenesis during neuronal differentiation by controlling the stability of Drosha and thus affecting miRNA production. Similar inferences were drawn after FUS/TLS silencing in human neuronal cell lines. FUS/TLS downregulation affects the biogenesis of a large class of miRNA and several of them have important roles in neuronal differentiation and synaptogenesis. Specific miRNAs, in particular miR-9, miR-125b, miR-132 and miR-143, are regulated by both TDP43 and FUS/TLS ALS-related proteins. In recent reports, TDP43 was shown to bind to and regulate the incorporation into the RISC complex of specific mature miRNAs, in both Drosophila and human systems. TDP43 interacting with miR-1/miR-206 family decreases the activity of these miRNAs, by the disruption of their association with the RISC complex. As this miRNA family is involved in muscle development and homeostasis, either depletion or overexpression of TDP43, by altering miR-1/miR-206 balance, might be involved in muscle pathogenesis of ALS. Nine specific miRNAs were selected and their levels were analysed in ALS patients, on the basis of their known misregulation after TDP43 depletion in cell lines. Samples of cerebrospinal fluid (CSF), serum and immortalized lymphoblastoid cell lines from fALS and sALS patients were analysed, and it was confirmed that there is dysregulation of miR-132, miR-143 and miR-574, whose processing is indeed regulated by TDP43 and/or FUS/TLS proteins. The sequencing of the 3′UTR region of the FUS/TLS gene in 420 ALS patients highlighted a mutation in two ALS patients with severe consequence, leading to FUS/TLS protein accumulation. This mutation maps to the seed sequence recognized by miR-141 and miR-200a in the 3′-UTR of FUS/TLS and that FUS/TLS is linked to these miRNAs by a feedforward regulatory loop, where FUS/TLS upregulates miR-141/200a, which in turn affects the FUS/TLS protein synthesis [21].

15. CNS-related miRNA dysregulations in ALS pathogenesis

miR-9, an evolutionarily conserved and multifunctional neuronal miRNA, is involved in the selection of neuronal precursors from the neuroepithelium in flies and in the specification of midbrain-hindbrain boundaries in vertebrates. Both miR-124 and miR-9 participates together in neuronal differentiation. Perturbation in their function results in the susceptibility to neuronal diseases. miR-9/miR-9* expression is significantly reduced in patients with Huntington's disease. miR-9 and miR-132 are downregulated in Alzheimer-affected brain. miR-9 has role in ALS also. There are several miRNAs, which are specific for neural cell fate and cell cycle regulation. After inducing neuronal differentiation, miR-9, miR-124a, miR-19a and miR-19b are differentially expressed in SOD1-G93A epSPCs, while miR-9 gets upregulated in SOD1-G93A differentiated cells, with respect to WT-SOD1 and control mice. Expression analysis of the predicted miRNA targets leads to identification of a functional network of Hes1. Pten, Socs1 and Stat3 genes are important for controlling epSPC fate and showing neurogenic potential in vitro. A time-course analysis and cellular distribution pattern of miR-9 were tested.

It was inferred that miR-9 expression is spatially and temporally controlled in SOD1-G93A spinal cord and there is upregulation at presymptomatic stage through early symptomatic stages, mainly in the ventral horns of grey matter, where neurodegeneration is known to occur. There is a role of miR-9 in pathogenesis in induced pluripotent stem cell differentiated into postmitotic neurons and derived from ALS patients with the TDP43 A90V and M337V mutations. In all these cases, the levels of miR-9 are decreased with respect to control neurons. In *Drosophila* TDP43 mutants, miR-9a expression is significantly inhibited; it supports the concept that TDP43 acts through miR-9a to control neuronal specification and to assure the robustness of genetic control programmes. The steady-state level of miR-9 is required for normal neuronal functions, as both up- and downregulation can lead to neurodegeneration. Mutant SOD1 deregulates neurofilament (NF) balance in motor neurons [63]. NF proteins are one of the major intermediate filaments of neuronal cytoskeleton. They provide the structural integrity of neurons and help in maintenance of cell shape and axonal calibre. In CSF of ALS patients, low-molecular-weight NF is in abundance, which leads to a significant correlation between CSF NFL levels and disease progression. NF might be used as a marker of disease progression in ALS [64]. In ALS spinal motor neurons undergo a selective reduction in the steady-state level of NFL mRNA, which results in alteration of the stoichiometry of NF expression [63]. miR-9 is an upstream regulator of NF mRNAs and there are no such evidences in determination of regulation of NFL by miR-9 in ALS [54]. The q-PCR of sALS ventral lumbar spinal cord tissue shows that a set of additional miRNAs, predicted to control NFL, was deregulated. miR-146a*, miR-524-5p and miR-582-3p are capable of interacting with NFL mRNA 3′ UTR in a manner that is steady with the suppressed steady-state mRNA levels observed for NFL in spinal motor neurons in ALS. This demonstrates the fact that miRNAs are involved in the suppression of NFL mRNA and ALS spinal motor neuron neurofilamentous form aggregates [65]. A recent study was performed on a RNA library derived from control and sALS spinal cords, and it was shown that a panel of novel miRNAs whose sequence is comprised in the miRNA response elements (MREs) within the NFL mRNA 3′ UTR was recognized to be differentially expressed in ALS, compared to control [66]. Functional analysis shows that miR-b1336 and miR-b2403 are significantly downregulated and both stabilise NFL mRNA. In motor neurons there are several miRNAs, which have the capability of controlling NF expression at post-transcriptional level. Dysregulation of miRNA expression occurs not only in motor neurons but also in spinal cord microglia isolated from SOD1-G93A mice. Scientists did whole expression profiling of miRNA and mRNA at presymptomatic stage and at onset of symptoms, and end stage of disease and pathway analysis was used to hypothesize a correlation between top ten altered inflammatory miRNAs and dysregulated inflammatory genes in ALS [65]. To characterize the relationship between miRNA/target deregulations functionally in ALS inflammation, microarray of miRNA from neonatal SOD1-G93A mouse brain primary microglia was done and it was found that the expression of mutant SOD1is able to increase about 50% of the expressed miRNAs [67]. There is significant increase in selected immune-enriched miRNAs, miR-22, miR-155, miR-125b and miR-146b amongst those most highly modulated. By luciferase assays and lentiviral infections, a group of researchers confirmed the increase in miR-365 and miR-125b, the last known to be involved in stimulation of pathogenic inflammatory responses and neurodegeneration by inhibiting neurotrophismrelevant genes. miR-365 and miR-125b suppress the IL-6/STAT3 pathway in ALS microglia, by targeting IL-6 and STAT3, respectively, and they have a role in overall increase of TNFα mRNA levels. TNFα treatment increases miR-125b levels in microglia; thus it results in abnormal TNFα release. IL-6, a marker of activated microglia, is downregulated after symptom onset in ALS animal models and TNFα is upregulated in G93A mice and in ALS patients. miR-365 and miR-125b dysregulations might have a hand in pathological cytokine profile of ALS. People suggest that the pathogenesis of ALS involves astroglial dysfunction, with a dramatic loss of the excitatory amino acid transporter-2/glial transporter1 (EAAT2/GLT1) in both ALS patients and animal models [68–71]. The EAAT2/GLT1, is an important atroglial transporter, dynamically regulated by neurons, and it is involved in maintenance of extracellular glutamate concentration below neurotoxic level [72, 73]. The exosomes containing miR-124a and released from neurons can be directly internalized into astrocytes, which results in increase in miR-124a and GLT1 protein levels. miR-124a is downregulated in spinal cord of mutant SOD1 mouse models at end stage of disease, and in vivo injection of miR-124a oligonucleotides into spinal cord of ALS mice results in 30% increase in EAAT2/GLT1 expression. There is very little information about miRNA expression in ALS-induced muscle impairment. There is miR-23 upregulation in skeletal muscle biopsies, collected from ALS patients, and it is correlated with reduction in peroxisome proliferator-activated receptor coactivator-1 (PGC-1alpha) mRNA and protein, observed in both mouse and human muscle diseased samples. This coactivator is involved in muscle mitochondrial biogenesis and function. There is reduction in skeletal muscle mitochondrial function in ALS. It has been suggested that there might be a relation in miR-23a inhibition of PGC-1α and its downstream signalling [74, 75].

16. Role of miR-206 in disease impediment

It was reported that miR-206, a skeletal muscle-specific miRNA, strongly induced in ALS mouse model is in coincidence with the onset of neurological symptoms. It is a modifier of disease pathogenesis. In G93A-SOD1 mice, loss of miR-206 expression does not affect disease onset apparently, but accelerates disease progression, by skeletal muscle atrophy, kyphosis and paralysis, and reduces survival. In miR-206$^{-/-}$/G93A-SOD1 mice, neuromuscular junctions (NMJs) are disorganized and reinnervation of denervated muscles by motor axons is postponed in the absence of miR-206. Transcript derived from the *miR-206/133b* locus, which was originally identified as a synapse-associated non-coding RNA called 7H4, has a role in encoding components of the postsynaptic apparatus. The reported 7H4 sequence does not include miR-206; RT-PCR shows that miR-206 sequences are included in this synapse-enriched transcript. Histone deacetylase 4 (HDAC4) mRNA is one of the strongest computationally predicted targets of miR-206. HDAC4 protein expression is upregulated in skeletal muscle of miR-206$^{-/-}$ animals in comparison with wild-type controls after denervation event. *Hdac4* mRNA levels remain unchanged in miR-206$^{-/-}$ mice. It suggests that miR-206 acts in this case by translational inhibition rather than by mRNA destabilization [21].

http://dx.doi.org/10.5772/63528

17. Side effects of our immune system

The immune system has a huge role in maintenance of physiological equilibrium within the CNS and in controlling neuronal cell death after adverse effects start. Butovsky et al. [65] performed a comparative analysis of miRNA expression profile of inflammatory monocytes and microglia from SOD1-G93A ALS mice to generate novel biomarkers and possible therapeutics. Spleen monocytes, Ly6Chi, are recruited to the spinal cord where they proliferate during disease progression. They have pronounced proinflammatory profile in both miRNA and gene expression profile. This type of miRNA profile was found maintained in ALS patients and is apparently unique for ALS, when compared with other neuroinflammatory diseases like multiple sclerosis [65]. De Felice et al. [75, 76] did a miRNA expression profile of circulating leukocytes in a small sample of sALS patients and detected variation of eight distinct miRNAs. miR-338-3p expression is upregulated in brain tissue from ALS patients [31]. miRNAs can circulate in cell-free forms in body fluids like serum and plasma and act as signalling molecule between cells [77, 78]. Ever-increasing evidences support the idea that serum circulating secretory vesicles, including exosomes and shedding microvesicles, can function as intercellular shuttles of RNA and miRNA [60]. Muscle-enriched miR-206 is upregulated not only in SOD1-G93A mice muscles but also there is symptomatic increase in circulation in those mice. The whole transcriptome analysis of both mRNA and miRNA of sALS fibroblasts is done, in order to confirm whether dysregulated processes in the CNS might be reproduced in cells from peripheral tissues. The microprocessor complex gene DGCR8, the gene encoding Dicer enzyme and the RISC proteins AGO1/2 are downregulated in sALS fibroblasts with consequent decrease of multiple miRNAs. This creates a new horizon for generating new diagnostic pool for ALS [21].

18. Hotspot identification

MicroRNAs can bind to the same complementary target sites or it can bind to proximally located sites adjacent to other miRNA target sites. A hotspot is a stretch of nucleotide sequence, which is prone to target of several groups of miRNAs. miRNAs are regulated and expressed spatially and temporally inside cell (**Figure 5**). This type of regulation and expression gives miRNAs power to play a plethora of roles in various different biological processes. All the miRNAs occupying position in "hotspot" may not regulate a gene in the same pattern. Generally, predominant miRNA competitively outcasts other miRNAs and plays as a potential repressor. There is no clear evidence of the cause behind competitive outcasting and variable effectiveness. Various researchers are trying to use different standards and parameters like the same chromosomal location for more than two miRNAs, the same orientation, phylogenetic relationships and absence of interfering transcription unit.

miRNA targets are generally predicted using miRanda and then further analysed for miRNA-prone regions in all the selected genes. Generally, a region is defined as hotspot, if it has a minimum of 10 nucleotides overlapping from the starting position and occurrence of three miRNA targets. It has been shown that there are 11 miRNA-prone regions in 35 genes associated to ALS. CYCS and MAP2K3 have one hotspot each in 3′ UTR, while single target site hotspot was in 5′ UTR in four genes (**Figure 5**), that is, BAX, DERL1, SLC1A2 and RAB5A. Studies have shown that MAP2K3 has two hotspots by miRNA cluster prediction. Target sites for three miRNAs, i.e. hsa-miR-107, hsa-miR-423-5p and hsa-miR-103, are congregated in another hotspot found in 3′ UTR. MAP2K3, having two such hotspots, is presumed to show more sensitivity towards gene regulation by microRNAs. The small number of hotspots makes the miRNAs more specific and stringent regulator. The variability in existence of such target site hotspots adds complexity in gene regulation [9] (**Figure 5**).

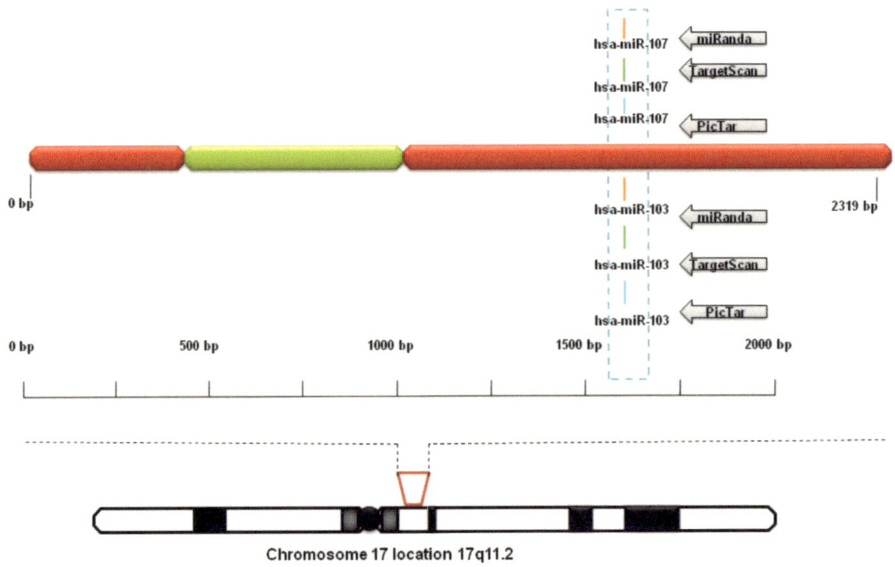

Figure 5. Schematic representation of susceptible 3′ hotspots of human MAP2K3 gene by various miRNAs like hsa-miR-107 and hsa-miR-103. To detect the susceptible sites on human MAP2K3 gene, bioinformatic tools like miRanda, TargetScan and PicTar were used (adapted from Ref. [9]).

19. Multifarious miRNA regulation

MicroRNA-mediated gene regulation adds multilayered complexity to gene expression. Distribution of target sites over several genes of one miRNA makes the picture more intricate. In principle, one miRNA can bind to more than one gene (multiplicity), and one gene can be controlled by more than one miRNA (cooperativity) [79]. Relaxed base pairing gives rise to multiplicity property. Target sites are rarely distributed on a gene. Generally they are scattered and the range of occurrence varies in numbers in a gene [80]. Often, presence of more target sites per gene indicates efficient regulation. Studies have shown that miRNAs, related to ALS, have multiple targets. After calculating multiplicity and cooperativity, scientists have shown that hsa-miR-370 showed maximum multiplicity as it showed 65 interactions with 30 gene sequences while no target site could be predicted in five genes, namely, *CASP1, GPX1, DERL1, CCS* and *SOD1.* It is highly expected that the degree of repression by hsa-miR-370 would be considerably high. It has been shown in the papers that hsa-miR-874 have 52 interactions with 29 genes and have no target in *CASP1, CHP, SOD1, RAC1, RAB5A* and *MAP2K6* genes. None of the above-mentioned miRNAs display any interaction with SOD1. Documented evidences show that SOD1 is one of the core factors for ALS that encodes the free radical scavenging enzyme copper zinc superoxide dismutase in ALS pathway. Then these miRNAs might not be involved in the regulation of *SOD1* activity. Scientists have reported that *PRPH* showed high cooperativity followed by *TNFRSF1A* and *TOMM40.* It is really difficult to interpret the complex picture presented by these multifaceted interactions. *PRPH* is regulated by 10 miRNAs at 23 positions, so first 10 miRNAs demonstrate high cooperativity towards *PRPH.* Relatively very low cooperativity was shown in *BID, MAP2K6* and *DERL1* genes. It might be inferred that there exists a low sensitivity of these genes towards microRNA-mediated gene regulation. Simple process of selection of microRNA targets is endowed with inherent complexity and this led to the development of a complex network by two phenomena, that is, multiplicity and cooperativity. The multiplicity and cooperativity might be the deciding factors for the mode of miRNA action. How these factors work is a matter of mystery [9].

20. Complex interrelationship

Figure 6 conveys interaction map of miRNA and selected 35 genes. Interactions amongst genes and miRNAs are depicted with arrows, where 1 = hsa-miR-370, 2 = hsa-miR-874, 3 = hsa-

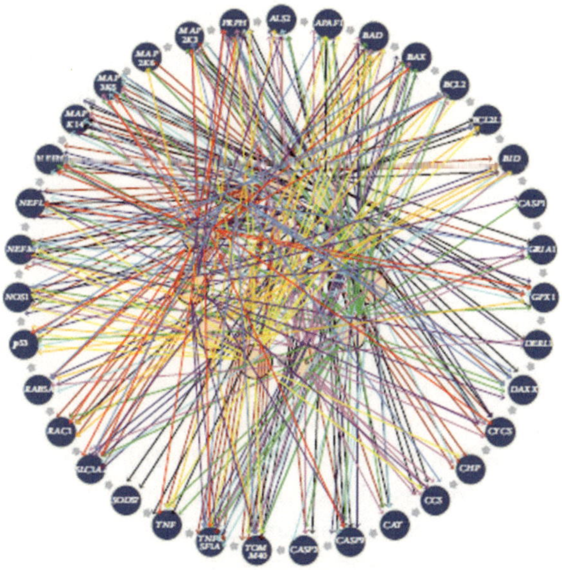

Figure 6. Interaction map of different miRNAs and selected 35 genes. Complex interrelationship amongst different genes and different miRNAs is depicted with the arrows. It is very evident from the diagram that one with miRNA can target 3′ UTR of several genes, thus adding layers to the gene regulation architecture (adapted from Ref. [9]).

miR-423-3p, 4 = hsa-miR-323-5p, 5 = hsa-miR-760, 6 = hsa-miR-149, 7 = hsa-miR-139-3p, 8 = hsa-miR-744, 9 = hsa-miR-324-3p, 10 = hsa-miR-339-3p and 11 = hsa-miR-654-5p. From **Figure 6** we can understand the multilayered regulation [9].

21. Usage of miRNAs in therapeutics

The human mind is not satisfied to know the causative factors of a disease. Our main target is to reduce ailment and to do that we need good diagnostic system along with good therapeutics. miRNAs are one of a kind. Being a regulator of gene expression, it has far-reaching effect on our physiology. They are dysregulated in several diseases. Researchers are now trying to generate therapeutic targets to treat ALS. Presently, riluzole is the only FDA-approved drug to treat ALS [81] and it modestly slows the disease progression. A phase I clinical trial of an antisense oligonucleotide [ISIS 333611] has been proven effective. This oligonucleotide targets SOD1 mRNA and represses the production of mutant SOD1 and this is effective when delivered to the CSF of patients with fALS [82]. The same kind of drug is there which targets the sense strand of the C9orf72 hexanucleotide repeat and reduces the toxicity by suppressing RNA foci formation both in vivo and in vitro [30, 33, 83]. Several delivery systems are being invented day in and day out to deliver miRNA formulations and drugs to the CNS through blood-brain barrier. The first miRNA-based therapeutic is the miR-122 antagonist SPC3649, which is currently being evaluated in phase II clinical trials. It targets the hepatitis C virus. So far, this agent has not exhibited any adverse effects.

There are two basic approaches of miRNA-based therapeutics. One is miRNA antagonists which impede endogenous miRNAs that have a harmful gain of function in diseased tissues and involve the use of an anti-miR – a chemically modified antisense RNA – to knockdown miRNA. In one of the first endeavours to use antagomirs in ALS, delivery of anti-miR-155 to *SOD1* Gly93Ala mice via ventricular osmotic pumps delayed mortality of the patients successfully. A downfall associated with this approach is the potential for nonspecific binding to other RNAs inside the cells. As one miRNA can regulate several mRNAs, it limits usage of miRNAs as therapeutics. In the second approach to miRNA therapeutics that involves miRNA mimics and miRNA replacement therapies, miRNAs are reintroduced into cells exhibiting downregulation, thus reactivating key pathways [84].

It is really difficult to dissect all the pathways, which are regulated by one miRNA. Before releasing drugs in clinics, there should be several clinical trials to eliminate any deleterious effect. Williams and group [85] showed that miRNA-206 delayed ALS progression and promoted regeneration of neuromuscular synapses effectively in mice. This group investigated pathological modifications in motor axons and nerve terminals that precede motor neuron degeneration and clinical symptoms and the role of the skeletal muscle-specific miR-206 in motor neuron-skeletal muscle fibre signalling. This miRNA is significantly upregulated in SOD1-G93A mouse model of ALS. The genetic ablation of miR-206 in these ALS mice accelerates the disease progression. miR26 might be needed for compensatory regeneration of

http://dx.doi.org/10.5772/63528

neuromuscular synapses after acute nerve injury and thus it decelerates ALS progression. miR-206 represses the translation of HDAC4 mRNA and counteracts its negative influence. This miRNA is also involved in neuromuscular gene expression and synapse formation. miR-206 decelerates ALS progression by detecting motor neuron injury and boosting compensatory regeneration of neuromuscular synapses by specifically inhibiting HDAC4 protein synthesis. HDAC4 has a deleterious role in ALS patients and it has been confirmed. It was shown in experiments that low progression rate in patients with ALS is associated to greater compensatory reinnervation and low HDAC4 levels. miR-133b is present in the same transcript encoding miR206, which is upregulated after denervation in the NMJs. The genetic ablation of miR-133b was studied in SOD1-G93A mice and it was noticed that the lack of miR-133b did not modify NMJ development or reinnervation after nerve injury and, overall, disease progression was not affected. miR-206 plays an important role in NMJ reinnervation specifically. miR-155 expression can be efficiently inhibited by anti-miR delivery to the CNS and periphery of SOD1-G93A mouse [86]. Inhibition of miR-155 can improve disease progression in ALS. Single intracerebro-ventricular injection of miR-29a-specific antagomir inhibiting CNS-related miR-29a expression in CNS can prolong the survival of ALS patients, thus suggesting miR-29a as a possible marker for disease progression. Anti-miR can be used as therapeutics in treating ALS but we should have an eye on the bystander effects [21].

22. Conclusion

Molecular neuropathology, genomics and proteomics related to it have made a real progress in the last few decades. Candidate genes and their involvement in molecular interactions and networks have opened new venues in therapeutics. ALS is polygenic and non-cell-autonomous disease. Due to the presence of many gene variants in this disease, it is difficult to predict the susceptible individuals. There is no such inheritance pattern. As miRNA population is dysregulated in ALS, candidate miRNAs can be used as biomarker and targets of therapeutics. Discoveries of ALS-related miRNAs are leading us to solve the intricate cellular network-related details. As of for now, we have drugs to slow down ALS. But we still have nothing to treat this disease completely. Intricacies in miRNA network are making the development of drug more difficult because of bystander effects. There are several scientist groups around the world trying to find out the possible therapeutics.

Truly, present write-ups address many milestones of biological consequences of microRNA that shed potential light on the in-depth mechanisms of ALS. It definitely explains the motor neuron development, thereby expanding our new knowledge of ALS post-transcriptionally. Apart from that, present knowledge laid a major foundation for development of therapeutic agents of ALS. Furthermore, covering specific miRNA signatures targeted by different genes of ALS are important for broad classification of ALS symptoms. This sectorization of microRNA expression might be important to improve the subclassification of ALS genes which provide a unique instructive role for therapeutic approaches.

Author details

Utpal Bhadra[1*], Anisha Pal[1], Jagamohan Chhatai[1] and Manika Pal Bhadra[2]

*Address all correspondence to: utpal@ccmb.res.in

1 Functional Genomics and Gene Silencing Group, Centre for Cellular and Molecular Biology, Hyderabad, India

2 Centre for Chemical Biology, Indian Institute for Chemical Technology, Hyderabad, India

References

[1] Howland DS, Liu J, She Y, Goad B, Maragakis NJ, Kim B, et al. Focal loss of the glutamate transporter EAAT2 in a transgenic rat model of SOD1 mutant-mediated amyotrophic lateral sclerosis [ALS]. Proc Natl Acad Sci U S A. 2002;99[3]:1604–9.

[2] Bruijn LI, Miller TM, Cleveland DW. Unraveling the mechanisms involved in motor neuron degeneration in ALS. Annu Rev Neurosci. 2004;27:723–49.

[3] Shabalina SA, Koonin EV. Origins and evolution of eukaryotic RNA interference. Trends Ecol Evol. 2008;23[10]:578–87.

[4] Martens-Uzunova ES, Olvedy M, Jenster G. Beyond microRNA – novel RNAs derived from small non-coding RNA and their implication in cancer. Cancer Lett. 2013;340[2]: 201–11.

[5] Davis BN, Hata A. Regulation of microRNA biogenesis: a miRiad of mechanisms. Cell Commun Signal. 2009;7:18.

[6] Riedmann LT, Schwentner R. miRNA, siRNA, piRNA and argonautes: news in small matters. RNA Biol. 2010;7[2]:133–9.

[7] Jacobsen A, Silber J, Harinath G, Huse JT, Schultz N, Sander C. Analysis of microRNA-target interactions across diverse cancer types. Nat Struct Mol Biol. 2013;20[11]:1325–32.

[8] Eulalio A, Huntzinger E, Izaurralde E. Getting to the root of miRNA-mediated gene silencing. Cell. 2008;132[1]:9–14.

[9] Shinde S, Arora N, Bhadra U. A complex network of microRNAs expressed in brain and genes associated with amyotrophic lateral sclerosis. Int J Genomics. 2013;2013:383024.

[10] Smrt RD, Zhao X. Epigenetic regulation of neuronal dendrite and dendritic spine development. Front Biol [Beijing]. 2010;5[4]:304–23.

[11] Alvarez JP, Pekker I, Goldshmidt A, Blum E, Amsellem Z, Eshed Y. Endogenous and synthetic microRNAs stimulate simultaneous, efficient, and localized regulation of multiple targets in diverse species. Plant Cell. 2006;18[5]:1134–51.

[12] Harries LW. MicroRNAs as mediators of the ageing process. Genes [Basel]. 2014;5[3]: 656–70.

[13] Lee RC, Feinbaum RL, Ambros V. The *C. elegans* heterochronic gene lin-4 encodes small RNAs with antisense complementarity to lin-14. Cell. 1993;75[5]:843–54.

[14] Reinhart BJ, Slack FJ, Basson M, Pasquinelli AE, Bettinger JC, Rougvie AE, et al. The 21-nucleotide let-7 RNA regulates developmental timing in *Caenorhabditis elegans*. Nature. 2000;403[6772]:901–6.

[15] Weaver R. Molecular Biology. McGraw-Hill Education; New York, NY10020, USA, 2011.

[16] Xing L, Kieff E. cis-Acting effects on RNA processing and Drosha cleavage prevent Epstein-Barr virus latency III BHRF1 expression. J Virol. 2011;85[17]:8929–39.

[17] Lee Y, Kim M, Han J, Yeom KH, Lee S, Baek SH, et al. MicroRNA genes are transcribed by RNA polymerase II. EMBO J. 2004;23[20]:4051–60.

[18] Valencia-Sanchez MA, Liu J, Hannon GJ, Parker R. Control of translation and mRNA degradation by miRNAs and siRNAs. Genes Dev. 2006;20[5]:515–24.

[19] Bartel DP. MicroRNAs: target recognition and regulatory functions. Cell. 2009;136[2]: 215–33.

[20] Hibio N, Hino K, Shimizu E, Nagata Y, Ui-Tei K. Stability of miRNA 5′ terminal and seed regions is correlated with experimentally observed miRNA-mediated silencing efficacy. Sci Rep. 2012;2:996.

[21] Volonte C, Apolloni S, Parisi C. MicroRNAs: newcomers into the ALS picture. CNS Neurol Disord Drug Targets. 2015;14[2]:194–207.

[22] Pillai RS. MicroRNA function: multiple mechanisms for a tiny RNA? RNA. 2005;11[12]: 1753–61.

[23] Bentwich I, Avniel A, Karov Y, Aharonov R, Gilad S, Barad O, et al. Identification of hundreds of conserved and nonconserved human microRNAs. Nat Genet. 2005;37[7]: 766–70.

[24] Winter J, Jung S, Keller S, Gregory RI, Diederichs S. Many roads to maturity: microRNA biogenesis pathways and their regulation. Nat Cell Biol. 2009;11[3]:228–34.

[25] Tomari Y, Zamore PD. MicroRNA biogenesis: drosha can't cut it without a partner. Curr Biol. 2005;15[2]:R61–4.

[26] Kiriakidou M, Tan GS, Lamprinaki S, De Planell-Saguer M, Nelson PT, Mourelatos Z. An mRNA m7G cap binding-like motif within human Ago2 represses translation. Cell. 2007;129[6]:1141–51.

[27] Chendrimada TP, Finn KJ, Ji X, Baillat D, Gregory RI, Liebhaber SA, et al. MicroRNA silencing through RISC recruitment of eIF6. Nature. 2007;447[7146]:823–8.

[28] Chan SP, Slack FJ. microRNA-mediated silencing inside P-bodies. RNA Biol. 2006;3[3]: 97–100.

[29] Duursma AM, Kedde M, Schrier M, le Sage C, Agami R. miR-148 targets human DNMT3b protein coding region. RNA. 2008;14[5]:872–7.

[30] Renton AE, Majounie E, Waite A, Simon-Sanchez J, Rollinson S, Gibbs JR, et al. A hexanucleotide repeat expansion in C9ORF72 is the cause of chromosome 9p21-linked ALS-FTD. Neuron. 2011;72[2]:257–68.

[31] Cortez MA, Bueso-Ramos C, Ferdin J, Lopez-Berestein G, Sood AK, Calin GA. MicroRNAs in body fluids – the mix of hormones and biomarkers. Nat Rev Clin Oncol. 2011;8[8]:467–77.

[32] Andersen PM, Al-Chalabi A. Clinical genetics of amyotrophic lateral sclerosis: what do we really know? Nat Rev Neurol. 2011;7[11]:603–15.

[33] DeJesus-Hernandez M, Mackenzie IR, Boeve BF, Boxer AL, Baker M, Rutherford NJ, et al. Expanded GGGGCC hexanucleotide repeat in noncoding region of C9ORF72 causes chromosome 9p-linked FTD and ALS. Neuron. 2011;72[2]:245–56.

[34] Sreedharan J, Brown RH, Jr. Amyotrophic lateral sclerosis: problems and prospects. Ann Neurol. 2013;74[3]:309–16.

[35] Yacila G, Sari Y. Potential therapeutic drugs and methods for the treatment of amyotrophic lateral sclerosis. Curr Med Chem. 2014;21[31]:3583–93.

[36] Appel SH, Beers DR, Henkel JS. T cell-microglial dialogue in Parkinson's disease and amyotrophic lateral sclerosis: are we listening? Trends Immunol. 2010;31[1]:7–17.

[37] Volonte C, Apolloni S, Carri MT, D'Ambrosi N. ALS: focus on purinergic signalling. Pharmacol Ther. 2011;132[1]:111–22.

[38] Hossaini M, Cardona Cano S, van Dis V, Haasdijk ED, Hoogenraad CC, Holstege JC, et al. Spinal inhibitory interneuron pathology follows motor neuron degeneration independent of glial mutant superoxide dismutase 1 expression in SOD1-ALS mice. J Neuropathol Exp Neurol. 2011;70[8]:662–77.

[39] McGown A, McDearmid JR, Panagiotaki N, Tong H, Al Mashhadi S, Redhead N, et al. Early interneuron dysfunction in ALS: insights from a mutant sod1 zebrafish model. Ann Neurol. 2013;73[2]:246–58.

[40] Chen K, Northington FJ, Martin LJ. Inducible nitric oxide synthase is present in motor neuron mitochondria and Schwann cells and contributes to disease mechanisms in ALS mice. Brain Struct Funct. 2010;214[2–3]:219–34.

[41] Clement AM, Nguyen MD, Roberts EA, Garcia ML, Boillee S, Rule M, et al. Wild-type nonneuronal cells extend survival of SOD1 mutant motor neurons in ALS mice. Science. 2003;302[5642]:113–7.

[42] Ilieva H, Polymenidou M, Cleveland DW. Non-cell autonomous toxicity in neurodegenerative disorders: ALS and beyond. J Cell Biol. 2009;187[6]:761–72.

[43] Boillee S, Vande Velde C, Cleveland DW. ALS: a disease of motor neurons and their nonneuronal neighbors. Neuron. 2006;52[1]:39–59.

[44] Di Giorgio FP, Carrasco MA, Siao MC, Maniatis T, Eggan K. Non-cell autonomous effect of glia on motor neurons in an embryonic stem cell-based ALS model. Nat Neurosci. 2007;10[5]:608–14.

[45] Castillo K, Nassif M, Valenzuela V, Rojas F, Matus S, Mercado G, et al. Trehalose delays the progression of amyotrophic lateral sclerosis by enhancing autophagy in motoneurons. Autophagy. 2013;9[9]:1308–20.

[46] Vargas MR, Pehar M, Cassina P, Beckman JS, Barbeito L. Increased glutathione biosynthesis by Nrf2 activation in astrocytes prevents p75NTR-dependent motor neuron apoptosis. J Neurochem. 2006;97[3]:687–96.

[47] Haidet-Phillips AM, Hester ME, Miranda CJ, Meyer K, Braun L, Frakes A, et al. Astrocytes from familial and sporadic ALS patients are toxic to motor neurons. Nat Biotechnol. 2011;29[9]:824–8.

[48] Eacker SM, Dawson TM, Dawson VL. Understanding microRNAs in neurodegeneration. Nat Rev Neurosci. 2009 Dec;10[12]:837–41.

[49] Lau P, de Strooper B. Dysregulated microRNAs in neurodegenerative disorders. Semin Cell Dev Biol. 2010;21[7]:768–73.

[50] Sonntag KC. MicroRNAs and deregulated gene expression networks in neurodegeneration. Brain Res. 2010;1338:48–57.

[51] Schaefer A, O'Carroll D, Tan CL, Hillman D, Sugimori M, Llinas R, et al. Cerebellar neurodegeneration in the absence of microRNAs. J Exp Med. 2007;204[7]:1553–8.

[52] Cuellar TL, Davis TH, Nelson PT, Loeb GB, Harfe BD, Ullian E, et al. Dicer loss in striatal neurons produces behavioral and neuroanatomical phenotypes in the absence of neurodegeneration. Proc Natl Acad Sci U S A. 2008;105[14]:5614–9.

[53] Xu Z, Yang C. TDP-43-The key to understanding amyotrophic lateral sclerosis. Rare Dis. 2014;2[1]:e944443.

[54] Haramati S, Chapnik E, Sztainberg Y, Eilam R, Zwang R, Gershoni N, et al. miRNA malfunction causes spinal motor neuron disease. Proc Natl Acad Sci U S A. 2010;107[29]:13111–6.

[55] Shin D, Shin JY, McManus MT, Ptacek LJ, Fu YH. Dicer ablation in oligodendrocytes provokes neuronal impairment in mice. Ann Neurol. 2009;66[6]:843–57.

[56] Tao J, Wu H, Lin Q, Wei W, Lu XH, Cantle JP, et al. Deletion of astroglial Dicer causes non-cell-autonomous neuronal dysfunction and degeneration. J Neurosci. 2011;31[22]: 8306–19.

[57] Pereira JA, Baumann R, Norrmen C, Somandin C, Miehe M, Jacob C, et al. Dicer in Schwann cells is required for myelination and axonal integrity. J Neurosci. 2010;30[19]: 6763–75.

[58] Verrier JD, Semple-Rowland S, Madorsky I, Papin JE, Notterpek L. Reduction of Dicer impairs Schwann cell differentiation and myelination. J Neurosci Res. 2010;88[12]: 2558–68.

[59] Gregory RI, Yan KP, Amuthan G, Chendrimada T, Doratotaj B, Cooch N, et al. The microprocessor complex mediates the genesis of microRNAs. Nature. 2004;432[7014]: 235–40.

[60] Kawahara Y, Mieda-Sato A. TDP-43 promotes microRNA biogenesis as a component of the Drosha and Dicer complexes. Proc Natl Acad Sci U S A. 2012;109[9]:3347–52.

[61] Buratti E, De Conti L, Stuani C, Romano M, Baralle M, Baralle F. Nuclear factor TDP-43 can affect selected microRNA levels. FEBS J. 2010;277[10]:2268–81.

[62] Ling SC, Albuquerque CP, Han JS, Lagier-Tourenne C, Tokunaga S, Zhou H, et al. ALS-associated mutations in TDP-43 increase its stability and promote TDP-43 complexes with FUS/TLS. Proc Natl Acad Sci U S A. 2010;107[30]:13318–23.

[63] Chen H, Qian K, Du Z, Cao J, Petersen A, Liu H, et al. Modeling ALS with iPSCs reveals that mutant SOD1 misregulates neurofilament balance in motor neurons. Cell Stem Cell. 2014;14[6]:796–809.

[64] Tortelli R, Ruggieri M, Cortese R, D'Errico E, Capozzo R, Leo A, et al. Elevated cerebrospinal fluid neurofilament light levels in patients with amyotrophic lateral sclerosis: a possible marker of disease severity and progression. Eur J Neurol. 2012;19[12]:1561–7.

[65] Butovsky O, Siddiqui S, Gabriely G, Lanser AJ, Dake B, Murugaiyan G, et al. Modulating inflammatory monocytes with a unique microRNA gene signature ameliorates murine ALS. J Clin Invest. 2012;122[9]:3063–87.

[66] Ishtiaq M, Campos-Melo D, Volkening K, Strong MJ. Analysis of novel NEFL mRNA targeting microRNAs in amyotrophic lateral sclerosis. PLoS One. 2014;9[1]:e85653.

[67] Parisi C, Arisi I, D'Ambrosi N, Storti AE, Brandi R, D'Onofrio M, et al. Dysregulated microRNAs in amyotrophic lateral sclerosis microglia modulate genes linked to neuroinflammation. Cell Death Dis. 2013;4:e959.

[68] Chiu IM, Chen A, Zheng Y, Kosaras B, Tsiftsoglou SA, Vartanian TK, et al. T lymphocytes potentiate endogenous neuroprotective inflammation in a mouse model of ALS. Proc Natl Acad Sci U S A. 2008;105[46]:17913–8.

[69] D'Ambrosi N, Finocchi P, Apolloni S, Cozzolino M, Ferri A, Padovano V, et al. The proinflammatory action of microglial P2 receptors is enhanced in SOD1 models for amyotrophic lateral sclerosis. J Immunol. 2009;183[7]:4648–56.

[70] Poloni M, Facchetti D, Mai R, Micheli A, Agnoletti L, Francolini G, et al. Circulating levels of tumour necrosis factor-alpha and its soluble receptors are increased in the blood of patients with amyotrophic lateral sclerosis. Neurosci Lett. 2000;287[3]:211–4.

[71] Hensley K, Fedynyshyn J, Ferrell S, Floyd RA, Gordon B, Grammas P, et al. Message and protein-level elevation of tumor necrosis factor alpha [TNF alpha] and TNF alpha-modulating cytokines in spinal cords of the G93A-SOD1 mouse model for amyotrophic lateral sclerosis. Neurobiol Dis. 2003;14[1]:74–80.

[72] Foran E, Trotti D. Glutamate transporters and the excitotoxic path to motor neuron degeneration in amyotrophic lateral sclerosis. Antioxid Redox Signal. 2009;11[7]:1587–602.

[73] Heath PR, Shaw PJ. Update on the glutamatergic neurotransmitter system and the role of excitotoxicity in amyotrophic lateral sclerosis. Muscle Nerve. 2002;26[4]:438–58.

[74] Russell AP, Wada S, Vergani L, Hock MB, Lamon S, Leger B, et al. Disruption of skeletal muscle mitochondrial network genes and miRNAs in amyotrophic lateral sclerosis. Neurobiol Dis. 2013;49:107–17.

[75] De Felice B, Guida M, Guida M, Coppola C, De Mieri G, Cotrufo R. A miRNA signature in leukocytes from sporadic amyotrophic lateral sclerosis. Gene. 2012;508[1]:35–40.

[76] Shioya M, Obayashi S, Tabunoki H, Arima K, Saito Y, Ishida T, et al. Aberrant microRNA expression in the brains of neurodegenerative diseases: miR-29a decreased in Alzheimer disease brains targets neurone navigator 3. Neuropathol Appl Neurobiol. 2010;36[4]:320–30.

[77] Reid G, Kirschner MB, van Zandwijk N. Circulating microRNAs: association with disease and potential use as biomarkers. Crit Rev Oncol Hematol. 2011;80[2]:193–208.

[78] Valadi H, Ekstrom K, Bossios A, Sjostrand M, Lee JJ, Lotvall JO. Exosome-mediated transfer of mRNAs and microRNAs is a novel mechanism of genetic exchange between cells. Nat Cell Biol. 2007;9[6]:654–9.

[79] Enright AJ, John B, Gaul U, Tuschl T, Sander C, Marks DS. MicroRNA targets in Drosophila. Genome Biol. 2003;5[1]:R1.

[80] John B, Enright AJ, Aravin A, Tuschl T, Sander C, Marks DS. Human microRNA targets. PLoS Biol. 2004;2[11]:e363.

[81] King IN, Yartseva V, Salas D, Kumar A, Heidersbach A, Ando DM, et al. The RNA-binding protein TDP-43 selectively disrupts microRNA-1/206 incorporation into the RNA-induced silencing complex. J Biol Chem. 2014;289[20]:14263–71.

[82] Miller TM, Pestronk A, David W, Rothstein J, Simpson E, Appel SH, et al. An antisense oligonucleotide against SOD1 delivered intrathecally for patients with SOD1 familial amyotrophic lateral sclerosis: a phase 1, randomised, first-in-man study. Lancet Neurol. 2013;12[5]:435–42.

[83] Lee YB, Chen HJ, Peres JN, Gomez-Deza J, Attig J, Stalekar M, et al. Hexanucleotide repeats in ALS/FTD form length-dependent RNA foci, sequester RNA binding proteins, and are neurotoxic. Cell Rep. 2013;5[5]:1178–86.

[84] Paez-Colasante X, Figueroa-Romero C, Sakowski SA, Goutman SA, Feldman EL. Amyotrophic lateral sclerosis: mechanisms and therapeutics in the epigenomic era. Nat Rev Neurol. 2015;11[5]:266–79.

[85] Williams AH, Valdez G, Moresi V, Qi X, McAnally J, Elliott JL, et al. MicroRNA-206 delays ALS progression and promotes regeneration of neuromuscular synapses in mice. Science. 2009;326[5959]:1549–54.

[86] Koval ED, Shaner C, Zhang P, du Maine X, Fischer K, Tay J, et al. Method for widespread microRNA-155 inhibition prolongs survival in ALS-model mice. Hum Mol Genet. 2013;22[20]:4127–35.

Chapter 9

Selective Vulnerability of Neuronal Subtypes in ALS: A Fertile Ground for the Identification of Therapeutic Targets

Cylia Rochat, Nathalie Bernard-Marissal and
Bernard L. Schneider

Additional information is available at the end of the chapter

http://dx.doi.org/10.5772/63703

Abstract

It is well defined that subpopulations of motoneurons have different vulnerability to the pathology causing amyotrophic lateral sclerosis (ALS). In the spinal cord, the fast fatigable motoneurons have been shown to be the first to degenerate, followed by fatigue-resistant and slow motoneurons. In contrast motoneurons located in the Onuf's and oculomotor nuclei appear to be resistant to disease. With a focus on research mainly done on mice overexpressing the mutated human superoxide dismutase (SOD1) protein, we review recent studies exploring the mechanisms that underlie the selective vulnerability of the various motoneuron subtypes. By comparing differences in gene expression between these populations, it has been possible to identify factors, which critically determine the survival of motoneurons and the neuromuscular function in the pathologic context of ALS. Furthermore, we discuss the contribution of non-cell autonomous processes, involving glial cells and the skeletal muscle, in the neurodegenerative process. Exploring the cause of neurodegeneration from the angle of the selective neuronal vulnerability has recently led to the identification of novel targets, which open opportunities for therapeutic intervention against ALS.

Keywords: motoneurons, SOD1, selective vulnerability, therapeutic target, ER stress

1. Introduction

Amyotrophic lateral sclerosis (ALS) primarily affects the motor system, which controls both voluntary and involuntary movements, including vital functions such as breathing, through

INTECH
open science | open minds

© 2016 The Author(s). Licensee InTech. This chapter is distributed under the terms of the Creative Commons Attribution License (http://creativecommons.org/licenses/by/3.0), which permits unrestricted use, distribution, and reproduction in any medium, provided the original work is properly cited. (cc) BY the activity of various types of motoneurons (MNs). Paralysis and death of the patients, which typically occurs within a few years after disease onset, is caused by the progressive dysfunction and degeneration of MNs in the cortex, brainstem and spinal cord. Remarkably, it has been established that the different types of MNs are not equally affected by ALS. This leads to contrasted effects on the motor system. For instance, with disease progression, patients lose their ability to speak, swallow and move, but they keep normal visual, sexual and bladder functions. Indeed, MNs located in the oculomotor and Onuf's nuclei are remarkably resistant to the disease [1]. In contrast, spinal MNs controlling voluntary movements, hypoglossal MNs important for swallowing and breathing, as well as the upper MNs, are typically among the first neurons to degenerate.

Upper MNs, also known as Betz cells or corticospinal MNs (CSMNs), are glutamatergic neurons located in the primary motor cortex and which activate lower MNs in the brainstem and spinal cord. Upon activation, the lower MNs induce muscle contraction via the release of the acetylcholine neurotransmitter in the neuromuscular junction (NMJ), a specialized synapse contacting the skeletal muscle fibers. The ensemble formed by lower MNs and the innervated muscle fiber is called the motor unit.

Spinal MNs are subdivided into α, β and γ MNs, depending on the type of muscle fibers they innervate (reviewed by [2]). In ALS, it is mainly α-MNs that degenerate. However, it is recognized that within the class of α-MNs, there is also a predictable variation in neuronal vulnerability to disease [3, 4]. It is therefore important to distinguish the following subtypes of α-MNs, defined by the contractile properties of the motor unit they are part of: the fast twitch fatigable (FF) MNs, the fast twitch fatigue-resistant (FR) MNs and the slow twitch fatigue-resistant (S) MNs [5]. This classification is also based on other characteristics, such as the size of the neuronal soma (FF MNs have larger cell bodies than S MNs), axonal conduction velocity (FF MNs are faster than S MNs), dendrite branching (FF MNs display a more complex dendritic tree than S MNs) [6], as well as the electrical properties of each of these MN subtypes [7].

The selective vulnerability observed between the different types of MNs provides a remarkable opportunity to explore the factors that specifically contribute to neurodegeneration. Until now, this approach has been mainly based on animal models overexpressing mutated forms of the superoxide dismutase 1 (SOD1) protein. Indeed, in more than 20% of the familial ALS cases (fALS), the SOD1 protein carries point mutations associated with autosomal dominant inheritance. Rodent models overexpressing mutated forms of SOD1 (mSOD1), often under the control of the human SOD1 promoter, faithfully replicate major clinical aspects of ALS [8–10]. Furthermore, MN subpopulations display a selective vulnerability pattern very similar to the one observed in humans [8]. These animal models are therefore instrumental to investigate the molecular and cellular mechanisms underlying the disease process. In this review, we will discuss how the research on ALS has identified novel therapeutic targets by comparing different MN subtypes in SOD1 models of fALS.

2. Comparing different populations of MNs

A careful analysis of disease progression in the high-copy $SOD1^{G93A}$ mouse models of ALS has allowed defining different stages of the disease. The first behavioral alterations occur as early as postnatal day 10 (P10), with a delay in the righting reflex and an increase in the number of mistakes observed in forelimb placement [11]. Around P50, subtle changes in mouse gait and muscle strength can be observed [12, 13] and by P80, clear impairments in the motor performance can be detected [14]. At 3 months of age, the animals reach disease onset, which is characterized by fine tremors, muscle atrophy and loss of body mass [15]. A severe paralysis of the hindlimbs is observed on average at P120 [16]. Soon after P135, the ALS mice become unable to right themselves when placed on their side, which is considered as the humane disease endpoint [15]. This highly reproducible course of the disease has been used to identify the corresponding neurodegenerative events in the mouse spinal cord. Thorough analysis has revealed a precise sequence in the loss of the different types of MNs, allowing for longitudinal studies to determine molecular and cellular correlates in the disease process.

2.1. Progression of the SOD1 pathology in mouse models of fALS

2.1.1. Spinal MNs

Spinal MNs are responsible for the control of voluntary movements. For instance, MNs located in the lumbar part of the spinal cord control the movement of the hindlimbs (**Figure 1**). These MNs innervate muscles, such as the *gastrocnemius*, which are composed of different types of muscle fibers. The type and the contractile properties of each muscle fiber are defined by the type of the innervating MN [5] (**Figure 2**). During the course of the disease observed in the high-copy $SOD1^{G93A}$ mice, the innervation of the *gastrocnemius* muscle undergoes dramatic changes that can be recorded by electromyography.

A significant decline of the compound muscle action potential (CMAP) is observed around P50 [17, 18], followed by a second decline seen around P100 [18, 19]. In line with the CMAP data, histological analysis has revealed an abrupt loss of muscle innervation at the age of approximately 50 days, corresponding to lower occupation of the NMJ in the fast twitch muscle [3, 14]. Therefore, SOD1 pathology leads first to a loss of the innervation of the type IIb muscle fibers by the FF MNs (**Figure 2B**). The second wave of denervation, which occurs at the late presymptomatic stage of the disease, is defined by the pruning of the FR axons innervating the type IIa muscle fibers [4] (**Figure 2C**). In contrast, the type I muscle fibers remain innervated by the S MNs almost until end stage [18]. Moreover, FR and S MNs have been shown to have a higher capacity for axonal sprouting compared to the FF MNs [3]. They may form new synapses on the denervated end plates [20] (**Figure 2B, C**). Although the loss of NMJs is typically observed early during the course of the pathology induced by mSOD1, the degeneration of MN cell bodies in the ventral horn starts at P100 and rapidly progresses, in line with the "dying back" process described by [14].

Overall, these studies highlight a predictable course of degeneration in the SOD1 mouse model, with evident differences in the vulnerability of the different subtypes of spinal MN. Whereas FF MNs are more sensitive to the pathology than FR MNs, the S MNs appear remarkably resistant to the disease. Saxena *et al.* identified these subtypes of MNs using a retrograde tracer locally injected either in the lateral compartment of the *gastrocnemius* muscle, mainly innervated by FF MNs [3], or in the *soleus* muscle innervated by FR and S MNs [13]. The labeled MNs were collected by laser microdissection and their transcriptome analyzed using Affymetrix microarrays. This advanced approach has revealed molecular mechanisms that were undetectable when analyzing the whole ventral spinal cord. In Section 3, we will discuss our current understanding of the mechanisms underlying the observed discrepancies in MN vulnerability.

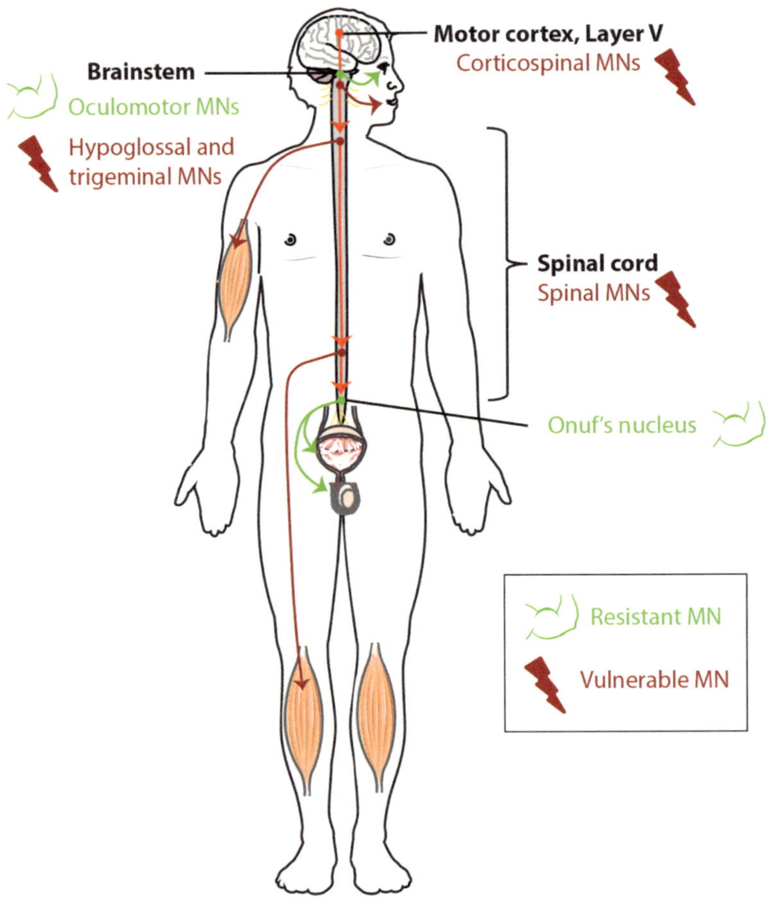

Figure 1. Transversal comparison of the vulnerability of different populations of motoneurons. Corticospinal, hypoglossal and spinal motoneurons (MNs), as well as neurons located in the trigeminal nucleus, progressively degenerate during the course of ALS. In contrast, the oculomotor neurons of the third cranial nerve, located in the brainstem, and which control eye movements, are resistant to disease. Motoneurons located in the Onuf's nucleus in the sacral region of the spinal cord, and which are responsible for the sexual and bladder functions, are also resistant to ALS.

http://dx.doi.org/10.5772/63703

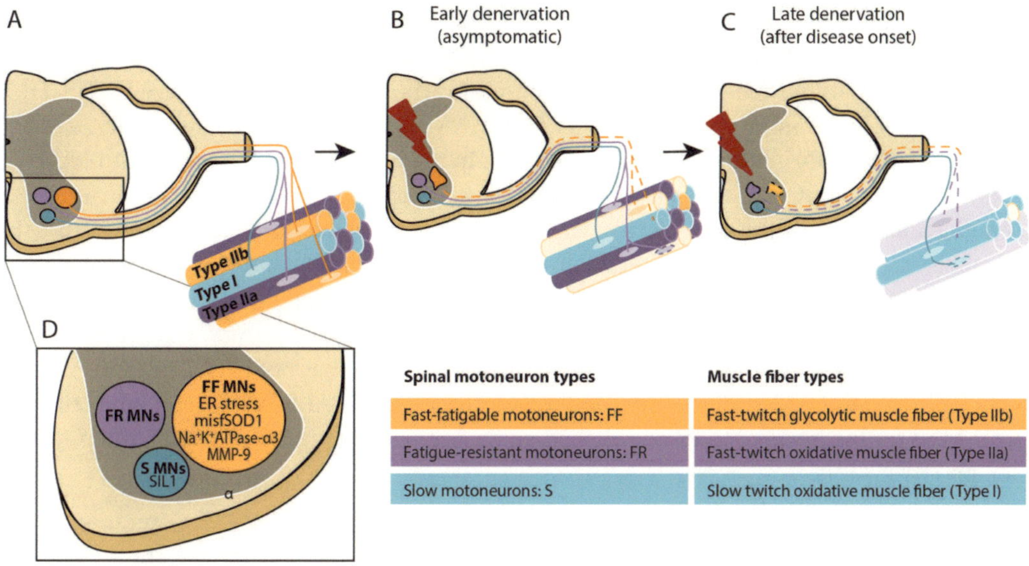

Figure 2. Longitudinal comparison of lumbar motoneurons during progression of the SOD1 pathology. (A) Organization of the motor units in the lumbar spinal cord. (B) The fast fatigable motoneurons (FF) are the first ones to degenerate in the SOD1 ALS mouse model. This degenerative event corresponds to the early denervation of the type IIb muscle fibers, before the onset of symptoms. (C) A second wave of denervation is observed when the fatigue-resistant motoneurons (FR) degenerate, mainly affecting the innervation of the type IIa muscle fibers and further progressing after symptom onset. Note that the axons of the resistant FR and S motoneurons can sprout and reinnervate the vacant neuromuscular junctions. The slow (S) motoneurons are resistant almost until disease end stage. (D) FF motoneurons are characterized by early ER stress and high amount of misfolded SOD1, and they abundantly express MMP-9 and the Na^+/K^+ ATPase-α3 pump. Disease-resistant S motoneurons are characterized by the expression of the ER chaperone SIL1.

2.1.2. Corticospinal MNs

The CSMNs localized in the layer V of the motor cortex are responsible for the initiation of the voluntary movement. These glutamatergic neurons collect, integrate, translate and transmit signals to lower MNs located in the spinal cord (**Figure 1**). CSMNs degenerate and die in ALS patients [21, 22]. There is also experimental evidence for the degeneration of CSMNs in the SOD1 animal models of fALS [23]. However, their role in the SOD1^{G93A} mouse model has been long overlooked; as without specific markers, it was difficult to discriminate these cells from other types of pyramidal neurons located in the layer V of the cortex. Retrograde tracers, as well as some adeno-associated viral (AAV) vectors able to retrogradely transduce neurons from their axonal projections, have proved their utility to study CSMNs [24]. Using retrograde tracers, a degeneration of the corticospinal tract and a loss of CSMNs were observed at end stage in SOD1^{G93A} fALS mice [25]. By combining retrograde tracers together with morphological and molecular approaches, Ozdinler *et al.* could demonstrate that CSMNs degenerate as soon as P30 in SOD1^{G93A} fALS mice [26]. Indeed, they observed a decrease in the size of CSMN somas, which were also found positive for markers of apoptosis. Already at P5, 2% of the neurons positive for CTIP2 (a transcription factor specific for CSMNs in layer V) display pyknosis. However, the most dramatic degeneration of the corticospinal tract is observed between P60 and P120, accompanied by astrogliosis and microgliosis in the neocortex at a later stage of the disease. Later, CSMNs could be easily identified in a transgenic mouse line expressing eGFP under the control of the ubiquitin carboxy-terminal hydrolase L1 (UCHL1) promoter [27]. By crossing these mice with SOD1^{G93A} mice, it was possible to analyze eGFP-expressing upper MNs in the context of ALS [28]. In the near future, this mouse model could be used for transcriptomic and proteomic analyses, which may provide further insight into the molecular mechanisms occurring in CSMNs during the course of ALS. A recent study by Gautam *et al.* [29] used the UCHL1-eGFP mice crossed with an Alsin KO mouse line to study in CSMNs the impact of ALS2, a gene involved in a small percentage of fALS cases. Intriguingly, Uchl1 null mice completely lacking UCHL1 activity show motor deficits, with a progressive and dramatic loss of CSMNs [30]. Although Uchl1 has not been linked to ALS yet, it will be interesting to further address the role of this gene in ALS. Moreover, analyzing the spinal MNs in this mouse model could shed some light on the impact of the CSMN degeneration on lower MNs.

However, it remains unclear what is the exact contribution of CSMN degeneration to the deficits observed in animal models of the SOD1 fALS pathology. Importantly, the silencing of mSOD1 in the cortex of SOD1^{G93A} rats can delay disease onset, and extends animal survival [31]. Even more, the treatment has neuroprotective effects on spinal MNs, preventing denervation of the NMJs. These data highlight the role of CSMNs in ALS, which may have been underestimated. Further longitudinal studies will be needed to explore the molecular mechanisms leading to CSMN degeneration in ALS and uncover potential therapeutic targets.

2.2. Transversal studies to compare motor nuclei

2.2.1. Onuf/oculomotor versus spinal/hypoglossal MNs

Pools of MNs located in the Onuf's and oculomotor nuclei are considered resistant to the disease. MNs located in the oculomotor nucleus are responsible for most of the eye movements. This function remains mostly intact in ALS patients, although slight defects can be detected toward end stage, in patients maintained with respiratory assist devices (reviewed by [32]). Similarly, the disease does not affect the survival of MNs in the Onuf's nucleus, which controls sexual and bladder functions [1]. In this nucleus, only few degenerating hallmarks have been observed, such as pyknotic nuclei or Bunina bodies [1]. The apparent resistance of the oculomotor and Onuf's nuclei contrasts with the progressive degeneration of spinal, hypoglossal and trigeminal MNs responsible for the locomotion, swallowing and the control of the jaw musculature, respectively [33, 34] (**Figure 1**).

Several research groups have taken advantage of the differential vulnerability between these motor nuclei to investigate the underlying molecular mechanisms [35–37]. These studies used techniques including the local injection of retrograde tracers, laser microdissection of cell subtypes and high-throughput analysis of gene expression.

Using microarrays, Kaplan *et al.* [38] determined in wild-type (WT) mice the gene expression profiles of the oculomotor and Onuf's nuclei, as compared to the vulnerable spinal MNs. A set of genes, including the matrix metalloproteinase 9 (MMP-9) and Hydroxysteroid (17-Beta) Dehydrogenase 2 (Hsd17b2), was found to be expressed at higher levels in the vulnerable spinal MNs, as compared to the resistant ones. Conversely, semaphorine3e (Sema3e) showed higher expression in the resistant MNs.

Another study compared oculomotor MNs, hypoglossal MNs and cervical spinal MNs in WT rats, and found that the pattern of expression of a set of genes was specific for each of these MN subpopulations [39]. Based on those results, protein levels were determined for six key genes, comparing their expression in WT and SOD1^{G93A} mice [40]. This study identified a protein expression signature specific to the disease-resistant oculomotor MNs, as compared to hypoglossal and spinal MNs. The GABA$_A$ receptor $\alpha1$, the guanylate cyclase soluble subunit $\alpha3$ and the parvalbumin protein were highly expressed in the resistant MNs. Conversely, vulnerable MNs displayed higher protein levels of dynein, peripherin and GABA$_A$ receptor $\alpha2$. These data suggest that differences in excitability, calcium handling and retrograde transport machinery may underlie the observed vulnerability pattern. Remarkably, these differences in protein expression were found to be conserved in the mouse and human species [40].

In an electrophysiological study using the high-copy SOD1^{G93A} mouse model, Venugopal *et al.* [41] compared the excitability of the vulnerable trigeminal MNs (TMNs) and the resistant oculomotor MNs *ex vivo*, at P8–12. Using a system based on the membrane properties of MNs, and a statistical clustering approach to predict the type of motor unit—i.e. FF, FR or S—, they could determine early perturbations of the firing threshold in the SOD1^{G93A} MNs. TMNs with low excitability had a decreased threshold, whereas the subpopulation of highly excitable TMNs had an increased firing threshold. Remarkably, no such electrophysiological effects of the SOD1^{G93A} pathology were observed in the oculomotor MNs.

Overall, despite the fact that these different pools of MNs have similar physiological roles, they display clear differences in their vulnerability to the ALS pathology. Transversal studies have already identified some of the mechanisms that may confer MN susceptibility to the disease.

3. Possible mechanisms implicated in selective motoneuron vulnerability

Here, we will summarize both intrinsic and extrinsic mechanisms, which may underlie the differences between subtypes of MNs in their ability to cope with the ALS pathology.

3.1. Intrinsic mechanisms

3.1.1. SOD1 misfolding and ER chaperones

One of the leading hypotheses for the cause of ALS is the gain of toxic properties resulting from the accumulation of misfolded proteins including SOD1. In normal conditions, the cytosolic SOD1 protein undergoes several maturation steps to acquire proper structure and function. These steps include the binding of copper and zinc and the formation of an intramolecular disulfide bond, to form an enzymatically active and stable homodimer [42]. When the SOD1 protein carries pathogenic mutations, it has an increased propensity to misfold (misfSOD1), leading to aggregation and accumulation in organelles such as the Endoplasmic Reticulum (ER) and the mitochondria [43]. Aggregation of SOD1 has been observed in patients with fALS [44, 45] and has also been reported in sporadic cases of ALS (sALS) [45, 46]. Using antibodies that specifically recognize misfSOD1 [47], Saxena *et al.* [7] found an accumulation of misfSOD1 in the FF MNs, as soon as P7 in the high-copy $SOD1^{G93A}$ mouse model (**Figure 2D**). In order to determine the changes in gene expression concomitant with the accumulation of misfSOD1, they performed a longitudinal study to compare the transcriptional profile of FF and FR/S MNs in the lumbar spinal cord [13]. Remarkably, the FF MNs are subjected to ER stress already at 3 weeks of age, which is 20 days before the initial denervation of the corresponding muscle in this animal model. It is only later, at about P50, that the more resistant FR MNs display similar gene expression changes indicative of ER stress. No such response is observed in the S MN almost until end stage, which is consistent with their apparent resistance to disease.

In-depth analysis showed that two ER chaperones have an important role in MN vulnerability: Calreticulin (CRT) and SIL1 (**Figure 2D**). CRT is a protein that binds Ca^{2+} ions. Interestingly CRT has been shown to be two-fold decreased in the FF MNs compared to S MNs, as soon as P38 [48]. *In vitro*, the authors showed that the lower CRT expression contributes to ER stress and calcium homeostasis disturbance, eventually leading to MN death. The role of CRT was confirmed *in vivo*, by crossing $SOD1^{G93A}$ mice with heterozygous $CRT^{+/-}$ mice [49]. The lower level of CRT expression accelerates the progression of the SOD1 pathology, prompting the initial loss of NMJ and leading to early muscle weakness. However, low CRT expression did affect neither the long-term survival of MNs nor animal survival, indicating that CRT is mainly implicated in the most vulnerable FF MNs during the early phase of the disease.

In an effort to find factors regulating the ER stress response in specific pools of MNs, Filézac de l'Etang *et al.* [50] analyzed in WT mice by real-time PCR the expression of a series of genes involved in protein folding, protein quality control and stress sensing, and compared the level of gene expression in FF and FR/S MNs. SIL1 was found to be six-times more expressed in S MNs than in FF MNs. SIL1 is a cochaperone protein, which increases the availability of the ER chaperone BiP by catalyzing the release of ADP from the ADP-BiP complex, and thereby facilitates the dissociation of BiP from its substrates. In the spinal cord of $Sil1^{-/+}$ mice, the ER unfolded protein response (UPR) is restricted to the FF MNs, whereas in Sil1 null mice, ER stress signaling is induced in all MNs. In the $SOD1^{G93A}$ ALS mice, SIL1 expression is reduced in FF MNs, compared to S MNs. However, when SIL1 is overexpressed in MNs using an AAV6 vector, UPR and ER stress signaling are reduced. Moreover, lifespan is prolonged by 84 days in the low-copy $SOD1^{G93A}$ mouse model, and 37 days in the high-copy $SOD1^{G93A}$ mouse model. Conversely, reduced SIL1 activity accelerates the ALS pathology in $Sil1^{-/+}$ $SOD1^{G93A}$ mice, and reduces the animal lifespan. Finally, both *in vitro* and *in vivo* experiments show that SIL1, coupled with BiP activity, controls ER homeostasis.

3.1.2. MMP-9

By comparing cranial and spinal MNs with the disease-resistant oculomotor and Onuf's nuclei in WT mice, the MMP-9 protein was found to be expressed only in the vulnerable MNs [38]. MMPs are zinc-dependent endopeptidases able to degrade extracellular matrix and basement membrane components. Although the role of MMP-9 in the context of ALS is still poorly understood, it might be involved in the disruption of the neuronal extracellular matrix interaction (reviewed by [51]). MMPs have also been shown to promote the inflammatory process [52]. Kaplan *et al.* [38] found that MMP-9 is highly expressed in the FF MNs, in contrast to the S MNs, which have undetectable MMP-9 levels (**Figure 2D**). Crossing SOD1^{G93A} mice with MMP-9 null mice [53] has significant effects on the disease process [38]. The denervation of the fast twitch *tibialis anterior* muscle is delayed by more than 80 days, and the mouse survival increased by 25%. Conversely, AAV6-mediated overexpression of MMP-9 in the FF MNs accelerates the denervation of the *tibialis anterior* in SOD1^{G93A} mice. However, MMP-9 overexpression in oculomotor neurons does not induce extraocular muscle denervation, suggesting that other factors may contribute to the resistance to disease in this population of MNs.

Although no mutations in MMP-9 gene have been linked to ALS yet, He *et al.* [54] found an association between the C(-1562)T polymorphism in the MMP-9 gene, and risk to develop Parkinson's disease and sALS.

3.1.3. Neuronal excitability

FF and S MNs also differ in their excitability profile. Because of their small soma size, the S MNs have high input resistance, and therefore need less synaptic activation to initiate an action potential. As compared to MNs with a larger soma size, the firing threshold is reached earlier in S MNs, followed by the FR and finally the FF MNs [55]. S MNs are therefore considered to be highly excitable, whereas FF MNs are poorly excitable. S MNs innervate slow twitch muscle fibers, which are typically part of the postural muscles, whereas the poorly excitable neurons control fast twitch fibers, highly present in phasic muscles, and which are used when strength or rapid response is needed. A recent study by Saxena *et al.* [7] explored how neuronal excitability might contribute to the vulnerability profile in each of these MN populations. They were able to genetically modulate MN excitability *in vivo* using a floxed pharmacologically selective actuator module (PSAM), coupled either to the 5HT3-receptor to induce neuronal depolarization, or to the glycine-receptor to induce neuronal hyperpolarization. By activating these channels with a specific ligand, they could show that enhancing neuronal excitability decreases accumulation of misfSOD1 and BiP in MNs, which reduces ALS pathology [7]. Conversely, the reduction of MN excitability enhanced accumulation of misfSOD1 and BiP, accelerating disease progression.

Recently, a study further explored the link between misfSOD1 accumulation and MN excitability. Ruegsegger *et al.* [56] found that misfSOD1 binds the Na^+/K^+ATPase-$\alpha3$ pump, impairing its ATPase activity. More specifically, misfSOD1 targets a 10 amino acid stretch, which is present in Na^+/K^+ATPase-$\alpha3$, and not in the closely related Na^+/K^+ATPase-$\alpha1$ isozyme. Remarkably, Na^+/K^+ATPase-$\alpha3$ is the main pump expressed in the vulnerable FF MNs. In contrast, FR MNs have similar expression of both Na^+/K^+ATPase-$\alpha1$ and $\alpha3$, whereas S MNs express almost exclusively Na^+/K^+ATPase-α1. Therefore, there could be a link between MN vulnerability and the expression of Na^+/K^+ATPase-α3, which may lead to ion imbalance when exposed to the deleterious effects of misfSOD1.

Le Masson *et al.* [57] used a computational model to demonstrate the dramatic effects that ion imbalance could have in MNs. The low excitable FF MNs have a high-energy demand to trigger action potentials, increasing their need for ATP. Ion pump deficiency caused by misfSOD1 will then consequently increase intracellular cation levels, leading to a constant MN depolarization. The induced burden on the mitochondrial function may affect ATP production, leading to a deficit in ATP used to restore ion homeostasis. Overall, the instability is increased, spreading ion imbalance within the MNs. Overall, these studies highlight the role of neuronal activity in each subpopulation of MNs exposed to the ALS pathology. These findings can be exploited to pinpoint key targets present in some neuronal subtypes to develop novel therapies.

3.2. Extrinsic mechanisms

3.2.1. CNS compartment

Over the 20 past years, it has been long debated whether ALS should be considered as a cell autonomous disease, mainly taking place in the MNs. It is now well established that astrocytes, oligodendrocytes and microglia also play a role in the pathology (reviewed by [58, 59]). Animal models of the SOD1 pathology have been intensively used to address this question. First, when the mSOD1 was selectively expressed in neurons using a panneuronal promoter, an ALS phenotype was observed only after 400 days [60]. It was next observed that expression of mSOD1 with a MN-specific promoter does not produce any ALS phenotype [61, 62]. Similarly, expression of mSOD1 only in astrocytes or microglia failed to produce any pathology [63, 64]. Next, several studies used fALS mice carrying a floxed mSOD1 transgene to selectively excise the transgene by expressing the Cre recombinase only in a given cell types. Using this approach, they could demonstrate that mSOD1 expression in MNs determines the time of disease onset. Expression of mSOD1 in either astrocytes or oligodendrocytes affects both disease onset and progression [65, 66], whereas the pathogenic contribution of mSOD1 in microglial cells is mainly observed during disease progression [67]. Similar effects have been observed with a different approach, using an AAV-based system to selectively express an artificial microRNA to target mSOD1 either in MNs or in astrocytes [68].

The majority of the vulnerable MNs are already degenerating before the clinical onset of the disease (**Figure 2**). When the resistant pool of MNs undergoes degenerative changes, they are typically exposed to a local environment containing reactive glial cells. Indeed, astrocytes and microglia become activated mainly in the late phase of the pathology. Several studies have shown their implication in the progression of the disease after the onset of the symptoms, most likely via their pathogenic interaction with the remaining MNs.

These findings point out the importance to investigate the role of broad range of cell types in the ALS pathology. Sun *et al.* [69] have recently addressed the temporal sequence of gene expression changes occurring in glial cells in the $SOD1^{G37R}$ mice. They applied the translating ribosome affinity purification (TRAP) technique [70], coupled with high-throughput RNA sequencing, to investigate the gene expression changes in MNs, astrocytes and oligodendrocytes. Just before disease onset, they observed the most prominent gene expression changes in MNs, mainly affecting the ER stress pathways. Later, astrocytes show changes in the expression of genes mostly involved in inflammation and metabolism. In oligodendrocytes, gene expression is most significantly changed at an early symptomatic stage. The observed dysregulation affects genes implicated in the myelination and lipid signaling pathways. This result somewhat contrasts with the delay in disease onset, which has been previously observed following the selective excision of mSOD1 in oligodendrocytes [65].

Oligodendrocytes are known to support the metabolic activity and the myelination of axons in the CNS (reviewed by [71]). Degenerating oligodendrocytes have been observed in ALS mice and patient tissues. Moreover, the pool of oligodendrocyte progenitors, identified by the expression of NG2, fails to properly differentiate, and they generate oligodendrocytes lacking expression of the myelin basic protein (MBP) and monocarboxylate transporter 1 (MCT1) [65, 72]. The loss of MCT1 may contribute to MN vulnerability, as this transporter is normally required for the supply of lactate, which is an important energy substrate for axonal support [73]. Remarkably, MCT4—another lactate transporter— is preferentially expressed in astrocytes and is reduced in ALS [74].

Although the role of astrocytes in ALS has raised a lot of interest, the mechanisms underlying astrocyte-mediated toxicity toward MNs are still incompletely resolved. The interaction between astrocytes and MNs has been mainly explored *in vitro*, using coculture systems. Recently, Meyer *et al.* [75] were able to differentiate "induced astrocytes" (i-astrocytes) from neuronal progenitor cells derived from the fibroblasts of ALS patients. In cocultures of MNs and i-astrocytes derived from SOD1 ALS, C9ORF72 ALS and sALS patients, the astrocytes are toxic to MNs, similarly to cocultures using astrocytes derived from the ALS spinal cord [9, 76]. This study suggests that astrocytes may convey toxic effects toward MNs, regardless of their tissue of origin. One of the first mechanisms proposed for astrocyte toxicity is the potential excitotoxicity caused by glutamate mishandling (reviewed by [77]). In ALS patients, there is reduced expression of the excitatory amino acid transporter 2 (EAAT2), which is the main glutamate transporter in astrocytes [78–80]. Inefficient removal of glutamate from the synaptic cleft may lead to MN hyperactivation and to a massive entry of calcium. Calcium influx into MNs can overload the storage capability of the ER and mitochondria, particularly in MNs where calcium storage could be already impaired [57, 81]. Several studies have highlighted the secretion of toxic factors by glial cells expressing mSOD1. Indeed, *in vitro* experiments have shown that activated astrocytes and microglia expressing mSOD1 secrete toxic factors such as FasL, nitric oxide (NO) and the IFN-γ cytokine. These factors can induce the death of MNs expressing mSOD1 (reviewed by [82]). In particular, the coculture with mSOD1 astrocytes leads to the selective death of MNs mediated through the LIGHT-lymphotoxin-β receptor death pathway [83].

Therefore, although glial cells are essential to support the function and metabolism of MNs in the healthy CNS, they are likely to play an active role in the disease process. Astrocytes, oligodendrocytes and microglial cells carrying ALS-causing mutations appear to malfunction, leading to the selective death of MNs.

The release of misfSOD1 is another major component, which may contribute to MN degeneration via extrinsic mechanisms. As mentioned before, misfSOD1 plays an important role in the degeneration of MNs and its toxicity has been implicated in many cellular dysfunctions (review by [58]). Most importantly, recent evidence suggests a role of misfSOD1 also in some sALS cases that are not related to SOD1 mutations. It has been demonstrated that misfSOD1 can convert WT SOD1 [84, 85] leading to the formation of fibrils and aggregates *in vitro* [86]. High expression of WT SOD1 can lead to an ALS-like phenotype in mice [87]. A prion-like mechanism of propagation of misfSOD1 from cell to cell has been highlighted in the past few years (reviewed by [88]). In ALS, exogenous mSOD1 protein [85], as well as the WT SOD1 protein [89], has been shown to penetrate the cell membrane of neuron-like cells by mechanisms related to macropinocytosis. Cell-to-cell transfer of misfSOD1 may also be mediated by the ER chaperone chromogranin or through exosomes [26, 90]. Importantly, disease onset occurs earlier in mSOD1 mice crossed with mice overexpressing chromogranin A, demonstrating that this mechanism may have an important role *in vivo* [91]. Basso *et al.* [90] highlight a potential role for astrocytes in mSOD1 propagation. Indeed, they compared *in vitro* the proteome and secretome of WT SOD1 and $SOD1^{G93A}$ astrocytes. Interestingly, these latter produced less protein than the WT SOD1 astrocytes. However, although fewer proteins are secreted by astrocytes expressing mSOD1, the amount of proteins shed via exosomes is increased. Furthermore, exosomes derived from astrocytes can transfer mSOD1 to MNs and induce cell death. It is proposed that astrocytes may secrete mSOD1 to limit the intracellular deposition of SOD1 aggregates. In turn, the released mSOD1 may exert toxic effects on neighboring cells. For example, exogenous forms of mSOD1 can be toxic to MNs *in vitro* via microglial activation [92].

Although experimental evidence for the propagation of misfSOD1 is still lacking *in vivo*, these results suggest that several cell types, including neurons, astrocytes and microglia, may contribute to the transfer of the protein and lead to toxic effects throughout the CNS. This pathogenic mechanism may participate in the cascade of events leading to MN degeneration, while the disease is progressing. With high level of SOD1 protein expression, and low levels of ER chaperones, MNs may be particularly vulnerable in case of exposure to misfSOD1.

3.2.2. PNS compartment

On top of the CNS components, it is also important to investigate the role of cells that may control the function of specific subtypes of MNs in the periphery, especially the Schwann cells and the skeletal muscle.

3.2.2.1. Schwann cells

The Schwann cells are the counterparts of oligodendrocytes in the peripheral nervous system (PNS), as they are the primary supporting and myelinating cells for the neurons in the PNS. Surprisingly, the suppression of mSOD1 in Schwann cells accelerates disease progression [93]. The terminal Schwann cells (TSCs) are also of particular interest as they play an important role in the maintenance, plasticity and regeneration of the NMJs (reviewed by [94]). Semaphorin 3A (Sema3a), a chemorepellent expressed by TSC, is involved in the repulsion of motor axons away from the end plate, leading to the denervation of the NMJ [95]. Remarkably, during reinnervation or toxin-induced paralysis of the *gastrocnemius* muscle, Sema3a is abundantly expressed by TSC located at the NMJ of type IIb/x muscle fibers, which are known to have low sprouting capacity [3, 96]. Even more intriguing is the upregulation of Sema3a in the TSC covering the motor nerve terminals innervating the type IIb/x muscle fibers in a mouse model of ALS [97]. Blocking the Sema3a receptor NRP1 was found to delay NMJ denervation in ALS mice, extending their lifespan [98], thus suggesting that Sema3a could contribute to the early loss of NMJ in these specific muscle fibers in ALS, and be implicated in their low sprouting capacity [3]. Moreover, a recent study has highlighted an increase of Sema3a levels in the motor cortex of ALS patients [99].

3.2.2.2. Muscle

One of the first changes observed in ALS patients and mouse models is the denervation of the NMJ, often long before the death of MNs. However, the role of the muscle in ALS is still debated (reviewed by [100]). Dobrowolny *et al.* [51] showed that overexpression of mSOD1 specifically in the muscle tissue leads to muscle atrophy and a loss of muscle strength. However, the shRNA-mediated silencing of mSOD1 in the muscle of SOD1 ALS mice, using either an AAV vector [101] or a lentiviral vector [102], does not provide any beneficial effect. The absence of any protective effect was confirmed using mice with Cre expression restricted to the skeletal muscle to suppress floxed mSOD1 in a tissue-specific manner [102]. Although these studies indicate that the skeletal muscle is not a primary site for the SOD1 pathology, it may have an important role in the maintenance of the neuromuscular connections. The neurite outgrowth inhibitor A (Nogo-A) is upregulated in the skeletal muscle of the mSOD1 mouse model and in ALS patients and this upregulation seems to occur specifically in the slow twitch muscle fibers [103]. Moreover, Nogo-A expression correlates with the severity of the clinical symptoms [104]. Overexpression of Nogo-A in the mouse muscle induces NMJ denervation, whereas crossing mSOD1 mice with Nogo-A KO mice protects the NMJ [105, 106]. Therapeutic approaches to block the action of Nogo-A have been proposed. Injection of an anti-Nogo-A antibody in $SOD1^{G93A}$ mice from the age of 70 days onward protects motor units and increases muscle strength in 90-day-old mice, although this protective effect seems to be lost at 120 days [107]. Ozanezumab, a humanized version of the anti-Nogo-A antibody, has been tested in ALS patients in a phase I clinical trial [108]. Overall, it appears that pathogenic processes taking place in the skeletal musculature can impact on the neuromuscular function, via mechanisms that may be specific to motor unit subtypes.

4. Identification and validation of therapeutic targets

Despite years of research and clinical testing, Riluzole remains the only FDA approved drug for ALS. It is therefore urgent to identify novel targets for therapeutic intervention against MN degeneration. The study of the different types of MNs highlights the fact that subpopulations of MNs can survive for long term and function in the context of the disease, which provides novel molecular targets for neuroprotective treatments.

One possibility is to identify factors that are active in the most vulnerable neurons, and design approaches to reduce their activity, with the hope to obtain neuroprotective effects in ALS. In SOD1 mice, MMP-9 has recently been shown to cause deleterious effects in the FF MNs, where it is preferentially expressed [38]. Edaravone is a free radical scavenger that inhibits MMP-9 upregulation [109]. This compound has been used since many years ago for the treatment of cerebral infarction or ischemic stroke. Edaravone has demonstrated therapeutic efficiency in the SOD1^{G93A} mouse model [110] as well as in the SOD1^{H46R} rat model [111], and more recently in the wobbler mice, which is often considered as a model for sALS [112]. A phase II clinical trial has shown that Edaravone can slow down the progression of the motor impairments in ALS patients, although this effect could not be statistically confirmed in a recent phase III trial [113]. Nevertheless, further analysis of the results has revealed the beneficial effects of the compound in a subgroup of ALS patients, according to the revised El Escorial diagnostic criteria, prompting the initiation of a new trial (http://www.alzforum.org/news/conference-coverage/does-free-radical-scavenger-edavarone-slow-als).(http://www.alzforum.org/news/conference-coverage/does-free-radical-scavenger-edavarone-slow-als). Of note, Edaravone is already approved in Japan for the treatment of ALS.

Another possibility is to identify proteins that are expressed only in the disease-resistant MNs. Here, factors implicated in the control of ER stress may play an important role in MNs (reviewed by [114]). Possible therapeutic approaches to relieve ER stress have been tested in the context of the ALS mice. For instance, Salubrinal has been shown to reduce ER stress [115]. In SOD1 mice, Salubrinal administration alleviates disease manifestation and slows down the progression of the disease [13]. However, Salubrinal as such cannot be used for treating ALS patients as it has been shown to affect long-term memory in mice [116]. Guanabenz is another FDA approved antihypertensive drug known to reduce ER stress. Its efficacy in ALS mice is however still controversial [117, 118]. It is therefore important to unravel targets that may be more specific to ALS. The discovery that the ER chaperones SIL1 and CRT are centrally involved in the most resistant populations of MNs has raised attention to these factors as potential specific targets [49, 50]. In particular, AAV-mediated overexpression of SIL1 in the MNs of ALS mice dramatically increases innervation of the NMJs and prolongs animal survival by 25—30%. However, it remains to be determined how to therapeutically target these factors in ALS patients, perhaps using adapted pharmacological approaches.

As the vulnerability of MNs could be caused by the accumulation of misfSOD1 in these cells, one potential therapeutic strategy is to prevent SOD1 toxicity by targeting the partially unfolded intermediates of the SOD1 protein that can later form aggregates. Israelson *et al.* [43] recently identified an ATP-independent protein chaperone called multifunctional macrophage migration inhibitory factor (MIF). This factor prevents the misfolding of SOD1, and decreases cell death in MNs expressing SOD1^{G93A} *in vitro.* Moreover, this chaperone is expressed only at low levels in MNs, which may contribute to their selective vulnerability.

Another approach to prevent SOD1 misfolding is to provide the metal cofactors that are critical for the proper folding and stability of the functional Cu/Zn SOD1 dimer (reviewed by [119, 120]). CuATSM is a chelator widely used for PET-imaging as it rapidly carries copper across the blood-brain barrier into the CNS. Preclinical studies in SOD1 mouse models have reported beneficial effects of CuATSM, including on animal survival [121, 122]. Recently, Williams *et al.* [123] used transgenic SOD1^{G93A} mice coexpressing the Copper-Chaperone-for-SOD (CCS) protein, which is normally expressed in humans but not in mice. Although these mice do not live longer than 2 weeks, the treatment with CuATSM delayed onset and slowed down the progression of the disease, dramatically extending the lifespan of these animals to 18 months [123]. A phase I clinical trial will be soon initiated to test the effects of CuATSM in ALS patients.

Other strategies directly target SOD1 to prevent its deleterious effects. The use of antibodies specific for misfSOD1 has been proposed [47, 124, 125]. On the other hand, gene therapy techniques can be used to reduce the overall level of SOD1 expression. This approach can be considered as SOD1 null mice are viable and do not show any obvious motor dysfunction (reviewed by [126]). Viral vectors delivering artificial shRNA or microRNA for RNA interference against SOD1 [68, 127–130], as well as antisense oligonucleotides targeting the SOD1 mRNA [131], are currently being investigated to suppress the expression of this protein. It remains however debated whether these techniques could be effective in patients other than those carrying SOD1 mutations, as the role of SOD1 in sALS remains unclear [132]. Nevertheless, some mechanisms contributing to SOD1 toxicity, such as ER stress and UPR, are likely to be implicated in a broad range of ALS cases, providing opportunities for largely applicable treatments.

5. Selective neuronal vulnerability in non-SOD1 ALS and other motoneuron diseases

Most of the studies described in this chapter have used the SOD1 mouse model to explore the selective vulnerability of MNs in ALS [13]. The pattern on MN vulnerability in ALS patients is still a matter of speculation. At the late stage of the disease, there is a dramatic degeneration of the MNs throughout the spinal cord. However, as the access to *post-mortem* tissue at various stages of the disease is obviously limited, it has not been possible to precisely determine how the ALS pathology affects the different subtypes of MNs in patients. Nevertheless, the preservation of the oculomotor and Onuf's nuclei in ALS patients has been confirmed by histological analysis [133].

It is also likely that differences exist between familial and sALS, as well as between the different genetic forms of ALS. This may also reduce the efficacy of therapies tested in the SOD1 model. SOD1 mutations are the cause of ALS only in a small fraction of the patients. In addition, the SOD1 pathology does not appear to be associated with Frontotemporal-Lobar degeneration, which is linked with other forms of ALS (FTLD-ALS) [134]. Therefore, there is an urgent need for other models of ALS to develop therapies better adapted to the different forms of the disease. During the past 10 years, genetic studies have identified ALS-causing mutations in several genes mainly involved in RNA metabolism, such as FUS, TARDBP and C9ORF72. FUS and TARDBP represent around 3 and 5% of fALS, respectively, whereas C9ORF72 cases are more prevalent and cover 30—50% of fALS as well as 5—7% of sALS [134]. Moreover, these genes have been found mutated in both ALS and FTLD-ALS patients, and TDP-43 positive inclusions are observed in non-SOD1 ALS patients [134]. Several research groups have generated rodents either overexpressing mutated forms of these genes or carrying gene deletions, with the objective to model the ALS pathology. Overall, the current rodent models for TDP-43-ALS or FUS-ALS display relatively mild MN degeneration. Axonal degeneration has been seen in the transgenic TDP-43 rat model, which seems to selectively affect the largest MNs [135]. This observation suggests that selective vulnerability is also likely to occur in the TDP-43 pathology.

Recently, more emphasis has been placed on modeling C9ORF72-ALS. Mouse lines generated with a bacterial artificial chromosome carrying a pathogenic hexanucleotide expansion in the full human C9ORF72 gene did not develop any behavioral symptoms in two independent studies [136, 137]. By contrast, using AAV vectors to express the G4C2 repeat expansion in the mouse CNS led to both histological and behavioral defects similar to the pathology observed in C9ORF72-ALS/FTLD patients [138]. Although 20% of neuron death was measured in the cortex, motor cortex and cerebellum of these mice, the number of spinal cord MNs was not reported. With the continuous development of ALS models, it will hopefully be possible to more accurately design therapeutic approaches against pathogenic pathways that may be common to different forms of ALS.

The recent development of mouse and human ES and iPS cells could provide an alternative to *in vivo* models. Several hundred lines with various mutations have been generated and are publicly available. In the context of SOD1, these models have been used to explore the non-cell autonomous pathogenic mechanisms. Survival of mES- or hES-derived MNs is decreased when the cells are grown on astrocytes differentiated from SOD1 or sporadic-ALS induced neural progenitors [76, 132]. MNs derived from patients carrying the C9ORF72 repeats display typical histopathological features, such as nuclear foci and the non-ATG translation of peptides encoded by the hexanucleotide repeats [139]. Remarkably, these neurons have an increased susceptibility to glutamate excitotoxicity. FUS, SOD1 and C9ORF72 ALS-derived MNs show electrophysiological abnormalities [140]. This technology presents the advantage to model a larger portion of ALS cases, allowing for comparative gene expression profiling experiments and testing of therapeutic compounds. However, it remains difficult to study the selective vulnerability of MN subtypes in such *in vitro* models, as they fail to replicate the differentiation into cellular subtypes and the precise architecture of the CNS tissue.

Lately, the transcriptome of the cerebellum and frontal cortex was analyzed *post mortem* in samples from C9ORF72-ALS and sALS patients [141]. The results show a prominent dysregulation of genes involved in the UPR and intracellular protein transport machinery in C9ORF72-ALS. In sALS, it is the genes involved in cytoskeleton organization and synaptic transmission, which are most affected. One should keep in mind that these molecular changes reflect only the late stage of the disease and in the future, it will be important to also access spinal cord tissue to perform similar transcriptome analysis.

More generally, it is tempting to speculate that the selective MN vulnerability observed in ALS may also apply to other MN disorders, such as spinal muscular atrophy (SMA) and Charcot-Marie-Tooth (CMT) diseases. In SMA patients, muscle biopsies show atrophy of the type II muscle fibers, with a compensatory hypertrophy of the type I fibers [142]. Moreover, the Onuf's nucleus is preserved, even in the most severely affected SMA type I patients. Even though atrophy is restricted to certain muscles in mouse models of the disease, it does not seem to be related to muscle fiber type or NMJ size [143]. However, the large size MNs innervating the proximal forelimb and axial muscles are specifically lost in presymptomatic Δ7 SMN mice [144]. This last observation could indicate a preferential vulnerability of some MN subtypes, although this will need to be confirmed with more specific markers to identify the FF or S MNs.

CMT is a heterogeneous group of genetic diseases affecting motor and/or sensory functions. Several genes have been identified linked to demyelinating CMT (CMT1) or axonal CMT (CMT2). Among the CMT2 cases, 20% are caused by mutations in the MFN2 gene encoding mitofusin 2 and are referred as CMT2A [145]. Several observations indicate a pattern of neurodegeneration, which may be very different from ALS. Biopsies of the *tibialis anterior* in CMT1 and CMT2 patients show atrophy of the type IIa muscle fibers and hypertrophy of the type I fibers [146]. Furthermore, in the late-onset CMT2A patients, the *soleus* muscle is affected before, and more severely than other leg muscles, including the *gastrocnemius* [147]. Few mouse models of CMT2 have been generated and are currently being studied. CMT2A mice based on the overexpression of $MFN2^{R94Q}$ develop motor deficits correlating with an overabundance of small axonal fibers in the sciatic nerve [148]. Further studies will be needed to characterize how CMT2A affects different subtypes of muscle fibers and MN populations, and leads to the observed neuromuscular impairments.

6. Conclusions

The identification of ALS-causing mutations in the SOD1 gene in 1993 has raised hopes in the ALS scientific community [10]. One year later, Gurney *et al.* [8] generated the well-known $SOD1^{G93A}$ mouse model, which reproduced most of the ALS features, and opened the way for exploring the causes of the disease and developing therapies. However, the challenge turned out to be more difficult than expected. Indeed, more than 20 years later, the identification of therapeutic targets in the mSOD1 mouse model has failed to bring any effective treatment to ALS patients.

Nevertheless, the characterization of mouse models overexpressing mutant forms of SOD1 has dramatically improved our understanding of the cellular processes leading to ALS. In particular, the very reproducible course of the disease observed in these mice has been instrumental to study the different stages of the disease, highlighting the fact that not all MNs are equally affected, and that glial cells are important actors in the pathogenic process. Recently, several research groups have identified critical factors, which determine MN vulnerability, providing novel targets for therapeutic intervention. One obvious difficulty in designing treatments for ALS is that at a given stage of the disease, the various pools of MNs or glial cells may face different toxic mechanisms, depending on their intrinsic vulnerability. This may limit the therapeutic efficacy of a single drug.

It remains unknown whether the observed MN vulnerability pattern is specific to mSOD1, and if the identified molecular mechanisms can be applied to other forms of ALS. To address this question, it is critical to further develop animal and cellular models of ALS, based on the genes, which have recently been linked to the disease. By comparing these models, it will be possible to pinpoint common pathogenic pathways, and with the development of more specific biomarkers, apply therapies when and where they are the most likely to succeed.

Acknowledgements

This work was supported by the Swiss National Science Foundation (Grant 310030L_156460) and by ERANET E-Rare FaSMALS (Grant 31ER30_160673). NBM is supported by the Neuromuscular Research Association Basel (NeRAB).

Author details

Cylia Rochat, Nathalie Bernard-Marissal and Bernard L. Schneider*

*Address all correspondence to: bernard.schneider@epfl.ch

Brain Mind Institute, Ecole polytechnique fédérale de Lausanne (EPFL), Lausanne, Switzerland

References

[1] Kihira T, Yoshida S, Yoshimasu F, Wakayama I, Yase Y. Involvement of Onuf's nucleus in amyotrophic lateral sclerosis. J Neurol Sci. 1997;147(1):81–8.

[2] Kanning KC, Kaplan A, Henderson CE. Motor neuron diversity in development and disease. Annu Rev Neurosci. 2010;33:409–40.

[3] Frey D, Schneider C, Xu L, Borg J, Spooren W, Caroni P. Early and selective loss of neuromuscular synapse subtypes with low sprouting competence in motoneuron diseases. J Neurosci. 2000;20(7):2534–42.

[4] Pun S, Santos AF, Saxena S, Xu L, Caroni P. Selective vulnerability and pruning of phasic motoneuron axons in motoneuron disease alleviated by CNTF. Nat Neurosci. 2006;9(3):408–19.

[5] Burke RE, Levine DN, Tsairis P, Zajac FE, 3rd. Physiological types and histochemical profiles in motor units of the cat gastrocnemius. J Physiol. 1973;234(3):723–48.

[6] Cullheim S, Fleshman JW, Glenn LL, Burke RE. Membrane area and dendritic structure in type-identified triceps surae alpha motoneurons. J Comp Neurol. 1987;255(1):68–81.

[7] Saxena S, Roselli F, Singh K, Leptien K, Julien JP, Gros-Louis F, et al. Neuroprotection through excitability and mTOR required in ALS motoneurons to delay disease and extend survival. Neuron. 2013;80(1):80–96.

[8] Gurney ME, Pu H, Chiu AY, Dal Canto MC, Polchow CY, Alexander DD, et al. Motor neuron degeneration in mice that express a human Cu,Zn superoxide dismutase mutation. Science. 1994;264(5166):1772–5.

[9] Nagai M, Re DB, Nagata T, Chalazonitis A, Jessell TM, Wichterle H, et al. Astrocytes expressing ALS-linked mutated SOD1 release factors selectively toxic to motor neurons. Nat Neurosci. 2007;10(5):615–22.

[10] Rosen DR, Siddique T, Patterson D, Figlewicz DA, Sapp P, Hentati A, et al. Mutations in Cu/Zn superoxide dismutase gene are associated with familial amyotrophic lateral sclerosis. Nature. 1993;362(6415):59–62.

[11] van Zundert B, Peuscher MH, Hynynen M, Chen A, Neve RL, Brown RH, Jr., et al. Neonatal neuronal circuitry shows hyperexcitable disturbance in a mouse model of the adult-onset neurodegenerative disease amyotrophic lateral sclerosis. J Neurosci. 2008;28(43):10864–74.

[12] Wooley CF. The US Army Center for Cardiovascular Diseases, 1918 US Army General Hospital No. 9, Lakewood, NJ. Am Heart Hosp J. 2005;3(2):118–9.

[13] Saxena S, Cabuy E, Caroni P. A role for motoneuron subtype-selective ER stress in disease manifestations of FALS mice. Nat Neurosci. 2009;12(5):627–36.

[14] Fischer LR, Culver DG, Tennant P, Davis AA, Wang M, Castellano-Sanchez A, et al. Amyotrophic lateral sclerosis is a distal axonopathy: evidence in mice and man. Exp Neurol. 2004;185(2):232–40.

[15] Chiu AY, Zhai P, Dal Canto MC, Peters TM, Kwon YW, Prattis SM, et al. Age-dependent penetrance of disease in a transgenic mouse model of familial amyotrophic lateral sclerosis. Mol Cell Neurosci. 1995;6(4):349–62.

[16] Nave KA. Myelination and support of axonal integrity by glia. Nature. 2010;468(7321): 244–52.

[17] Kennel PF, Finiels F, Revah F, Mallet J. Neuromuscular function impairment is not caused by motor neurone loss in FALS mice: an electromyographic study. Neuroreport. 1996;7(8):1427–31.

[18] Hegedus J, Putman CT, Gordon T. Time course of preferential motor unit loss in the SOD1 G93A mouse model of amyotrophic lateral sclerosis. Neurobiol Dis. 2007;28(2): 154–64.

[19] Azzouz M, Leclerc N, Gurney M, Warter JM, Poindron P, Borg J. Progressive motor neuron impairment in an animal model of familial amyotrophic lateral sclerosis. Muscle Nerve. 1997;20(1):45–51.

[20] Schaefer AM, Sanes JR, Lichtman JW. A compensatory subpopulation of motor neurons in a mouse model of amyotrophic lateral sclerosis. J Comp Neurol. 2005;490(3):209–19.

[21] Rosler KM, Truffert A, Hess CW, Magistris MR. Quantification of upper motor neuron loss in amyotrophic lateral sclerosis. Clin Neurophysiol. 2000;111(12):2208–18.

[22] Stewart HG, Andersen PM, Eisen A, Weber M. Corticomotoneuronal dysfunction in ALS patients with different SOD1 mutations. Clin Neurophysiol. 2006;117(8):1850–61.

[23] Ozdinler PH, Benn S, Yamamoto TH, Guzel M, Brown RH, Jr., Macklis JD. Corticospinal motor neurons and related subcerebral projection neurons undergo early and specific neurodegeneration in hSOD1G(9)(3)A transgenic ALS mice. J Neurosci. 2011;31(11): 4166–77.

[24] Jara JH, Villa SR, Khan NA, Bohn MC, Ozdinler PH. AAV2 mediated retrograde transduction of corticospinal motor neurons reveals initial and selective apical dendrite degeneration in ALS. Neurobiol Dis. 2012;47(2):174–83.

[25] Zang DW, Cheema SS. Degeneration of corticospinal and bulbospinal systems in the superoxide dismutase 1(G93A G1H) transgenic mouse model of familial amyotrophic lateral sclerosis. Neurosci Lett. 2002;332(2):99–102.

[26] Urushitani M, Sik A, Sakurai T, Nukina N, Takahashi R, Julien JP. Chromogranin-mediated secretion of mutant superoxide dismutase proteins linked to amyotrophic lateral sclerosis. Nat Neurosci. 2006;9(1):108–18.

[27] Yasvoina MV, Genc B, Jara JH, Sheets PL, Quinlan KA, Milosevic A, et al. eGFP expression under UCHL1 promoter genetically labels corticospinal motor neurons and a subpopulation of degeneration-resistant spinal motor neurons in an ALS mouse model. J Neurosci. 2013;33(18):7890–904.

[28] Genc B, Lagrimas AK, Kuru P, Hess R, Tu MW, Menichella DM, et al. Visualization of sensory neurons and their projections in an upper motor neuron reporter line. PLoS One. 2015;10(7):e0132815.

[29] Gautam M, Jara JH, Sekerkova G, Yasvoina MV, Martina M, Ozdinler PH. Absence of alsin function leads to corticospinal motor neuron vulnerability via novel disease mechanisms. Hum Mol Genet. 2016.

[30] Jara JH, Genc B, Cox GA, Bohn MC, Roos RP, Macklis JD, et al. Corticospinal motor neurons are susceptible to increased ER stress and display profound degeneration in the absence of UCHL1 function. Cereb Cortex. 2015;25(11):4259–72.

[31] Thomsen GM, Gowing G, Latter J, Chen M, Vit JP, Staggenborg K, et al. Delayed disease onset and extended survival in the SOD1G93A rat model of amyotrophic lateral sclerosis after suppression of mutant SOD1 in the motor cortex. J Neurosci. 2014;34(47): 15587–600.

[32] Sharma R, Hicks S, Berna CM, Kennard C, Talbot K, Turner MR. Oculomotor dysfunction in amyotrophic lateral sclerosis: a comprehensive review. Arch Neurol. 2011;68(7): 857–61.

[33] Smittkamp SE, Spalding HN, Brown JW, Gupte AA, Chen J, Nishimune H, et al. Measures of bulbar and spinal motor function, muscle innervation, and mitochondrial function in ALS rats. Behav Brain Res. 2010;211(1):48–57.

[34] Kashlan ON, Kashlan BN, Oh SS, McGinley LM, Chen KS, Kupfer R, et al. Histological Bulbar Manifestations in the ALS Rat. Neurodegener Dis. 2015;15(2):121–6.

[35] Alexianu ME, Ho BK, Mohamed AH, La Bella V, Smith RG, Appel SH. The role of calcium-binding proteins in selective motoneuron vulnerability in amyotrophic lateral sclerosis. Ann Neurol. 1994;36(6):846–58.

[36] Obal I, Engelhardt JI, Siklos L. Axotomy induces contrasting changes in calcium and calcium-binding proteins in oculomotor and hypoglossal nuclei of Balb/c mice. J Comp Neurol. 2006;499(1):17–32.

[37] Laslo P, Lipski J, Nicholson LF, Miles GB, Funk GD. Calcium binding proteins in motoneurons at low and high risk for degeneration in ALS. Neuroreport. 2000;11(15): 3305–8.

[38] Kaplan A, Spiller KJ, Towne C, Kanning KC, Choe GT, Geber A, et al. Neuronal matrix metalloproteinase-9 is a determinant of selective neurodegeneration. Neuron. 2014;81(2):333–48.

[39] Hedlund E, Karlsson M, Osborn T, Ludwig W, Isacson O. Global gene expression profiling of somatic motor neuron populations with different vulnerability identify molecules and pathways of degeneration and protection. Brain. 2010;133(Pt 8):2313–30.

[40] Comley L, Allodi I, Nichterwitz S, Nizzardo M, Simone C, Corti S, et al. Motor neurons with differential vulnerability to degeneration show distinct protein signatures in health and ALS. Neuroscience. 2015;291:216–29.

[41] Venugopal S, Hsiao CF, Sonoda T, Wiedau-Pazos M, Chandler SH. Homeostatic dysregulation in membrane properties of masticatory motoneurons compared with oculomotor neurons in a mouse model for amyotrophic lateral sclerosis. J Neurosci. 2015;35(2):707–20.

[42] Chattopadhyay M, Valentine JS. Aggregation of copper-zinc superoxide dismutase in familial and sporadic ALS. Antioxid Redox Signal. 2009;11(7):1603–14.

[43] Israelson A, Ditsworth D, Sun S, Song S, Liang J, Hruska-Plochan M, et al. Macrophage migration inhibitory factor as a chaperone inhibiting accumulation of misfolded SOD1. Neuron. 2015;86(1):218–32.

[44] Kato S, Takikawa M, Nakashima K, Hirano A, Cleveland DW, Kusaka H, et al. New consensus research on neuropathological aspects of familial amyotrophic lateral sclerosis with superoxide dismutase 1 (SOD1) gene mutations: inclusions containing

SOD1 in neurons and astrocytes. Amyotroph Lateral Scler Other Motor Neuron Disord. 2000;1(3):163–84.

[45] Forsberg K, Andersen PM, Marklund SL, Brannstrom T. Glial nuclear aggregates of superoxide dismutase-1 are regularly present in patients with amyotrophic lateral sclerosis. Acta Neuropathol. 2011;121(5):623–34.

[46] Lobsiger CS, Boillee S, Cleveland DW. Toxicity from different SOD1 mutants dysregulates the complement system and the neuronal regenerative response in ALS motor neurons. Proc Natl Acad Sci U S A. 2007;104(18):7319–26.

[47] Gros-Louis F, Soucy G, Lariviere R, Julien JP. Intracerebroventricular infusion of monoclonal antibody or its derived Fab fragment against misfolded forms of SOD1 mutant delays mortality in a mouse model of ALS. J Neurochem. 2010;113(5):1188–99.

[48] Bernard-Marissal N, Moumen A, Sunyach C, Pellegrino C, Dudley K, Henderson CE, et al. Reduced calreticulin levels link endoplasmic reticulum stress and Fas-triggered cell death in motoneurons vulnerable to ALS. J Neurosci. 2012;32(14):4901–12.

[49] Bernard-Marissal N, Sunyach C, Marissal T, Raoul C, Pettmann B. Calreticulin levels determine onset of early muscle denervation by fast motoneurons of ALS model mice. Neurobiol Dis. 2015;73:130–6.

[50] Filezac de L'Etang A, Maharjan N, Cordeiro Brana M, Ruegsegger C, Rehmann R, Goswami A, et al. Marinesco-Sjogren syndrome protein SIL1 regulates motor neuron subtype-selective ER stress in ALS. Nat Neurosci. 2015;18(2):227–38.

[51] Dobrowolny G, Aucello M, Molinaro M, Musaro A. Local expression of mIgf-1 modulates ubiquitin, caspase and CDK5 expression in skeletal muscle of an ALS mouse model. Neurol Res. 2008;30(2):131–6.

[52] Millers EK, Masci PP, Lavin MF, de Jersey J, Guddat LW. Crystallization and preliminary X-ray analysis of a Kunitz-type inhibitor, textilinin-1 from Pseudonaja textilis textilis. Acta Crystallogr Sect F Struct Biol Cryst Commun. 2006;62(Pt 7):642–5.

[53] Vu TH, Shipley JM, Bergers G, Berger JE, Helms JA, Hanahan D, et al. MMP-9/gelatinase B is a key regulator of growth plate angiogenesis and apoptosis of hypertrophic chondrocytes. Cell. 1998;93(3):411–22.

[54] He X, Zhang L, Yao X, Hu J, Yu L, Jia H, et al. Association studies of MMP-9 in Parkinson's disease and amyotrophic lateral sclerosis. PLoS One. 2013;8(9):e73777.

[55] Jokic D, Boudon C, Pognon G, Bonin M, Schenk KJ, Gross M, et al. Structural and binding features of cofacial bis-porphyrins with calixarene spacers: pac-man porphyrins that can chew. Chemistry. 2005;11(14):4199–209.

[56] Ruegsegger C, Maharjan N, Goswami A, Filezac de L'Etang A, Weis J, Troost D, et al. Aberrant association of misfolded SOD1 with Na(+)/K(+)ATPase-alpha3 impairs its

http://dx.doi.org/10.5772/63703

activity and contributes to motor neuron vulnerability in ALS. Acta Neuropathol. 2016;131(3):427–51.

[57] Le Masson G, Przedborski S, Abbott LF. A computational model of motor neuron degeneration. Neuron. 2014;83(4):975–88.

[58] Ilieva H, Polymenidou M, Cleveland DW. Non-cell autonomous toxicity in neurodegenerative disorders: ALS and beyond. J Cell Biol. 2009;187(6):761–72.

[59] Komine O, Yamanaka K. Neuroinflammation in motor neuron disease. Nagoya J Med Sci. 2015;77(4):537–49.

[60] Jaarsma D, Teuling E, Haasdijk ED, De Zeeuw CI, Hoogenraad CC. Neuron-specific expression of mutant superoxide dismutase is sufficient to induce amyotrophic lateral sclerosis in transgenic mice. J Neurosci. 2008;28(9):2075–88.

[61] Lino MM, Schneider C, Caroni P. Accumulation of SOD1 mutants in postnatal motoneurons does not cause motoneuron pathology or motoneuron disease. J Neurosci. 2002;22(12):4825–32.

[62] Pramatarova A, Laganiere J, Roussel J, Brisebois K, Rouleau GA. Neuron-specific expression of mutant superoxide dismutase 1 in transgenic mice does not lead to motor impairment. J Neurosci. 2001;21(10):3369–74.

[63] Beers DR, Henkel JS, Xiao Q, Zhao W, Wang J, Yen AA, et al. Wild-type microglia extend survival in PU.1 knockout mice with familial amyotrophic lateral sclerosis. Proc Natl Acad Sci U S A. 2006;103(43):16021–6.

[64] Gong YH, Parsadanian AS, Andreeva A, Snider WD, Elliott JL. Restricted expression of G86R Cu/Zn superoxide dismutase in astrocytes results in astrocytosis but does not cause motoneuron degeneration. J Neurosci. 2000;20(2):660–5.

[65] Kang SH, Li Y, Fukaya M, Lorenzini I, Cleveland DW, Ostrow LW, et al. Degeneration and impaired regeneration of gray matter oligodendrocytes in amyotrophic lateral sclerosis. Nat Neurosci. 2013;16(5):571–9.

[66] Yamanaka K, Boillee S, Roberts EA, Garcia ML, McAlonis-Downes M, Mikse OR, et al. Mutant SOD1 in cell types other than motor neurons and oligodendrocytes accelerates onset of disease in ALS mice. Proc Natl Acad Sci U S A. 2008;105(21):7594–9.

[67] Boillee S, Yamanaka K, Lobsiger CS, Copeland NG, Jenkins NA, Kassiotis G, et al. Onset and progression in inherited ALS determined by motor neurons and microglia. Science. 2006;312(5778):1389–92.

[68] Dirren E, Aebischer J, Rochat C, Towne C, Schneider BL, Aebischer P. SOD1 silencing in motoneurons or glia rescues neuromuscular function in ALS mice. Ann Clin Transl Neurol. 2015;2(2):167–84.

[69] Sun S, Sun Y, Ling SC, Ferraiuolo L, McAlonis-Downes M, Zou Y, et al. Translational profiling identifies a cascade of damage initiated in motor neurons and spreading to

glia in mutant SOD1-mediated ALS. Proc Natl Acad Sci U S A. 2015;112(50):E6993–7002.

[70] Heiman M, Schaefer A, Gong S, Peterson JD, Day M, Ramsey KE, et al. A translational profiling approach for the molecular characterization of CNS cell types. Cell. 2008;135(4):738–48.

[71] Nave KA. Myelination and the trophic support of long axons. Nat Rev Neurosci. 2010;11(4):275–83.

[72] Philips T, Bento-Abreu A, Nonneman A, Haeck W, Staats K, Geelen V, et al. Oligodendrocyte dysfunction in the pathogenesis of amyotrophic lateral sclerosis. Brain. 2013;136(Pt 2):471–82.

[73] Lee Y, Morrison BM, Li Y, Lengacher S, Farah MH, Hoffman PN, et al. Oligodendroglia metabolically support axons and contribute to neurodegeneration. Nature. 2012;487(7408):443–8.

[74] Ferraiuolo L, Higginbottom A, Heath PR, Barber S, Greenald D, Kirby J, et al. Dysregulation of astrocyte-motoneuron cross-talk in mutant superoxide dismutase 1-related amyotrophic lateral sclerosis. Brain. 2011;134(Pt 9):2627–41.

[75] Meyer K, Ferraiuolo L, Miranda CJ, Likhite S, McElroy S, Renusch S, et al. Direct conversion of patient fibroblasts demonstrates non-cell autonomous toxicity of astrocytes to motor neurons in familial and sporadic ALS. Proc Natl Acad Sci U S A. 2014;111(2):829–32.

[76] Haidet-Phillips AM, Hester ME, Miranda CJ, Meyer K, Braun L, Frakes A, et al. Astrocytes from familial and sporadic ALS patients are toxic to motor neurons. Nat Biotechnol. 2011;29(9):824–8.

[77] King AE, Woodhouse A, Kirkcaldie MT, Vickers JC. Excitotoxicity in ALS: overstimulation, or overreaction? Exp Neurol. 2016;275 Pt 1:162–71.

[78] Fray AE, Ince PG, Banner SJ, Milton ID, Usher PA, Cookson MR, et al. The expression of the glial glutamate transporter protein EAAT2 in motor neuron disease: an immunohistochemical study. Eur J Neurosci. 1998;10(8):2481–9.

[79] Rothstein JD. Excitotoxicity and neurodegeneration in amyotrophic lateral sclerosis. Clin Neurosci. 1995;3(6):348–59.

[80] Sasaki S, Komori T, Iwata M. Excitatory amino acid transporter 1 and 2 immunoreactivity in the spinal cord in amyotrophic lateral sclerosis. Acta Neuropathol. 2000;100(2):138–44.

[81] Jaiswal MK. Selective vulnerability of motoneuron and perturbed mitochondrial calcium homeostasis in amyotrophic lateral sclerosis: implications for motoneurons specific calcium dysregulation. Mol Cell Ther. 2014;2:26.

[82] Aebischer J, Bernard-Marissal N, Pettmann B, Raoul C. Death receptors in the selective degeneration of motoneurons in amyotrophic lateral sclerosis. J Neurodegener Dis. 2013;2013:746845.

[83] Aebischer J, Cassina P, Otsmane B, Moumen A, Seilhean D, Meininger V, et al. IFNgamma triggers a LIGHT-dependent selective death of motoneurons contributing to the non-cell-autonomous effects of mutant SOD1. Cell Death Differ. 2011;18(5):754–68.

[84] Grad LI, Guest WC, Yanai A, Pokrishevsky E, O'Neill MA, Gibbs E, et al. Intermolecular transmission of superoxide dismutase 1 misfolding in living cells. Proc Natl Acad Sci U S A. 2011;108(39):16398–403.

[85] Munch C, O'Brien J, Bertolotti A. Prion-like propagation of mutant superoxide dismutase-1 misfolding in neuronal cells. Proc Natl Acad Sci U S A. 2011;108(9):3548–53.

[86] Chia R, Tattum MH, Jones S, Collinge J, Fisher EM, Jackson GS. Superoxide dismutase 1 and tgSOD1 mouse spinal cord seed fibrils, suggesting a propagative cell death mechanism in amyotrophic lateral sclerosis. PLoS One. 2010;5(5):e10627.

[87] Graffmo KS, Forsberg K, Bergh J, Birve A, Zetterstrom P, Andersen PM, et al. Expression of wild-type human superoxide dismutase-1 in mice causes amyotrophic lateral sclerosis. Hum Mol Genet. 2013;22(1):51–60.

[88] Grad LI, Fernando SM, Cashman NR. From molecule to molecule and cell to cell: prion-like mechanisms in amyotrophic lateral sclerosis. Neurobiol Dis. 2015;77:257–65.

[89] Grad LI, Yerbury JJ, Turner BJ, Guest WC, Pokrishevsky E, O'Neill MA, et al. Intercellular propagated misfolding of wild-type Cu/Zn superoxide dismutase occurs via exosome-dependent and -independent mechanisms. Proc Natl Acad Sci U S A. 2014;111(9):3620–5.

[90] Basso M, Pozzi S, Tortarolo M, Fiordaliso F, Bisighini C, Pasetto L, et al. Mutant copper-zinc superoxide dismutase (SOD1) induces protein secretion pathway alterations and exosome release in astrocytes: implications for disease spreading and motor neuron pathology in amyotrophic lateral sclerosis. J Biol Chem. 2013;288(22):15699–711.

[91] Ezzi SA, Lariviere R, Urushitani M, Julien JP. Neuronal over-expression of chromogranin A accelerates disease onset in a mouse model of ALS. J Neurochem. 2010;115(5):1102–11.

[92] Zhao W, Beers DR, Henkel JS, Zhang W, Urushitani M, Julien JP, et al. Extracellular mutant SOD1 induces microglial-mediated motoneuron injury. Glia. 2010;58(2):231–43.

[93] Lobsiger CS, Boillee S, McAlonis-Downes M, Khan AM, Feltri ML, Yamanaka K, et al. Schwann cells expressing dismutase active mutant SOD1 unexpectedly slow disease progression in ALS mice. Proc Natl Acad Sci U S A. 2009;106(11):4465–70.

[94] Balice-Gordon RJ. Dynamic roles at the neuromuscular junction. Schwann cells. Curr Biol. 1996;6(9):1054–6.

[95] Pasterkamp RJ, Giger RJ. Semaphorin function in neural plasticity and disease. Curr Opin Neurobiol. 2009;19(3):263–74.

[96] Duchen LW. Changes in motor innervation and cholinesterase localization induced by botulinum toxin in skeletal muscle of the mouse: differences between fast and slow muscles. J Neurol Neurosurg Psychiatry. 1970;33(1):40–54.

[97] De Winter F, Vo T, Stam FJ, Wisman LA, Bar PR, Niclou SP, et al. The expression of the chemorepellent Semaphorin 3A is selectively induced in terminal Schwann cells of a subset of neuromuscular synapses that display limited anatomical plasticity and enhanced vulnerability in motor neuron disease. Mol Cell Neurosci. 2006;32(1–2):102–17.

[98] Venkova K, Christov A, Kamaluddin Z, Kobalka P, Siddiqui S, Hensley K. Semaphorin 3A signaling through neuropilin-1 is an early trigger for distal axonopathy in the SOD1G93A mouse model of amyotrophic lateral sclerosis. J Neuropathol Exp Neurol. 2014;73(7):702–13.

[99] Korner S, Boselt S, Wichmann K, Thau-Habermann N, Zapf A, Knippenberg S, et al. The axon guidance protein semaphorin 3A is increased in the motor cortex of patients with amyotrophic lateral sclerosis. J Neuropathol Exp Neurol. 2016.

[100] Loeffler JP, Picchiarelli G, Dupuis L, Gonzalez De Aguilar JL. The role of skeletal muscle in amyotrophic lateral sclerosis. Brain Pathol. 2016.

[101] Towne C, Raoul C, Schneider BL, Aebischer P. Systemic AAV6 delivery mediating RNA interference against SOD1: neuromuscular transduction does not alter disease progression in fALS mice. Mol Ther. 2008;16(6):1018–25.

[102] Miller TM, Kim SH, Yamanaka K, Hester M, Umapathi P, Arnson H, et al. Gene transfer demonstrates that muscle is not a primary target for non-cell-autonomous toxicity in familial amyotrophic lateral sclerosis. Proc Natl Acad Sci U S A. 2006;103(51):19546–51.

[103] Jokic N, Gonzalez de Aguilar JL, Pradat PF, Dupuis L, Echaniz-Laguna A, Muller A, et al. Nogo expression in muscle correlates with amyotrophic lateral sclerosis severity. Ann Neurol. 2005;57(4):553–6.

[104] Bruneteau G, Bauche S, Gonzalez de Aguilar JL, Brochier G, Mandjee N, Tanguy ML, et al. Endplate denervation correlates with Nogo-A muscle expression in amyotrophic lateral sclerosis patients. Ann Clin Transl Neurol. 2015;2(4):362–72.

[105] Jokic N, Gonzalez de Aguilar JL, Dimou L, Lin S, Fergani A, Ruegg MA, et al. The neurite outgrowth inhibitor Nogo-A promotes denervation in an amyotrophic lateral sclerosis model. EMBO Rep. 2006;7(11):1162–7.

[106] Simonen M, Pedersen V, Weinmann O, Schnell L, Buss A, Ledermann B, et al. Systemic deletion of the myelin-associated outgrowth inhibitor Nogo-A improves regenerative and plastic responses after spinal cord injury. Neuron. 2003;38(2):201–11.

[107] Bros-Facer V, Krull D, Taylor A, Dick JR, Bates SA, Cleveland MS, et al. Treatment with an antibody directed against Nogo-A delays disease progression in the SOD1G93A mouse model of Amyotrophic lateral sclerosis. Hum Mol Genet. 2014;23(16):4187–200.

[108] Meininger V, Pradat PF, Corse A, Al-Sarraj S, Rix Brooks B, Caress JB, et al. Safety, pharmacokinetic, and functional effects of the nogo-a monoclonal antibody in amyotrophic lateral sclerosis: a randomized, first-in-human clinical trial. PLoS One. 2014;9(5):e97803.

[109] Yagi K, Kitazato KT, Uno M, Tada Y, Kinouchi T, Shimada K, et al. Edaravone, a free radical scavenger, inhibits MMP-9-related brain hemorrhage in rats treated with tissue plasminogen activator. Stroke. 2009;40(2):626–31.

[110] Ito H, Wate R, Zhang J, Ohnishi S, Kaneko S, Ito H, et al. Treatment with edaravone, initiated at symptom onset, slows motor decline and decreases SOD1 deposition in ALS mice. Exp Neurol. 2008;213(2):448–55.

[111] Aoki M, Warita H, Mizuno H, Suzuki N, Yuki S, Itoyama Y. Feasibility study for functional test battery of SOD transgenic rat (H46R) and evaluation of edaravone, a free radical scavenger. Brain Res. 2011;1382:321–5.

[112] Ikeda K, Iwasaki Y. Edaravone. A free radical scavenger, delayed symptomatic and pathological progression of motor neuron disease in the Wobbler mouse. PLoS One. 2015;10(10):e0140316.

[113] Abe K, Itoyama Y, Sobue G, Tsuji S, Aoki M, Doyu M, et al. Confirmatory double-blind, parallel-group, placebo-controlled study of efficacy and safety of edaravone (MCI-186) in amyotrophic lateral sclerosis patients. Amyotroph Lateral Scler Frontotemporal Degener. 2014;15(7–8):610–7.

[114] Saxena S, Caroni P. Selective neuronal vulnerability in neurodegenerative diseases: from stressor thresholds to degeneration. Neuron. 2011;71(1):35–48.

[115] Boyce M, Bryant KF, Jousse C, Long K, Harding HP, Scheuner D, et al. A selective inhibitor of eIF2alpha dephosphorylation protects cells from ER stress. Science. 2005;307(5711):935–9.

[116] Costa-Mattioli M, Gobert D, Stern E, Gamache K, Colina R, Cuello C, et al. eIF2alpha phosphorylation bidirectionally regulates the switch from short- to long-term synaptic plasticity and memory. Cell. 2007;129(1):195–206.

[117] Vieira FG, Ping Q, Moreno AJ, Kidd JD, Thompson K, Jiang B, et al. Guanabenz treatment accelerates disease in a mutant SOD1 mouse model of ALS. PLoS One. 2015;10(8):e0135570.

[118] Wang L, Popko B, Tixier E, Roos RP. Guanabenz, which enhances the unfolded protein response, ameliorates mutant SOD1-induced amyotrophic lateral sclerosis. Neurobiol Dis. 2014;71:317–24.

[119] Kayatekin C, Zitzewitz JA, Matthews CR. Zinc binding modulates the entire folding free energy surface of human Cu,Zn superoxide dismutase. J Mol Biol. 2008;384(2):540–55.

[120] Trumbull KA, Beckman JS. A role for copper in the toxicity of zinc-deficient superoxide dismutase to motor neurons in amyotrophic lateral sclerosis. Antioxid Redox Signal. 2009;11(7):1627–39.

[121] McAllum EJ, Lim NK, Hickey JL, Paterson BM, Donnelly PS, Li QX, et al. Therapeutic effects of CuII(atsm) in the SOD1-G37R mouse model of amyotrophic lateral sclerosis. Amyotroph Lateral Scler Frontotemporal Degener. 2013;14(7–8):586–90.

[122] Roberts BR, Lim NK, McAllum EJ, Donnelly PS, Hare DJ, Doble PA, et al. Oral treatment with Cu(II)(atsm) increases mutant SOD1 in vivo but protects motor neurons and improves the phenotype of a transgenic mouse model of amyotrophic lateral sclerosis. J Neurosci. 2014;34(23):8021–31.

[123] Williams JR, Trias E, Beilby PR, Lopez NI, Labut EM, Bradford CS, et al. Copper delivery to the CNS by CuATSM effectively treats motor neuron disease in SOD mice co-expressing the Copper-Chaperone-for-SOD. Neurobiol Dis. 2016;89:1–9.

[124] Liu HN, Tjostheim S, Dasilva K, Taylor D, Zhao B, Rakhit R, et al. Targeting of monomer/misfolded SOD1 as a therapeutic strategy for amyotrophic lateral sclerosis. J Neurosci. 2012;32(26):8791–9.

[125] Patel P, Kriz J, Gravel M, Soucy G, Bareil C, Gravel C, et al. Adeno-associated virus-mediated delivery of a recombinant single-chain antibody against misfolded superoxide dismutase for treatment of amyotrophic lateral sclerosis. Mol Ther. 2014;22(3):498–510.

[126] Turner BJ, Talbot K. Transgenics, toxicity and therapeutics in rodent models of mutant SOD1-mediated familial ALS. Prog Neurobiol. 2008;85(1):94–134.

[127] Foust KD, Salazar DL, Likhite S, Ferraiuolo L, Ditsworth D, Ilieva H, et al. Therapeutic AAV9-mediated suppression of mutant SOD1 slows disease progression and extends survival in models of inherited ALS. Mol Ther. 2013;21(12):2148–59.

[128] Ralph GS, Radcliffe PA, Day DM, Carthy JM, Leroux MA, Lee DC, et al. Silencing mutant SOD1 using RNAi protects against neurodegeneration and extends survival in an ALS model. Nat Med. 2005;11(4):429–33.

[129] Raoul C, Abbas-Terki T, Bensadoun JC, Guillot S, Haase G, Szulc J, et al. Lentiviral-mediated silencing of SOD1 through RNA interference retards disease onset and progression in a mouse model of ALS. Nat Med. 2005;11(4):423–8.

[130] Wang H, Yang B, Qiu L, Yang C, Kramer J, Su Q, et al. Widespread spinal cord transduction by intrathecal injection of rAAV delivers efficacious RNAi therapy for amyotrophic lateral sclerosis. Hum Mol Genet. 2014;23(3):668–81.

[131] Miller TM, Pestronk A, David W, Rothstein J, Simpson E, Appel SH, et al. An antisense oligonucleotide against SOD1 delivered intrathecally for patients with SOD1 familial amyotrophic lateral sclerosis: a phase 1, randomised, first-in-man study. Lancet Neurol. 2013;12(5):435–42.

[132] Re DB, Le Verche V, Yu C, Amoroso MW, Politi KA, Phani S, et al. Necroptosis drives motor neuron death in models of both sporadic and familial ALS. Neuron. 2014;81(5): 1001–8.

[133] Mannen T, Iwata M, Toyokura Y, Nagashima K. The Onuf's nucleus and the external anal sphincter muscles in amyotrophic lateral sclerosis and Shy-Drager syndrome. Acta Neuropathol. 1982;58(4):255–60.

[134] Lattante S, Ciura S, Rouleau GA, Kabashi E. Defining the genetic connection linking amyotrophic lateral sclerosis (ALS) with frontotemporal dementia (FTD). Trends Genet. 2015;31(5):263–73.

[135] McGoldrick P, Joyce PI, Fisher EM, Greensmith L. Rodent models of amyotrophic lateral sclerosis. Biochim Biophys Acta. 2013;1832(9):1421–36.

[136] O'Rourke JG, Bogdanik L, Muhammad AK, Gendron TF, Kim KJ, Austin A, et al. C9orf72 BAC Transgenic mice display typical pathologic features of ALS/FTD. Neuron. 2015;88(5):892–901.

[137] Peters TL, Fang F, Weibull CE, Sandler DP, Kamel F, Ye W. Severe head injury and amyotrophic lateral sclerosis. Amyotroph Lateral Scler Frontotemporal Degener. 2013;14(4):267–72.

[138] Chew J, Gendron TF, Prudencio M, Sasaguri H, Zhang YJ, Castanedes-Casey M, et al. Neurodegeneration. C9ORF72 repeat expansions in mice cause TDP-43 pathology, neuronal loss, and behavioral deficits. Science. 2015;348(6239):1151–4.

[139] Donnelly CJ, Zhang PW, Pham JT, Haeusler AR, Mistry NA, Vidensky S, et al. RNA toxicity from the ALS/FTD C9ORF72 expansion is mitigated by antisense intervention. Neuron. 2013;80(2):415–28.

[140] Wainger BJ, Kiskinis E, Mellin C, Wiskow O, Han SS, Sandoe J, et al. Intrinsic membrane hyperexcitability of amyotrophic lateral sclerosis patient-derived motor neurons. Cell Rep. 2014;7(1):1–11.

[141] Prudencio M, Belzil VV, Batra R, Ross CA, Gendron TF, Pregent LJ, et al. Distinct brain transcriptome profiles in C9orf72-associated and sporadic ALS. Nat Neurosci. 2015;18(8):1175–82.

[142] Dubowitz V. Muscle disorders in childhood. Major Probl Clin Pediatr. 1978;16:iii-xiii, 1–282.

[143] Thomson SR, Nahon JE, Mutsaers CA, Thomson D, Hamilton G, Parson SH, et al. Morphological characteristics of motor neurons do not determine their relative susceptibility to degeneration in a mouse model of severe spinal muscular atrophy. PLoS One. 2012;7(12):e52605.

[144] d'Errico P, Boido M, Piras A, Valsecchi V, De Amicis E, Locatelli D, et al. Selective vulnerability of spinal and cortical motor neuron subpopulations in delta7 SMA mice. PLoS One. 2013;8(12):e82654.

[145] Feely SM, Laura M, Siskind CE, Sottile S, Davis M, Gibbons VS, et al. MFN2 mutations cause severe phenotypes in most patients with CMT2A. Neurology. 2011;76(20):1690–6.

[146] Ericson U, Ansved T, Borg K. Charcot-Marie-Tooth disease—muscle biopsy findings in relation to neurophysiology. Neuromuscul Disord. 1998;8(3–4):175–81.

[147] Chung KW, Suh BC, Shy ME, Cho SY, Yoo JH, Park SW, et al. Different clinical and magnetic resonance imaging features between Charcot-Marie-Tooth disease type 1A and 2A. Neuromuscul Disord. 2008;18(8):610–8.

[148] Cartoni R, Arnaud E, Medard JJ, Poirot O, Courvoisier DS, Chrast R, et al. Expression of mitofusin 2(R94Q) in a transgenic mouse leads to Charcot-Marie-Tooth neuropathy type 2A. Brain. 2010;133(Pt 5):1460–9.

Chapter 10

Neuronal Intermediate Filaments in Amyotrophic Lateral Sclerosis

Philippe Codron, Julien Cassereau, Joël Eyer and Franck Letournel

Additional information is available at the end of the chapter

http://dx.doi.org/10.5772/63161

Abstract

Neuronal intermediate filaments (NIFs) are the most abundant cytoskeletal element in mature neurons. They are composed of different protein subunits encoded by separate genes such as neurofilament light chain (NFL), neurofilament medium chain (NFM), neurofilament heavy chain (NFH), α-internexin and peripherin. NIFs are dynamic structures playing important functions in cell architecture and differentiation, interactions between proteins or subcellular organelles, and in axonal calibre determination and myelination. Consequently, their presence modulates electrophysiological properties of axons. NIFs have long been assigned a role in the pathogenesis of amyotrophic lateral sclerosis (ALS). Indeed, accumulation and abnormal phosphorylation of NIF subunits in motor neuron are one of the major pathological features in both sporadic and familial forms of the disease. Moreover, mutations in the NFH and peripherin genes and elevated cerebrospinal fluid NIF levels reported in ALS cases, associated with studies in transgenic mice, provided the evidence that primary defects in NIFs could be causative for motor neuron disease. However, the processes leading to the NIF abnormalities and the links to the pathogenesis of ALS remain unclear, leaving a challenging open field for further investigations in this highly disabilitating disease. Here, we review the main characteristics of these NIFs and their involvement in the pathomechanisms of ALS.

Keywords: Intermediate filaments, Neurofilaments, cytoskeleton, amyotrophic lateral sclerosis, tubulin, microtubules, axonal transport

INTECH
open science | open minds

© 2016 The Author(s). Licensee InTech. This chapter is distributed under the terms of the Creative Commons Attribution License (http://creativecommons.org/licenses/by/3.0), which permits unrestricted use, distribution, and reproduction in any medium, provided the original work is properly cited.

1. Neuronal intermediate filaments

1.1. Characteristics

Intermediate filaments (IFs) are components of the cytoskeleton, together with microtubules (MTs) and microfilaments. IFs are defined by their diameter when examined by transmission electronic microscopy (10 nm), which is intermediate between microtubules (15 nm) and microfilaments (6 nm). They also differ from these two structures by the various sizes and primary organisation of their constitutive proteins, their non-polar architecture and their relative insolubility. Intermediate filaments form a large family of proteins; they are classified into five types according to their gene organisation, size, structure and cell-type expression (**Table 1**). IFs expressed in neurons of the central and peripheral nervous systems are called neuronal intermediate filaments (NIFs) and include nestin, synemin, vimentin, α-internexin, peripherin and neurofilaments (NFs) that are composed of three subunits, neurofilament light chain (NFL), neurofilament medium chain (NFM) and neurofilament heavy chain (NFH) (for low-, medium-, and high-molecular-weight NFs) [1–5].

Neurons express differentially IF proteins depending on their developing stage and their localisation in the nervous system. While nestin, synemin and vimentin are mainly expressed during the neuronal development, NFs, peripherin and α-internexin are the main intermediate filament subunits in mature neurons from the central and peripheral nervous system [6]. In this chapter, we focus on those three subtypes of NIFs.

Type	Name	Cell/tissue
I	Acid keratins	Epithelia
II	Basic keratins	Epithelia
III	Desmin	Muscle
	GFAP	Astroglia
	Peripherin	PNS neurons
	Vimentin	Mesenchyme
IV	Neurofilaments (NFL, NFM, NFH)	PNS and CNS neurons
	α-Internexin	CNS neurons
	Nestin	CNS stem cells
V	Nuclear lamins	Nucleus

IFs found in mature neurons are NFL, NFM, NFH, peripherin and α-internexin. Abbreviations: GFAP, glial fibrillary acidic protein; CNS, central nervous system; PNS, peripheral nervous system [7].

Table 1. Classification of intermediate filaments.

1.2. Expression and post-translational modifications

Genes coding for NFL and NFM (*NEFL* and *NEFM*) are closely linked on chromosome 8 (8p21), while NFH gene (*NEFH*) is located on chromosome 22 (22q12.2) [8–10]. Peripherin is encoded

http://dx.doi.org/10.5772/63161

by *PRPH* located on chromosome 12 (q12–q13) [11], and α-internexin is encoded by *INA* located on chromosome 10 (10q24.33) [3]. As for other IFs, NFs, peripherin and α-internexin share a common tripartite structure, with non-helical amino- and carboxy-terminal regions (head and tail domains) flanking a 46-nm-long central α-helical rod domain composed of approximately 310 highly conserved amino acids [9, 10, 12] (**Figure 1**). These segments are joined by short non-helical linker sequences, aligning the individual IF subunits prior to filament assembly. While peripherin and NFL have a short-tail domain, those of NFM and NFH are longer and contain numerous KSP (Lys-Ser-Pro) repeats that can be phosphorylated on serine (S) residues. These sites are frequently modified by phosphorylation, glycosylation, nitration, oxidation and ubiquitination, which can impact NIF interactions and dynamics [6].

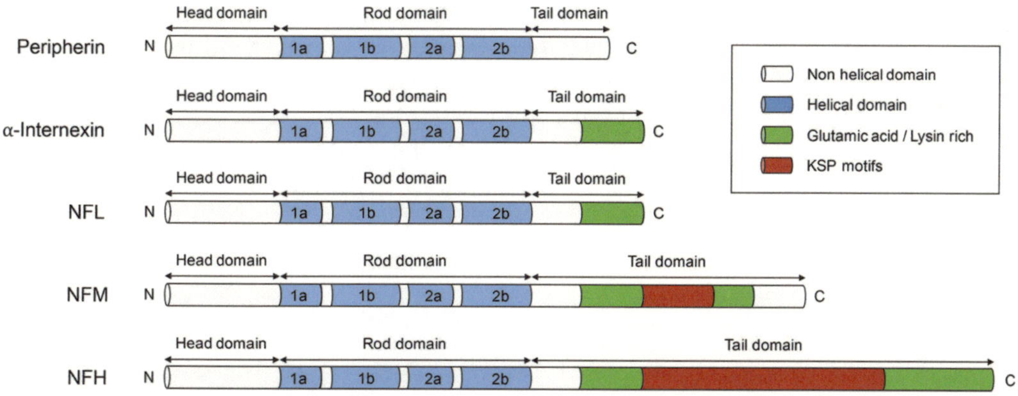

Figure 1. Schematic representation of adult neuronal IF subunits. All NIF subunits share a highly conserved central helical domain of 310 amino acid residues involved in the formation of coiled-coil structures. Flanking this central rod domain are the amino- and the carboxy-terminal domains conferring functional specificity to the different types of NIF proteins. The NFM and NFH carboxy-terminal regions contain Lys-Ser-Pro (KSP) repeats, which can be phosphorylated. Abbreviations: NF, neurofilament; NFL, NF-light; NFM, NF-medium; NFH, NF-heavy; C, carboxy-terminal; N, amino-terminal.

Multiple aspects of IF biology are regulated by their post-translational modifications. The phosphorylation state of NIF proteins depends on a dynamic balance between the activities of kinases and phosphatases. Phosphorylation of the head domain by secondary-messenger-dependent protein kinase A (PKA) and protein kinase C (PKC) prevents NIF subunits assembly or leads to the disassembly of pre-existing filaments [13, 14]. Phosphorylation of the KSP motifs on NFM and NFH tail domains by cyclin-kinase Cdk5 and microtubule-associated protein (MAP) kinase promotes the formation of cross-bridges with MTs and slows NF axonal transport [15, 16]. Phosphorylation of the head and tail domains is closely related; indeed, phosphorylation of NFM head domain by PKA reduces the phosphorylation of tail domain by MAP kinases [17]. This mechanism could be a way to protect neurons from abnormal accumulation of phosphorylated NIFs in perikarya. NIF dephosphorylation is mainly catalysed by phosphatase 2A; dephosphorylation of the head domain is necessary to allow NIF polymerization and transport into the axon, while dephosphorylation of the tail domain facilitates their interaction with other cytoskeletal proteins and their degradation [18, 19].

NIFs are also post-translationally modified by glycosylation and nitration. Glycosylation resides on attachment of *O*-linked *N*-acetyl glucosamine (O-GlcNAc) to S and threonine (T) residues; the precise function of glycosylation is still unknown, but several clues suggest a role in the NIF assembly [20]. NIF nitration is catalysed by superoxide dismutase 1 (SOD1) on tyrosine residues; the nitration of NIFs changes hydrophobic residues into negatively charged hydrophilic residues, thereby disrupting their assembly and stability.

1.3. Transport, assembly and degradation

Following their synthesis in the cell body, NIF proteins are assembled into filamentous structures and transported into the axons. They are transported bidirectionally in the axon along microtubules using kinesin (anterograde) or dynein (retrograde) motor proteins [21, 22]. Studies analysing the transport of green-fluorescent protein (GFP)-tagged NIF subunits have shown that NIFs are transported intermittently in axons, their movements being interrupted by prolonged pauses. Only a small fraction of NIFs moves at any given time and direction, and approximately 97% of NIFs spent their time pausing [23–25]. The direction of NIF transport is modulated by their phosphorylation status, since phosphorylation promotes their release from kinesin and increases their affinity for dynein [22, 26].

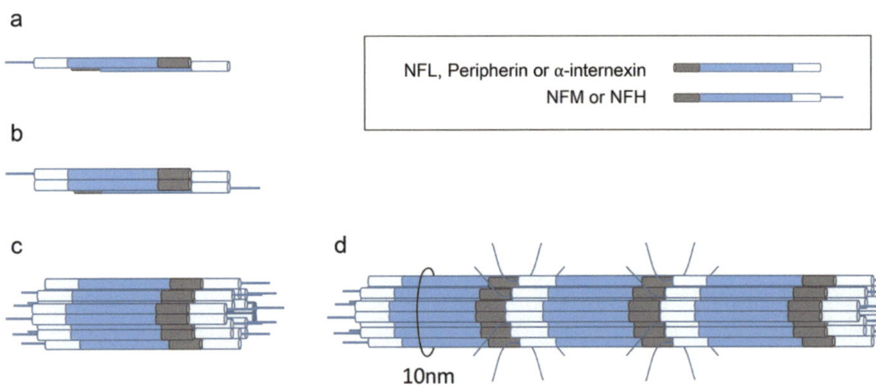

Figure 2. Schematic model of IF assembly in mature neurons. Two NIF subunits (NFL and either NFH or NFM) form head-to-tail coiled-coil dimers (a), anti-parallel half-staggered tetramers (b), protofilaments (c) and 10-nm NF (d). C-terminal domains of NFM and NFH form lateral projections and participate in the stabilisation of the filament network [33].

NIF subunits can assemble into filaments as soon as they are expressed in neurons, depending on their post-translational modifications. Subunits can also disassemble and reassemble during their transport. NIF assembly does not require nucleotide binding or hydrolysis. The first step of the filament formation is the dimerisation of an NFL subunit with either an NFM or an NFH subunit, via the association of their rod domains to form parallel side-to-side coiled-coil dimers. Two coiled-coil dimers line up in a half-staggered manner, forming an anti-parallel tetramer. Tetramers combine to form protofilaments, which finally assemble to constitute the final 10-nm filament [27, 28] (**Figure 2**). The C-terminal domains of NFM and NFH form lateral projections extending from the filament core [29]. Those projections participate to the stabilisation of the filament network and interact with other filament structures and subcellular organelles. Peripherin and α-internexin can co-assemble with NFL, NFM and NFH to form NIFs in mature neurons, respectively, in the peripheral and in the central nervous system [30–32]. Thus, NIFs are heteropolymers composed of different subunits, with a ratio changing during neuronal development and activity. This stoichiometry is particularly important and can lead to severe NF disorganisation when unbalanced.

In normal neurons, non-phosphorylated NIFs are found primarily in the soma and proximal axons, while phosphorylated NIFs are located more distal in axons and in terminals [34]. Inside the axon, NIFs are organised into a three-dimensional array interconnected with the other components of the cytoskeleton by several cross-bridges. NIFs, microtubules and actin filaments are interlinked by proteins of the plakin family including, among others, plectin, bullous pemphigoid antigen-1 protein (BPAG1), actin cross-linking factor 7 (ACF7), desmoplakin, envoplakin and periplakin [35–38]. Lateral projections of NFH and NFM tails also fasten adjacent structures (**Figure 3**).

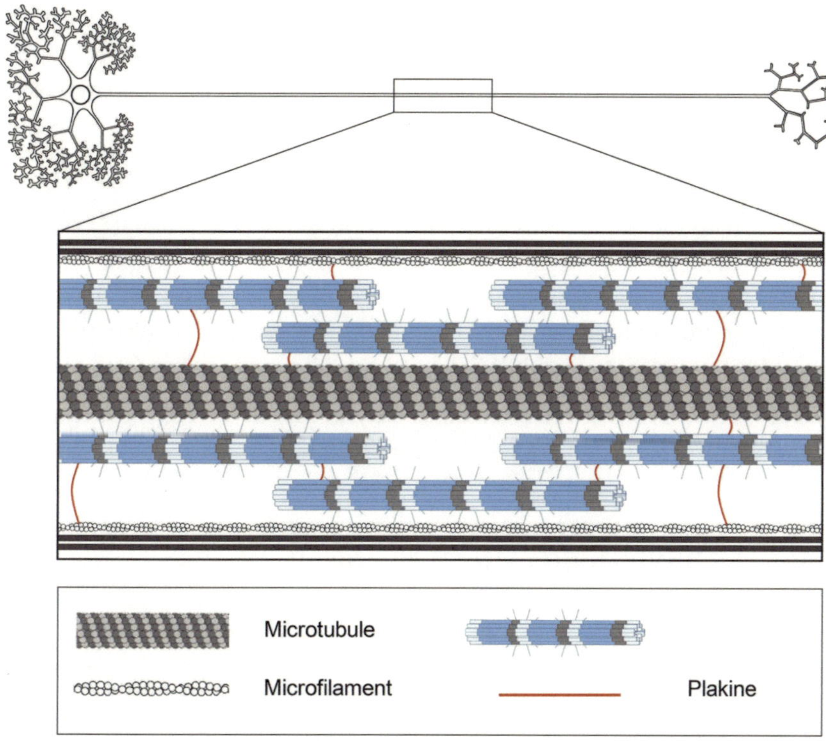

Figure 3. Schematic representation of the cytoskeleton organisation in axons. The components of the axoplasm are organised into a three-dimensional array interconnected by NFM and NFH tails and plakin-family proteins [39].

Following their synthesis, assembly and disassembly, NIFs are slowly transported towards the nerve terminal where they are degraded by specific calcium-activated proteases, such as calpain I, and neutral proteases. NIFs are also degraded by non-specific proteases like cathepsin D, trypsin and α-chymotrypsin. As mentioned above, post-translational modifications regulate NIF degradation: for example, phosphorylation protects NIFs from proteolysis, while ubiquitination facilitates their degradation [40, 41].

1.4. Roles

As members of the cytoskeletal system, NIFs work together with microtubules and microfilaments to enhance structural integrity and cell shape [42]. In the last decades, it has become increasingly apparent that IFs, instead of being inert, are in fact highly dynamic structures [43] relaying signals from the plasma membrane to the nucleus [44], orchestrating the position and function of cellular organelles [45] and regulating protein synthesis [46]. These interactions are principally mediated through NIF-associated proteins that can modulate NIF structure and function. Linker proteins such as Fodrin, Hamartin or MAP2 are responsible for NIF interactions with filaments and organelles [29, 47, 48], whereas enzymes (principally kinases and phosphatases) modulate their architecture, assembly and spacing.

Another major role recognised for NIFs is to modulate the calibre of axons, with a direct repercussion on the axonal conduction velocity, myelin thickness and inter-nodal length. Indeed, NIF density is correlated with axonal calibre in sciatic nerve fibres of rats and mice [49]. Moreover, the axonal radial growth during axonal development or regeneration coincides with the entry of NFs into axons [50]. In the same way, triple heterozygous knockout mice (NFL±, NFM± and NFH±), with a reduction of NF content but with a normal structure and stoichiometry of the NIF network, exhibit a 50% decrease of the axonal diameter in L5 ventral root [51]. Finally, the disruption of the NFM gene expression or the deletion of its carboxy-terminal domain in mice reduces the inter-filament spacing and axonal calibre, illustrating the preponderant role of NFM in determining axonal diameter [52, 53]. The phosphorylation state of NFM and NFH carboxy-terminal domains might be linked to axon calibre control by regulating NF transport and inter-filament spacing, but the exact mechanisms remain unknown.

Thus, NIFs have a central role in cell architecture, dynamics of the organelles, axon structure and calibre. Therefore, defects in their metabolism could lead to neurodegenerative processes.

2. Implication in amyotrophic lateral sclerosis

2.1. Clinical features

Amyotrophic lateral sclerosis (ALS) is a progressive neurodegenerative disease characterised by the loss of motor neurons of the spinal cord, brain stem and motor cortex. Common clinical symptoms of the disease are progressive paralysis, muscle atrophy and death within 2–5 years usually from respiratory failure [54]. Although most cases are sporadic (sALS), approximately 10% of ALS patients have a positive family history (fALS). To date, there is no curative treatment of the disease.

Primary evidence for a contribution of NIFs in ALS pathogenesis came from neuropathological observations. Most of all, ALS is characterised by the loss and degeneration of upper motor

http://dx.doi.org/10.5772/63161

neurons in the motor cortex (Betz cells), and lower motor neurons in the brainstem (cranial motor nuclei) and spinal cord (anterior horn) [55]. One of the hallmarks of both sporadic and familial ALS is the presence of inclusion bodies in the perikarya of degenerating motor neurons, described as Lewy body-like inclusions (LBLIs), Skein-like inclusions (SLIs) or hyaline conglomerate inclusions (HCIs). Other typical images observed in the disease are motor neurons with swollen argyrophilic perikarya, and large swellings of the proximal part of the axons called spheroids. In immunocytochemical studies, these abnormalities have been shown to contain several proteins, such as ubiquitin or stable tubule-only polypeptide (STOP) [56], but they are particularly reactive for neurofilament subunits [57, 58] and peripherin [59, 60] (**Figure 4**). Interestingly, NIF inclusions in the cell body and the proximal axon are hyperphosphorylated, while as mentioned above in normal neurons NIFs are dephosphorylated in those sites and only phosphorylated in more distal part of the axon.

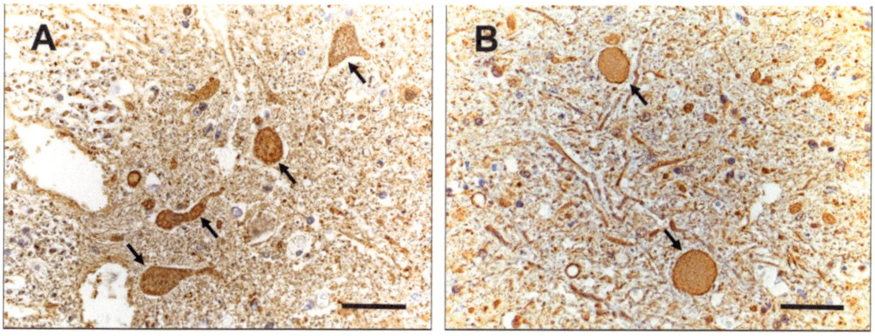

Figure 4. Neuropathological features in ALS. Immunohistochemistry for neurofilaments subunit (phosphorylated form): diffuse labelling in neuronal swelling perikarya (a) and axonal spheroids (b) in ventral horn of cervical spine. Scale bars, 20 μm.

Evidence for the involvement of NIFs in the pathogenesis of ALS has been reinforced in the last 20 years by the discovery of NIF gene mutations linked to the disease. Indeed, codon deletions and insertions in *PRPH* and *NEFH* genes have been identified in several sporadic ALS patients [61–64]. Although these mutations are not considered as a cause of familial ALS, they could be a risk factor for sporadic ALS occurrence.

Other evidences came from several studies showing that cerebrospinal fluid NIF levels are significantly higher in ALS patients than in patients with other neurodegenerative diseases, especially for those with rapidly progressive disease [65, 66]. Although their contributions to ALS pathogenesis remain unclear, all these clinical and neuropathological features suggest that NIFs represent a component of the pathological mechanisms of the disease.

2.2. Animal model contributions

On the basis of these findings, several animal models have been developed, including mice knockout for NIF genes, and mice expressing mouse, human and modified NIF subunits. While deletions of NIF genes have limited phenotype and thus are not extensively used to study ALS pathogenesis, the axonal calibre reduction seen in knockout mice for NFL, NFM and NFH genes demonstrated that neurofilaments play an important role in the radial growth of axons (**Table 2**). Interestingly, transgenic mice overexpressing either NFL, NFM, NFH, human NFH, peripherin or a mutated NFL show clinical and/or neuropathological alterations similar to those found in ALS (**Table 3**). Finally, in order to investigate NF dynamics, NFH-LacZ and NFH-GFP mice have been generated; while NFs are retained in cell bodies and deficient in axons in NFH-LacZ mice, the fluorescent fusion protein is normally transported along axons in NFH-GFP mice, suggesting that β-galactosidase reporter alters the fusion protein dynamics whereas GFP does not [67, 68]. All these animal models are therefore very useful to study the processes underlying NIF accumulation and their role in motor neuron death.

Mice	Motor dysfunction	Axonal calibre reduction	References
NFL -/-	No	>50%	[69]
NFM -/-	No	>50%	[70]
NFH -/-	No	10%	[71]
α-Internexin -/-	No	No	[72]
Peripherin -/-	No	No	[73]

Table 2. Knockout mice for NIF genes.

Mice	Motor dysfunction	NF inclusions	References
Mouse NFL	Yes	Spinal motor neurons and DRG	[74]
Mouse NFM	No	Spinal motor neurons and DRG	[75]
Mouse NFH	No	Spinal motor neurons and DRG	[76]
Human NFL	No	Thalamus and cortex	[77]
Human NFM	No	Cortex and forebrain	[78]
Human NFH	Yes	Spinal motor neurons and DRG	[79]
Mutated NFL (tail)	Yes	Spinal motor neurons and DRG	[80]
α-Internexin	No	Purkinje cells	[81]
Peripherin	Yes	Spinal motor neurons	[82]

Table 3. Mice overexpressing neuronal IF genes or expressing mutated neuronal IF proteins.

2.3. Pathophysiological hypotheses

Accumulation of neurofilaments in motor neurons undeniably participates in the pathogenesis of ALS, breaking perikarya and axonal structures, disrupting organelles dynamics and interactions, and affecting axonal transport. However, it is still difficult to determine whether

http://dx.doi.org/10.5772/63161

NIF aggregations are the cause or consequence of the disease. For example, the motor neuron loss caused by SOD1G85R mutation is still present despite the absence of NFL in transgenic mice [83, 84], but the animal's lifespan is prolonged by approximately 15%, suggesting an increased neuron toxicity when NFs are present in SOD1-mediated disease.

The mechanisms governing the formation of IF aggregates in ALS remain unclear because multiple factors can potentially induce the accumulation of NIFs. Firstly, these accumulations could result from perturbations of NIF transport through their abnormal phosphorylation, leading to accumulation in cell bodies and in proximal axons. Glutamate excitotoxicity could be involved in this process by activating mitogen-activated protein kinases and protein kinase N1 [85, 86]. Direct disruption of the transport motors themselves could also result in NIF accumulation, as it has been demonstrated in transgenic mice harbouring mutations or modified expression in kinesin and dynein genes [87]. Finally, one of the emerging hypotheses is that the aggregation of NIFs in ALS could result from their altered stoichiometry. Indeed, overexpression of NFL, NFM or NFH in mice provokes NF aggregations and morphological alterations similar to those found in ALS [74–76]. Remarkably, the motor neuron disease caused by excess of human NFH in transgenic mice can be rescued by a correct stoichiometry with the co-expression of human NFL transgene in a dosage-dependent fashion [88]. In a similar way, the onset of peripherin-mediated disease in transgenic mice overexpressing *PRPH* is accelerated by the deficiency of *NEFL* [82], peripherin interacting with NFM and NFH to form disorganised NIF structures. Another interesting point supporting this hypothesis is that NFL mRNA level is 70% decreased in degenerating motor neurons from ALS patients [89]. This could be due to reduced transcript stability, with a possible involvement of mutated SOD1 and TAR DNA-binding protein (TDP-43) that can bind and destabilise NFL mRNA [90, 91].

2.4. The paradox concerning perikaryal versus axonal aggregation of NIF, and the protective effect of perycarial NFH accumulation

Transgenic mice carrying mutant SOD1 transgenes develop neuronal, clinical and pathological features similar to those observed in ALS [92]. Surprisingly, the removal of axonal NIF by crossing the SOD1 transgenic mice with the NFH-LacZ transgenic mice does not affect the pathogenesis induced by SOD1 suggesting that axonal neurofilament aggregation is not the cause of ALS [93]. On the other side, overexpression of mouse NFL and NFH in SOD1G93A mice and overexpression of human NFH in SOD1G37R mice increase their lifespan by, respectively, 15 and 65%, associated with an increase of perycarial NF inclusions and a decrease of axonal spheroids (**Table 4**). Taken together, these last results suggest a protective effect of perikaryal accumulation of NFH proteins in motor neuron disease caused by mutant SOD1. Several hypotheses have been proposed to explain this protective effect. One possibility is that NF proteins may act as calcium chelators thanks to their multiple calcium-binding sites [94]. It also cannot be excluded that the accumulation of NFs could interfere with glutamate receptors and prevent glutamate excitotoxicity [95]. Finally, NF inclusions may act as a phosphorylation sink for cyclin-dependent kinase 5 or for toxic oxygen radical species induced by mutant SOD1, thereby reducing damage to other essential cellular components [96].

Mice	Lifespan	Perycarial NF inclusions	References
SODG85R – NFL -/-	Increased by 15%	No change	[84]
SODG93A – NFL overexpression	Increased by 15%	Increased	[97]
SODG93A – NFH overexpression	Increased by 15%	Increased	[97]
SODG37R – human NFH overexpression	Increased by 65%	Increased	[98]

Table 4. Effects of NF changes in SOD1-mediated disease.

3. Future directions

Implications of NIF abnormalities in the pathogenesis of ALS remain unclear. Despite extensive studies over the past 20 years, it is still unknown how these abnormalities occur and what are their exact contributions to the disease pathogenesis. Understanding how they are formed remains an important objective in the study of both sporadic and familial forms of the disease. Perhaps, the analysis of future generation of mouse models with new familial ALS mutations or conditional control of abnormal NIF proteins will help to address this issue.

Author details

Philippe Codron[1,2,3], Julien Cassereau[2,3], Joël Eyer[4*] and Franck Letournel[1,4]

*Address all correspondence to: joel.eyer@univ-angers.fr

1 Neurobiology and Neuropathology Laboratory, University Hospital of Angers, Angers, France

2 Department of Neurology, University Hospital of Angers, Angers, France

3 UMR INSERM, U771-CNRS6214, University Hospital of Angers, Angers, France

4 UPRES-EA3143, University Hospital of Angers, Angers, France

References

[1] Izmiryan A, Cheraud Y, Khanamiryan L, Leterrier JF, Federici T, Peltekian E, et al. Different expression of synemin isoforms in glia and neurons during nervous system development. Glia. 2006 Aug 15;54(3):204–13.

[2] Julien JP, Mushynski WE. Neurofilaments in health and disease. Prog Nucleic Acid Res Mol Biol. 1998;61:1–23.

[3] Kaplan MP, Chin SS, Fliegner KH, Liem RK. Alpha-internexin, a novel neuronal intermediate filament protein, precedes the low molecular weight neurofilament protein (NF-L) in the developing rat brain. J Neurosci. 1990 Aug;10(8):2735–48.

[4] Lendahl U, Zimmerman LB, McKay RD. CNS stem cells express a new class of intermediate filament protein. Cell. 1990 Feb 23;60(4):585–95.

[5] Portier MM, de Néchaud B, Gros F. Peripherin, a new member of the intermediate filament protein family. Dev Neurosci. 1983–1984;6(6):335–44.

[6] Perrot R, Berges R, Bocquet A, Eyer J. Review of the multiple aspects of neurofilament functions, and their possible contribution to neurodegeneration. Mol Neurobiol. 2008 Aug;38(1):27–65.

[7] Liu Q, Xie F, Siedlak SL, Nunomura A, Honda K, Moreira PI, et al. Neurofilament proteins in neurodegenerative diseases. Cell Mol Life Sci. 2004 Dec;61(24):3057–75.

[8] Hurst J, Flavell D, Julien JP, Meijer D, Mushynski W, Grosveld F. The human neurofilament gene (NEFL) is located on the short arm of chromosome 8. Cytogenet Cell Genet. 1987;45(1):30–2.

[9] Lees JF, Shneidman PS, Skuntz SF, Carden MJ, Lazzarini RA. The structure and organization of the human heavy neurofilament subunit (NF-H) and the gene encoding it. EMBO J. 1988 Jul;7(7):1947–55.

[10] Myers MW, Lazzarini RA, Lee VM, Schlaepfer WW, Nelson DL. The human mid-size neurofilament subunit: a repeated protein sequence and the relationship of its gene to the intermediate filament gene family. EMBO J. 1987 Jun;6(6):1617–26.

[11] Moncla A, Landon F, Mattei MG, Portier MM. Chromosomal localisation of the mouse and human peripherin genes. Genet Res. 1992 Apr;59(2):125–9.

[12] Foley J, Ley CA, Parysek LM. The structure of the human peripherin gene (PRPH) and identification of potential regulatory elements. Genomics. 1994 Jul 15;22(2):456–61.

[13] Hisanaga S, Gonda Y, Inagaki M, Ikai A, Hirokawa N. Effects of phosphorylation of the neurofilament L protein on filamentous structures. Cell Regul. 1990 Jan;1(2):237–48.

[14] Sihag RK, Jaffe H, Nixon RA, Rong X. Serine-23 is a major protein kinase A phosphorylation site on the amino-terminal head domain of the middle molecular mass subunit of neurofilament proteins. J Neurochem. 1999 Feb;72(2):491–9.

[15] Ackerley S, Thornhill P, Grierson AJ, Brownlees J, Anderton BH, Leigh PN, et al. Neurofilament heavy chain side arm phosphorylation regulates axonal transport of neurofilaments. J Cell Biol. 2003 May 12;161(3):489–95.

[16] Nixon RA, Brown BA, Marotta CA. Posttranslational modification of a neurofilament protein during axoplasmic transport: implications for regional specialization of CNS axons. J Cell Biol. 1982 Jul;94(1):150–8.

[17] Zheng Y-L, Li B-S, Veeranna null, Pant HC. Phosphorylation of the head domain of neurofilament protein (NF-M): a factor regulating topographic phosphorylation of NF-M tail domain KSP sites in neurons. J Biol Chem. 2003 Jun 27;278(26):24,026–32.

[18] Saito T, Shima H, Osawa Y, Nagao M, Hemmings BA, Kishimoto T, et al. Neurofilament-associated protein phosphatase 2A: its possible role in preserving neurofilaments in filamentous states. Biochemistry. 1995 Jun 6;34(22):7376–84.

[19] Veeranna null, Shetty KT, Link WT, Jaffe H, Wang J, Pant HC. Neuronal cyclin-dependent kinase-5 phosphorylation sites in neurofilament protein (NF-H) are dephosphorylated by protein phosphatase 2A. J Neurochem. 1995 Jun;64(6):2681–90.

[20] Dong DL, Xu ZS, Chevrier MR, Cotter RJ, Cleveland DW, Hart GW. Glycosylation of mammalian neurofilaments. Localization of multiple O-linked N-acetylglucosamine moieties on neurofilament polypeptides L and M. J Biol Chem. 1993 Aug 5;268(22): 16,679–87.

[21] Shah JV, Flanagan LA, Janmey PA, Leterrier JF. Bidirectional translocation of neurofilaments along microtubules mediated in part by dynein/dynactin. Mol Biol Cell. 2000 Oct;11(10):3495–508.

[22] Yabe JT, Pimenta A, Shea TB. Kinesin-mediated transport of neurofilament protein oligomers in growing axons. J Cell Sci. 1999 Nov;112(Pt 21):3799–814.

[23] Roy S, Coffee P, Smith G, Liem RK, Brady ST, Black MM. Neurofilaments are transported rapidly but intermittently in axons: implications for slow axonal transport. J Neurosci. 2000 Sep 15;20(18):6849–61.

[24] Trivedi N, Jung P, Brown A. Neurofilaments switch between distinct mobile and stationary states during their transport along axons. J Neurosci. 2007 Jan 17;27(3):507–16.

[25] Wang L, Ho CL, Sun D, Liem RK, Brown A. Rapid movement of axonal neurofilaments interrupted by prolonged pauses. Nat Cell Biol. 2000 Mar;2(3):137–41.

[26] Motil J, Chan WK-H, Dubey M, Chaudhury P, Pimenta A, Chylinski TM, et al. Dynein mediates retrograde neurofilament transport within axons and anterograde delivery of NFs from perikarya into axons: regulation by multiple phosphorylation events. Cell Motil Cytoskeleton. 2006 May;63(5):266–86.

[27] Angelides KJ, Smith KE, Takeda M. Assembly and exchange of intermediate filament proteins of neurons: neurofilaments are dynamic structures. J Cell Biol. 1989 Apr;108(4): 1495–506.

[28] Heins S, Wong PC, Müller S, Goldie K, Cleveland DW, Aebi U. The rod domain of NF-L determines neurofilament architecture, whereas the end domains specify filament assembly and network formation. J Cell Biol. 1993 Dec;123(6 Pt 1):1517–33.

[29] Hirokawa N, Glicksman MA, Willard MB. Organization of mammalian neurofilament polypeptides within the neuronal cytoskeleton. J Cell Biol. 1984 Apr;98(4):1523–36.

[30] Beaulieu JM, Robertson J, Julien JP. Interactions between peripherin and neurofilaments in cultured cells: disruption of peripherin assembly by the NF-M and NF-H subunits. Biochem Cell Biol. 1999;77(1):41–5.

[31] Yuan A, Sasaki T, Kumar A, Peterhoff CM, Rao MV, Liem RK, et al. Peripherin is a subunit of peripheral nerve neurofilaments: implications for differential vulnerability of CNS and PNS axons. J Neurosci. 2012 Jun 20;32(25):8501–8.

[32] Yuan A, Rao MV, Sasaki T, Chen Y, Kumar A, Veeranna null, et al. Alpha-internexin is structurally and functionally associated with the neurofilament triplet proteins in the mature CNS. J Neurosci. 2006 Sep 27;26(39):10,006–19.

[33] Szaro BG, Strong MJ. Post-transcriptional control of neurofilaments: new roles in development, regeneration and neurodegenerative disease. Trends Neurosci. 2010 Jan; 33(1):27–37.

[34] Sternberger LA, Sternberger NH. Monoclonal antibodies distinguish phosphorylated and nonphosphorylated forms of neurofilaments in situ. Proc Natl Acad Sci USA. 1983 Oct;80(19):6126–30.

[35] Kowalczyk AP, Bornslaeger EA, Norvell SM, Palka HL, Green KJ. Desmosomes: intercellular adhesive junctions specialized for attachment of intermediate filaments. Int Rev Cytol. 1999;185:237–302.

[36] Ruhrberg C, Hajibagheri MA, Simon M, Dooley TP, Watt FM. Envoplakin, a novel precursor of the cornified envelope that has homology to desmoplakin. J Cell Biol. 1996 Aug;134(3):715–29.

[37] Stappenbeck TS, Green KJ. The desmoplakin carboxyl terminus coaligns with and specifically disrupts intermediate filament networks when expressed in cultured cells. J Cell Biol. 1992 Mar;116(5):1197–209.

[38] Yang Y, Dowling J, Yu QC, Kouklis P, Cleveland DW, Fuchs E. An essential cytoskeletal linker protein connecting actin microfilaments to intermediate filaments. Cell. 1996 Aug 23;86(4):655–65.

[39] Lariviere RC, Julien J-P. Functions of intermediate filaments in neuronal development and disease. J Neurobiol. 2004 Jan;58(1):131–48.

[40] Goldstein ME, Sternberger NH, Sternberger LA. Phosphorylation protects neurofilaments against proteolysis. J Neuroimmunol. 1987 Mar;14(2):149–60.

[41] Gou JP, Leterrier JF. Possible involvement of ubiquitination in neurofilament degradation. Biochem Biophys Res Commun. 1995 Dec 14;217(2):529–38.

[42] Fuchs E, Cleveland DW. A structural scaffolding of intermediate filaments in health and disease. Science. 1998 Jan 23;279(5350):514–9.

[43] Helfand BT, Chang L, Goldman RD. Intermediate filaments are dynamic and motile elements of cellular architecture. J Cell Sci. 2004 Jan 15;117(Pt 2):133–41.

[44] Chang L, Goldman RD. Intermediate filaments mediate cytoskeletal crosstalk. Nat Rev Mol Cell Biol. 2004 Aug;5(8):601–13.

[45] Toivola DM, Tao G-Z, Habtezion A, Liao J, Omary MB. Cellular integrity plus: organelle-related and protein-targeting functions of intermediate filaments. Trends Cell Biol. 2005 Nov;15(11):608–17.

[46] Kim S, Wong P, Coulombe PA. A keratin cytoskeletal protein regulates protein synthesis and epithelial cell growth. Nature. 2006 May 18;441(7091):362–5.

[47] Frappier T, Stetzkowski-Marden F, Pradel LA. Interaction domains of neurofilament light chain and brain spectrin. Biochem J. 1991 Apr 15;275(Pt 2):521–7.

[48] Haddad LA, Smith N, Bowser M, Niida Y, Murthy V, Gonzalez-Agosti C, et al. The TSC1 tumor suppressor hamartin interacts with neurofilament-L and possibly functions as a novel integrator of the neuronal cytoskeleton. J Biol Chem. 2002 Nov 15;277(46):44,180–6.

[49] Friede RL, Samorajski T. Axon caliber related to neurofilaments and microtubules in sciatic nerve fibers of rats and mice. Anat Rec. 1970 Aug;167(4):379–87.

[50] Hoffman PN, Griffin JW, Price DL. Control of axonal caliber by neurofilament transport. J Cell Biol. 1984 Aug;99(2):705–14.

[51] Nguyen MD, Larivière RC, Julien JP. Reduction of axonal caliber does not alleviate motor neuron disease caused by mutant superoxide dismutase 1. Proc Natl Acad Sci USA. 2000 Oct 24;97(22):12,306–11.

[52] Elder GA, Friedrich VL, Bosco P, Kang C, Gourov A, Tu PH, et al. Absence of the midsized neurofilament subunit decreases axonal calibers, levels of light neurofilament (NF-L), and neurofilament content. J Cell Biol. 1998 May 4;141(3):727–39.

[53] Rao MV, Campbell J, Yuan A, Kumar A, Gotow T, Uchiyama Y, et al. The neurofilament middle molecular mass subunit carboxyl-terminal tail domains is essential for the radial growth and cytoskeletal architecture of axons but not for regulating neurofilament transport rate. J Cell Biol. 2003 Dec 8;163(5):1021–31.

[54] Kiernan MC, Vucic S, Cheah BC, Turner MR, Eisen A, Hardiman O, et al. Amyotrophic lateral sclerosis. Lancet. 2011 Mar 12;377(9769):942–55.

[55] Hirano A. Neuropathology of ALS An overview. Neurology. 1996 Oct 1;47(4 Suppl 2): 63S–66S.

[56] Letournel F, Bocquet A, Dubas F, Barthelaix A, Eyer J. Stable tubule only polypeptides (STOP) proteins co-aggregate with spheroid neurofilaments in amyotrophic lateral sclerosis. J Neuropathol Exp Neurol. 2003 Dec;62(12):1211–9.

[57] Munoz DG, Greene C, Perl DP, Selkoe DJ. Accumulation of phosphorylated neurofilaments in anterior horn motoneurons of amyotrophic lateral sclerosis patients. J Neuropathol Exp Neurol. 1988 Jan;47(1):9–18.

[58] Troost D, Sillevis Smitt PA, de Jong JM, Swaab DF. Neurofilament and glial alterations in the cerebral cortex in amyotrophic lateral sclerosis. Acta Neuropathol. 1992;84(6): 664–73.

[59] Corbo M, Hays AP. Peripherin and neurofilament protein coexist in spinal spheroids of motor neuron disease. J Neuropathol Exp Neurol. 1992 Sep;51(5):531–7.

[60] He CZ, Hays AP. Expression of peripherin in ubiquinated inclusions of amyotrophic lateral sclerosis. J Neurol Sci. 2004 Jan 15;217(1):47–54.

[61] Al-Chalabi A, Andersen PM, Nilsson P, Chioza B, Andersson JL, Russ C, et al. Deletions of the heavy neurofilament subunit tail in amyotrophic lateral sclerosis. Hum Mol Genet. 1999 Feb;8(2):157–64.

[62] Figlewicz DA, Krizus A, Martinoli MG, Meininger V, Dib M, Rouleau GA, et al. Variants of the heavy neurofilament subunit are associated with the development of amyotrophic lateral sclerosis. Hum Mol Genet. 1994 Oct;3(10):1757–61.

[63] Gros-Louis F, Larivière R, Gowing G, Laurent S, Camu W, Bouchard J-P, et al. A frameshift deletion in peripherin gene associated with amyotrophic lateral sclerosis. J Biol Chem. 2004 Oct 29;279(44):45,951–6.

[64] Leung CL, He CZ, Kaufmann P, Chin SS, Naini A, Liem RKH, et al. A pathogenic peripherin gene mutation in a patient with amyotrophic lateral sclerosis. Brain Pathol. 2004 Jul;14(3):290–6.

[65] Boylan KB, Glass JD, Crook JE, Yang C, Thomas CS, Desaro P, et al. Phosphorylated neurofilament heavy subunit (pNF-H) in peripheral blood and CSF as a potential prognostic biomarker in amyotrophic lateral sclerosis. J Neurol Neurosurg Psychiatr. 2013 Apr;84(4):467–72.

[66] Tortelli R, Ruggieri M, Cortese R, D'Errico E, Capozzo R, Leo A, et al. Elevated cerebrospinal fluid neurofilament light levels in patients with amyotrophic lateral sclerosis: a possible marker of disease severity and progression. Eur J Neurol. 2012 Dec; 19(12):1561–7.

[67] Eyer J, Peterson A. Neurofilament-deficient axons and perikaryal aggregates in viable transgenic mice expressing a neurofilament-beta-galactosidase fusion protein. Neuron. 1994 Feb;12(2):389–405.

[68] Letournel F, Bocquet A, Perrot R, Dechaume A, Guinut F, Eyer J, et al. Neurofilament high molecular weight-green fluorescent protein fusion is normally expressed in neurons and transported in axons: a neuronal marker to investigate the biology of neurofilaments. Neuroscience. 2006;137(1):103–11.

[69] Zhu Q, Couillard-Després S, Julien JP. Delayed maturation of regenerating myelinated axons in mice lacking neurofilaments. Exp Neurol. 1997 Nov;148(1):299–316.

[70] Elder GA, Friedrich VL, Margita A, Lazzarini RA. Age-related atrophy of motor axons in mice deficient in the mid-sized neurofilament subunit. J Cell Biol. 1999 Jul 12;146(1): 181–92.

[71] Jacomy H, Zhu Q, Couillard-Després S, Beaulieu JM, Julien JP. Disruption of type IV intermediate filament network in mice lacking the neurofilament medium and heavy subunits. J Neurochem. 1999 Sep;73(3):972–84.

[72] Levavasseur F, Zhu Q, Julien JP. No requirement of alpha-internexin for nervous system development and for radial growth of axons. Brain Res Mol Brain Res. 1999 May 21;69(1):104–12.

[73] Larivière RC, Nguyen MD, Ribeiro-da-Silva A, Julien J-P. Reduced number of unmyelinated sensory axons in peripherin null mice. J Neurochem. 2002 May;81(3):525–32.

[74] Xu Z, Cork LC, Griffin JW, Cleveland DW. Increased expression of neurofilament subunit NF-L produces morphological alterations that resemble the pathology of human motor neuron disease. Cell. 1993 Apr 9;73(1):23–33.

[75] Wong PC, Marszalek J, Crawford TO, Xu Z, Hsieh ST, Griffin JW, et al. Increasing neurofilament subunit NF-M expression reduces axonal NF-H, inhibits radial growth, and results in neurofilamentous accumulation in motor neurons. J Cell Biol. 1995 Sep; 130(6):1413–22.

[76] Marszalek JR, Williamson TL, Lee MK, Xu Z, Hoffman PN, Becher MW, et al. Neurofilament subunit NF-H modulates axonal diameter by selectively slowing neurofilament transport. J Cell Biol. 1996 Nov;135(3):711–24.

[77] Julien JP, Tretjakoff I, Beaudet L, Peterson A. Expression and assembly of a human neurofilament protein in transgenic mice provide a novel neuronal marking system. Genes Dev. 1987 Dec;1(10):1085–95.

[78] Gama Sosa MA, Friedrich VL, DeGasperi R, Kelley K, Wen PH, Senturk E, et al. Human midsized neurofilament subunit induces motor neuron disease in transgenic mice. Exp Neurol. 2003 Nov;184(1):408–19.

[79] Côté F, Collard JF, Julien JP. Progressive neuronopathy in transgenic mice expressing the human neurofilament heavy gene: a mouse model of amyotrophic lateral sclerosis. Cell. 1993 Apr 9;73(1):35–46.

[80] Lee MK, Marszalek JR, Cleveland DW. A mutant neurofilament subunit causes massive, selective motor neuron death: implications for the pathogenesis of human motor neuron disease. Neuron. 1994 Oct;13(4):975–88.

[81] Ching GY, Chien CL, Flores R, Liem RK. Overexpression of alpha-internexin causes abnormal neurofilamentous accumulations and motor coordination deficits in transgenic mice. J Neurosci. 1999 Apr 15;19(8):2974–86.

[82] Beaulieu JM, Nguyen MD, Julien JP. Late onset of motor neurons in mice overexpressing wild-type peripherin. J Cell Biol. 1999 Nov 1;147(3):531–44.

[83] Larivière RC, Beaulieu J-M, Nguyen MD, Julien J-P. Peripherin is not a contributing factor to motor neuron disease in a mouse model of amyotrophic lateral sclerosis caused by mutant superoxide dismutase. Neurobiol Dis. 2003 Jul;13(2):158–66.

[84] Williamson TL, Bruijn LI, Zhu Q, Anderson KL, Anderson SD, Julien JP, et al. Absence of neurofilaments reduces the selective vulnerability of motor neurons and slows disease caused by a familial amyotrophic lateral sclerosis-linked superoxide dismutase 1 mutant. Proc Natl Acad Sci USA. 1998 Aug 4;95(16):9631–6.

[85] Ackerley S, Grierson AJ, Brownlees J, Thornhill P, Anderton BH, Leigh PN, et al. Glutamate slows axonal transport of neurofilaments in transfected neurons. J Cell Biol. 2000 Jul 10;150(1):165–76.

[86] Manser C, Stevenson A, Banner S, Davies J, Tudor EL, Ono Y, et al. Deregulation of PKN1 activity disrupts neurofilament organisation and axonal transport. FEBS Lett. 2008 Jun 25;582(15):2303–8.

[87] Chevalier-Larsen E, Holzbaur ELF. Axonal transport and neurodegenerative disease. Biochim Biophys Acta. 2006 Dec;1762(11–12):1094–108.

[88] Meier J, Couillard-Després S, Jacomy H, Gravel C, Julien JP. Extra neurofilament NF-L subunits rescue motor neuron disease caused by overexpression of the human NF-H gene in mice. J Neuropathol Exp Neurol. 1999 Oct;58(10):1099–110.

[89] Wong NK, He BP, Strong MJ. Characterization of neuronal intermediate filament protein expression in cervical spinal motor neurons in sporadic amyotrophic lateral sclerosis (ALS). J Neuropathol Exp Neurol. 2000 Nov;59(11):972–82.

[90] Ge W-W, Wen W, Strong W, Leystra-Lantz C, Strong MJ. Mutant copper-zinc superoxide dismutase binds to and destabilizes human low molecular weight neurofilament mRNA. J Biol Chem. 2005 Jan 7;280(1):118–24.

[91] Strong MJ, Volkening K, Hammond R, Yang W, Strong W, Leystra-Lantz C, et al. TDP43 is a human low molecular weight neurofilament (hNFL) mRNA-binding protein. Mol Cell Neurosci. 2007 Jun;35(2):320–7.

[92] Tu PH, Raju P, Robinson KA, Gurney ME, Trojanowski JQ, Lee VM. Transgenic mice carrying a human mutant superoxide dismutase transgene develop neuronal cytoskeletal pathology resembling human amyotrophic lateral sclerosis lesions. Proc Natl Acad Sci USA. 1996 Apr 2;93(7):3155–60.

[93] Eyer J, Cleveland DW, Wong PC, Peterson AC. Pathogenesis of two axonopathies does not require axonal neurofilaments. Nature. 1998 Feb 5;391(6667):584–7.

[94] Roy J, Minotti S, Dong L, Figlewicz DA, Durham HD. Glutamate potentiates the toxicity of mutant Cu/Zn-superoxide dismutase in motor neurons by postsynaptic calcium-dependent mechanisms. J Neurosci. 1998 Dec 1;18(23):9673–84.

[95] Ehlers MD, Fung ET, O'Brien RJ, Huganir RL. Splice variant-specific interaction of the NMDA receptor subunit NR1 with neuronal intermediate filaments. J Neurosci. 1998 Jan 15;18(2):720–30.

[96] Nguyen MD, Larivière RC, Julien JP. Deregulation of Cdk5 in a mouse model of ALS: toxicity alleviated by perikaryal neurofilament inclusions. Neuron. 2001 Apr;30(1):135–47.

[97] Kong J, Xu Z. Overexpression of neurofilament subunit NF-L and NF-H extends survival of a mouse model for amyotrophic lateral sclerosis. Neurosci Lett. 2000 Mar 3;281(1):72–4.

[98] Couillard-Després S, Zhu Q, Wong PC, Price DL, Cleveland DW, Julien JP. Protective effect of neurofilament heavy gene overexpression in motor neuron disease induced by mutant superoxide dismutase. Proc Natl Acad Sci USA. 1998 Aug 4;95(16):9626–30.

Chapter 11

Trophic Factors in the Therapeutic Challenge Against ALS: Current Research Directions

Anna Sobuś and Bogusław Machaliński

Additional information is available at the end of the chapter

http://dx.doi.org/10.5772/63428

Abstract

Amyotrophic lateral sclerosis (ALS) is a fatal neurodegenerative disorder, which up to date remains incurable. Multiple experimental approaches toward finding an effective way of reducing ALS progression and improving patients' condition have been proposed but none of them brought significant desired effects. In recent years, studies focused on stem cells (SCs) have proven that not only cells themselves but also trophic factors, which they secrete, may cause positive effects on neural tissue environment. Crucial issues that have to be considered in any study implementing SC's secreted trophic factors are administration route and type of administered cells. Furthermore, the understanding of trophic factor function, secretion manner, and their potential influence on damaged cells may be immensely beneficial. This chapter focuses on recent studies exploiting trophic factors to improve ALS patients and animal ALS models' condition.

Keywords: amyotrophic lateral sclerosis, trophic factors, neurotrophins, BDNF, GDNF, VEGF, IGF-1, GLP-1

1. Introduction

Amyotrophic lateral sclerosis (ALS), also known as Lou Gehrig's disease, is a fatal neurodegenerative disease, characterized by progressive loss of motor neuron functions in the spinal cord, cortex, and brainstem [1]. ALS was first described in the 1870s by the French neurologist Jean-Marie Charcot. The incidence of ALS ranges from 1 to 4 new cases per year. Typical first symptoms, which occur because of gradual loss of neuron functions, are muscle weakness, impaired reflexes, and speech difficulties. Patients in the later stages of the disease

INTECH
open science | open minds

© 2016 The Author(s). Licensee InTech. This chapter is distributed under the terms of the Creative Commons Attribution License (http://creativecommons.org/licenses/by/3.0), which permits unrestricted use, distribution, and reproduction in any medium, provided the original work is properly cited.

may also suffer from cognitive impairments, among which aphasia and semantic dementia are the most frequently reported [2]. Eventually, in most cases, weakening of respiratory muscles results in death caused by asphyxiation within 3–5 years after diagnosis. From a pathophysiologic point of view, two forms of ALS are widely described—familial ALS (fALS) and sporadic ALS (sALS). fASL affects approximately 10% of patients, whereas sALS is responsible for the other 90%. Mutations in *SOD1* gene, which encodes Cu/Zn superoxide dismutase 1, are common among patients with fALS, and more than 160 different mutations in *SOD1* have been described to date [2]. However, recent studies have reported potential relationships between other genes and fALS, including those encoding transactive response DNA-binding protein (TARDBP), fused in sarcoma (FUS) and c90RF72 [3]. The precise cause of sALS has not been identified, but environmental factors, lifestyle, and genetic predispositions are considered as key factors in the disease development [4]. Evidence has demonstrated that especially exposure to tobacco smoke and the quantity of cigarettes smoked are significantly correlated with ALS [5]. Pathophysiological mechanisms that result in neurodegeneration involve protein aggregation, mitochondrial dysfunction, generation of free radicals, excitotoxicity, disrupted axonal transport, and dysregulation of neurotrophic factor levels [6]. Notably, no effective cure for ALS has been discovered, leaving newly diagnosed patients with no chance for complete recovery. The only remedy approved by the Food and Drug Administration (FDA) is riluzole, an antiglutamatergic agent, which may cause excitotoxicity reduction and, therefore, extend survival by up to few months [7]. Because of the lack of an effective treatment and the relatively late manifestation of first symptoms, often when neuron loss is already in an advanced stage, the search for new ways to manage ALS turns to stem cell (SC)-based therapy. SCs are considered to be a promising tool of modern medicine because of their ability to transform into almost any other cell type and their capability of an infinite divisions number. Two main directions in SC-based therapies for ALS are considered – "structural" cell replacement and humoral neuroprotection via secretion of trophic factors. The main issues that must be considered in all forms of SC-based therapies are the proper administration method, the optimal type of administered cells, and the identification of factors that are crucial for the survival and differentiation of transplanted cells [8]. Recently, the greatest effect evidenced from the studies implementing various types of SCs is their ability to improve neural tissue microenvironment and provide soluble neurotrophic factors rather than structural replacement of lost cells [9]. Accordingly, this review focuses on the role of trophic factors in ALS progression and the chance of implementing therapies that take advantage of their properties.

Two different types of adult SCs are under extensive investigation in the perspective of ALS therapy: mesenchymal stem cells (MSCs) and SCs connected with the organization of nerve tissue. MSCs are an attractive source for potential therapeutic approaches for several reasons. Firstly, MSCs are characterized by great plasticity [10] and can be easily obtained from different sources, including bone marrow [bone marrow stem cells (BMSCs)], adipose tissue [adipocyte stem cells (ASCs)], or umbilical cord blood [11]. Moreover, MSCs can differentiate into cells of all three germ layers (ectoderm, endoderm, and mesoderm) when cultured under specific conditions [12], and their expansion in vitro does not involve any changes in function or chromosome structure, as observed in cells obtained from ALS patients [13]. It has been also found that MSCs can support regeneration of damaged parenchymal cells by scavenging toxic inflammatory cytokines and secreting trophic cytokines that are involved in neuroprotection [14]. Cells connected with nerve tissue organization are also being used in ALS research, including neural progenitor cells (NPCs), astrocyte precursor cells [15], and olfactory ensheathing stem cells (OESCs), which have been recently used in treatment of spinal cord injury [16]. Embryonic SCs have also been extensively investigated, but their implementation raises major clinical and ethical concerns. Although the physiological relevance of pluripotency is of significant importance, induced pluripotent stem cells (iPSCs) have been demonstrated to differentiate into a variety of cell types, including muscle, cardiac muscle, and hepatocyte cells. All of the abovementioned cell types might present different advantages when used in ALS management. Because ALS affects motor neurons at different levels and in various ways, attention is focusing more on restoring neuronal tissue homeostasis than on cell replacement. In addition, conditions in the adult spine do not favor the differentiation of transplanted cells into neural ones. However, it has been observed that the environment in spinal cord fluid from ALS patients stimulates transplanted MSCs to secrete factors that relieve ALS symptoms [17].

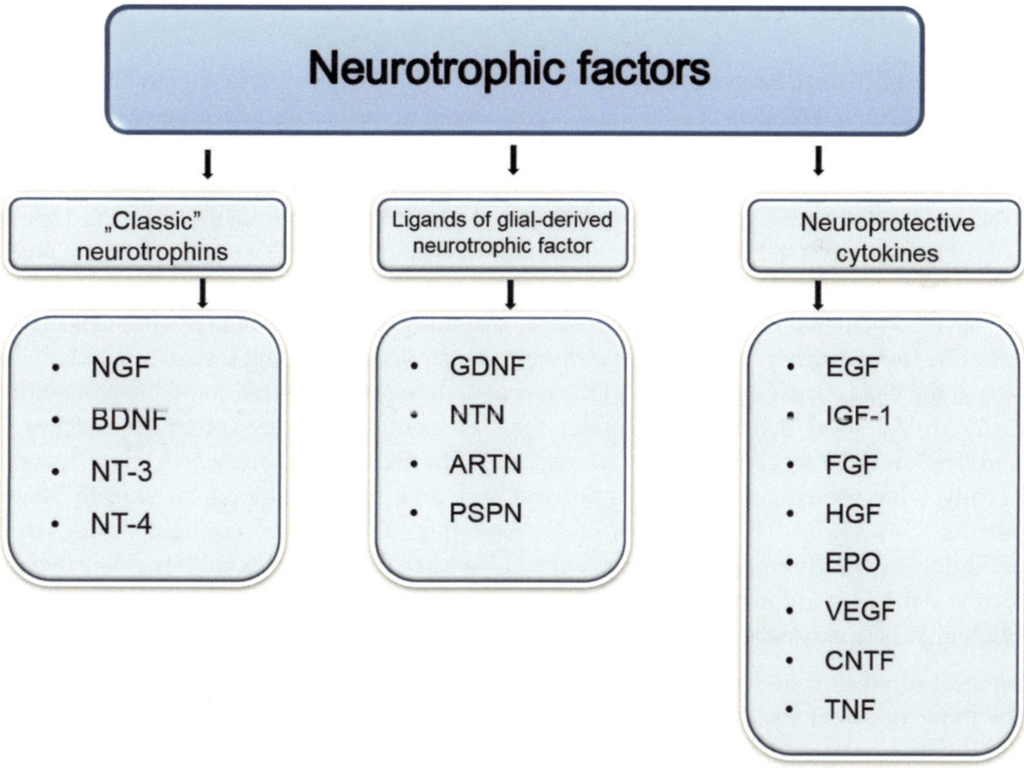

Figure 1. Classification of neurotrophic factors according to their structure and function. NGF, nerve growth factor; BDNF, brain-derived neurotrophic factor; NT-3, neurotrophin-3; NT-4, neurotrophin-4; GDNF, glial-derived neurotrophic factor; NTN, neurturin; ARTN, artemin; PSPN, persephin; EGF, epidermal growth factor; IGF-1, insulin-like growth factor; FGF, fibroblast growth factor; HGF, hepatocyte growth factor; EPO, erythropoietin; VEGF, vascular endothelial growth factor; CNTF, ciliary neurotrophic factor; TNF, tumor necrosis factor.

These factors are mainly neurotrophins, proteins synthesized and secreted by the brain, spinal cord, and other cells that are dependent on peripheral sensory neurons.

Neurotrophins are responsible for nerve growth and survival, synapse formation, and axonal growth [18]. In general, neurotrophins provide neuroprotection, thus slowing down neurodegeneration. Neurotrophins also prevent oxidative stress and inhibit apoptosis [19]. Neurotrophic factors can be categorized in different ways based on their activities in preventing neuronal cell death [19] or by their structural and functional affiliations (**Figure 1**). Accordingly, "classic" neurotrophins, ligands of glial-derived neurotrophic factor (GDNF), and neuroprotective cytokines can be distinguished. The group of classic neurotrophins includes nerve growth factor (NGF), brain-derived neurotrophic factor (BDNF), neurotrophin-3 (NT-3), and neurotrophin-4 (NT-4) [20]. Furthermore, factors that are connected with more than just neural cells, such as IGF-1, also demonstrate potential as ALS therapies. Growth factors involved in vasculogenesis, such as vascular endothelial growth factor (VEGF), basic fibroblast growth factor, and angiopoietin, might also be correlated with ALS progression.

2. Trophic factors correlated with ALS

Previous studies have investigated the expression patterns of trophic factors in both in vitro cultures and animal models of ALS. Data accumulated in the last decade suggest that trophic factors are notable not only for monitoring ALS therapy and disease progression but also for potentially helping in ALS diagnosis. SCs, particularly MSCs, exhibit higher levels of NGF, BDNF, and VEGF expression after stimulation with protein extracts from the brains and spinal cords of transgenic SOD1 (G93A) rats (an animal ALS model) [21]. The fact of changing levels of these proteins at various disease stages demonstrates that they might be essential during ALS development and progression. Therefore, exploiting their potential in treatment is highly desirable. Unfortunately, their pharmacokinetic constraints, including their restricted ability to cross the blood-brain barrier (BBB) [22] and penetrate gray matter, limited bioavailability, and relatively short half-life [23], hinder their efficient use. Hence, other approaches of neurotrophin delivery, e.g., with viral vectors or by SCs grafts, are worth investigation. Recently, it has been reported that SCs derived from umbilical cord blood, an ethically sound source of SCs, express higher levels of neurotrophic factors when cultured under stress conditions [24]. Furthermore, in patients with ALS who received autologous transplant of bone marrow-derived stem/progenitor cells, slower disease progression was positively correlated with higher NTs expression levels [25].

The most promising studies aimed at assessing the involvement of neurotrophins and other growth factors in ALS and their potentials in ALS treatment are summarized below.

3. Brain-derived neurotrophic factor

BDNF was discovered in 1982 by purification from pig brain as a protein responsible for promoting survival of sensory neurons [26]. BDNF is considered to be the best characterized neurotrophic factor in the central nervous system (CNS), mainly because of its crucial role in the maintenance of normal brain function. Similar to other neurotrophins, BDNF may interact via a common p75NTR receptor or a specific tropomyosin-related kinase receptor, TrkB [27]. After binding of BDNF to TrkB and autophosphorylation of the receptor, three signaling pathways are activated: the phosphatidylinositol 3-kinase pathway (PI3K), mitogen-activated protein kinase/extracellular signal-regulated protein kinase pathway (MAPK/ERK), and phospholipase Cγ pathway (PLCγ) [28]. Expression of BDNF is increased in the hippocampus, cerebral cortex, cerebellum, and amygdala of the brain [29]. BDNF has many functions during both the development and normal function of the mature human brain, such as promoting the elongation and growth of neurites and initiating axon formation [30]. Notably, effects exerted by BDNF on neural cells differ depending on the method of stimulation. Dendritic cells exposed to increasing levels of neurotrophin for a certain time exhibit enlarged branching, whereas acute, transient elevation of BDNF concentrations results in neurite elongation and spine head enlargement [31]. BDNF is also involved in the formation, stabilization, and modulation of synaptic connections [32, 33]. Consequently, BDNF is deeply associated with normal CNS functions and exerts a plethora of actions that are crucial for neural tissue survival. Therefore, impaired expression of BDNF appears to be implicated in many diseases connected with the nervous system, including ALS.

Preclinical studies performed on a mice model of ALS, SOD1 (G93A), demonstrated that BDNF promotes the survival of neuronal cells [18]. A study conducted in wobbler mutant mice (another ALS model) injected with recombinant human BDNF resulted in a slower rate of grip strength decrease and greater muscle tensions compared with control animals [34]. However, clinical trials based on BDNF injections in humans, both subcutaneous and intrathecal, have not demonstrated noticeable improvements in ALS patients' conditions [35, 36]. Clinical trials with intrathecal delivery of BDNF were conducted in 2003 and 2005 but failed to demonstrate any meaningful effect of BDNF on motor function because of small study sizes [37, 38]. Recently, it has been reported that muscle progenitor cells (MPCs) expressing BDNF, GDNF, and insulin-like growth factor (IGF-1) injected into the legs of SOD1 mice delayed disease onset and even prolonged the lifespans of treated animals by 13 days. Decreases in neuromuscular junction degeneration and increased axonal survival were also observed [39]. However, another study observed no prolonged lifespan in ALS mutant rats after intramuscular transplantations of human mesenchymal stem cells (hMSCs) modified by lentiviral infection to express BDNF. The same study reported that infection of the same hMSCs expressing GDNF and VEGF into the muscle tissue of SOD1 (G93A) rats caused improvement in survival and motor function of the subjects [40], suggesting that the positive effects observed in different studies implementing neurotrophins against ALS were exerted by trophic factors other than BDNF.

4. Glial-derived neurotrophic factor

GDNF was first isolated as a factor promoting the survival of dopaminergic neurons in embryonic ventral midbrain cell cultures [41]. GDNF also improves motor neuron functions

[42] and decreases the rate of apoptotic dopamine neurons in vitro [43] and in vivo after an ischemic stroke [44]. In ALS patients, the levels of GDNF in the cerebrospinal fluid and muscle biopsies are increased [45, 46]. Compared with other NTFs (including BDNF, NT-3, and NT-4), GDNF exhibits almost 100 times higher efficacy in supporting the survival of spinal motor neurons [47]. GDNF also has beneficial effects on neuronal cells in SOD-1 (G93A) mice. NPCs expressing GDNF decreased the loss of motor neurons and stimulated changes in trophic factor expression in motor neurons of the spinal cord [23]. However, the same study did not observe any correlation between the presence of GDNF and the integration of neuromuscular junctions or disease progression [23]. In another study, hMSCs were genetically engineered to express GDNF and subsequently injected into three muscle groups. The injected cells were able to survive, graft, and further secrete GDNF. Moreover, an increase in the number of neuromuscular connections and motor neuron cell bodies in the spinal cord was also observed. As a result, hMSC-GDNF increased the lifespan of SOD-1 rats by up to 28 days [48]. Other studies using intramuscular injections of cells expressing GDNF from adenoviral transduction have also observed beneficial effects of GDNF on neurons in ALS animal models [49, 50]. These effects may be exerted by preventing apoptosis by preserving the Akt signaling pathway [51]. Taken together, GDNF seems to be a promising candidate for ALS treatment. However, there remain no clinical studies with this trophic factor in ALS patients. Moreover, GDNF may not have the ability to cross BBB [52], which compels the need to consider other routes of administration to the CNS, such as intracerebroventricularly.

5. Vascular endothelial growth factor

The first member of VEGF protein family was described from the discovery of vascular permeability factor (VPF), which is responsible for increasing tumor-induced vascular permeability [53]. VPF has also been observed in other cell types and named VEGF (now it is known as VEGF-A). VEGF is produced by many cell types, including macrophages, platelets, keratinocytes, and renal mesangial cells. Expression of VEGF initiates during gastrulation and is crucial for vasculogenesis and angiogenesis [54, 55]. In addition to the established roles of the VEGF family in angiogenesis and lymphangiogenesis, it has also been suggested that these proteins have prominent neurotrophic effects. VEGF family members are also involved in nerve migration [56] and axonal guidance [57] and protect cells from the effects of damaging agents, such as hypoxia, excitotoxicity, mechanical trauma, and serum deprivation [58–59]. In 2001, it was found that mice with deletion of the HIF-response (HIF - Hypoxia-Inducible Factor) element in the VEGF promoter present adult-onset progressive degeneration of motor neurons, similar to that encountered in ALS [60]. There have been several gene therapy approaches using VEGF in animal models of ALS. In one of the first studies, delivery of VEGF into the diaphragm, intercostal, facial, and tongue muscles before initial symptoms resulted in delayed ALS onset. Furthermore, improved motor function and prolonged survival were observed [61]. In another study, expression of VEGF was increased by the use of a zinc-finger protein (transcription factor) delivered with an adenoviral vector to primary motor neurons. It has been shown that increased VEGF expression in those cells increased stimulated axon outgrowth and enhanced nerve regeneration overall [62]. Despite the fact that the abovementioned study was conducted in rats that underwent nerve-crush injuries and not in the SOD-1 (G93A) ALS model, their method of delivery has potential as an approach to regenerate neural cells in ALS therapy. To date, the only study which implemented zinc-finger proteins as transcription modulating factors in SOD-1 rats was based on the delivery of plasmid DNA to a single muscle and did not result in any difference in lifespan between treated and control animals. However, after six injections (one per week), better performance in behavioral tests was observed in the treated SOD-1 (G93A) group [63]. Of note, SCs have also been implemented as a method of VEGF delivery. Intrathecal transplantation of human neural stem cells (NSCs), which were modified to overexpress VEGF, significantly delayed disease onset and prolonged lifespan in ALS model mice [64]. Transplanted cells have also exhibited the ability to migrate to gray matter, integrate into the spinal cord anterior horn, and transform into motor neurons [64]. Further examination of the expression levels of proteins associated with apoptosis revealed that neuroprotective mechanisms might have been caused by apoptotic regulation. In control animals injected with PBS, expression levels of proapoptotic Bax and caspase 3 were significantly higher than antiapoptotic Bcl-2 and Bcl-xL, whereas the opposite effect was observed in subjects injected with NSCs expressing VEGF [64]. Intracerebroventricular delivery of recombinant VEGF in an ALS rat model improved motor performance and prolonged the survival of treated animals by up to 22 days [65]. VEGF also has the ability to protect the innervation of neuromuscular junctions (NMJs) in ALS [66]. Currently, there is one ongoing clinical trial that is based on intracerebroventricular administration of sNN0029 (rhVEGF165). To date, no results from this trial have been published.

6. Insulin-like growth factor 1

IGF-1 was discovered in 1957 as a factor stimulating the incorporation of sulfate into rat cartilage [67]. IGF-1's insulin-like activity was described later [68], and the growth factor mediator of anabolic and mitogenic function was named insulin-like growth factor. IGF-1 is secreted mostly by the liver and acts as an endocrine hormone after transportation to other tissues [69]. The effects of IGF-1 on neural cells were first reported in 1987 when the expression of IGF-1 receptors was observed in CNS neural cells. Afterward, other studies have reported that IGF-1 is involved in signaling between developing muscle and motor neurons in spinal cord and induces proliferation and nerve sprouting in adult muscle [70]. Moreover, IGF-1 promotes GDNF actions and stimulates neuroprotection [71]. Preclinical studies testing IGF-1 in animal models have validated these abilities. SOD-1 (G93A) mice injected with an adeno-associated virus 2 (AAV2)-based vector encoding IGF-1 into their spinal cords presented delayed disease onset, slower weight loss, and increased survival in treated objects [72]. A similar study conducted in a rat ALS model employing AAV2 to deliver IGF-1 into the spinal cord reported a reduced loss of motor neurons [73]. In 2008, a clinical trial on IGF-1 with ALS patients was performed. In this study, 330 patients were subjected to subcutaneous injections of recombinant human IGF-1 daily for 2 years [74]. After 2 years, no differences in muscle function or survival rate were observed between treated patients and the placebo group. The authors concluded that IGF-1 does not provide benefits for ALS patients. No preclinical studies have demonstrated any beneficial effects of subcutaneously administered IGF-1 either. Positive outcomes were only observed after intrathecal injections or when the trophic factor was delivered with a viral vector, indicating that the method of administration might be crucial for successful treatment. Another study conducted on nine ALS patients intrathecally injected with IGF-1 every 2 weeks for 40 weeks reported that their method of administration caused modest but significant beneficial effects [75].

7. Glucagon-like peptide 1

GLP-1 is an endogenous peptide responsible for controlling plasma glucose levels by stimulating insulin synthesis and its secretion from pancreatic β cells [76]. So far, little is known regarding the role of GLP-1 in the physiology of neural tissue. However, GLP-1 receptors have been observed on the neurons of various brain regions, including the hippocampus, cerebellum, and cerebral cortex [77], indicating that it is involved in proper neuronal function. GLP-1 protects neural cells from excitotoxicity [78] and participates in learning and memory processes [79]. All of these features make GLP-1 a potentially useful factor to investigate for ALS therapy. An in vitro study using motor neurons derived from Sod-1 (G93A) transgenic mice that were exposed to kainite (excitotoxic stimulus) reported that a synthetic analogue of GLP-1 exhibited neuroprotective effects [80]. The neuroprotective potential of GLP-1 has also been tested in a mouse model of ALS. Human MSCs were transfected with a plasmid vector encoding *GLP-1*, encapsulated and subsequently injected into the cerebral ventricle [81]. This method of treatment significantly prolonged the lifespans of treated animals (by 13 days), delayed symptom onsets, decreased weight loss, and caused improvements in motor performance tests. These data suggest that GLP-1 may become a new target for ALS therapeutic research. However, further in vivo studies optimizing administration route and delivery methods should be conducted in animal models before effective use in any clinical trial.

8. Conclusions

As long as the exact cause of ALS remains elusive, it will be hard to propose any fully effective and accurately targeted form of therapy. Therefore, clinical trials should consider the broadest spectrum of neuroprotection possible. However, the methods employed have not always been standardized based on the results of preclinical research in animal models, resulting in ambiguous results in different studies performed in ALS patients. Since trophic factors have the ability to support survival and strengthen the functions of neural cells, further, more extensive studies are required to precisely investigate the real role of humoral activity in the natural history of ALS. To date, the most promising effects appear to be those obtained in studies employing VEGF and GDNF; however, clinical trials conducted on large numbers of patients remain lacking.

Acknowledgements

This is supported by the National Centre for Research and Development Grant STRAT-EGMED1/234261/2NCBR/2014.

Author details

Anna Sobuś and Bogusław Machaliński*

*Address all correspondence to: machalin@pum.edu.pl

Department of General Pathology, Pomeranian Medical University, Szczecin, Poland

References

[1] Zinman L., Cudkowicz M., Emerging targets and treatments in amyotrophic lateral sclerosis, *Lancet Neurol*, 2011; 10(5), 481–490.

[2] Gordon P., Amyotrophic lateral sclerosis: an update for 2013 clinical features, pathophysiology, management and therapeutic trials, *Aging Dis*, 2013; 4(5): 295–310.

[3] Millecamps S., Salachas F., Cazeneuve C., Gordon P., Bricka B., Camuzat A. et al., SOD1, ANG, VAPB, TARDBP, and FUS mutations in familial amyotrophic lateral sclerosis: genotype-phenotype correlations, *J Med Genet*, 2010; 47(8): 554–560.

[4] Morren J.A., Galvez-Jimenez N., Current and prospective disease-modifying therapies for amyotrophic lateral Sclerosis, *Expert Opin Investig Drugs*, 2012; 21: 297–320.

[5] Wang H., O'Reilly E.J., Weisskopf M.G., Logroscino G., McCullough M.L., Thun M.J., et al., Smoking and risk of amyotrophic lateral sclerosis: a pooled analysis of 5 prospective cohorts, *Arch Neurol*, 2011; 68: 207–213.

[6] Rothstein J.D., Current hypotheses for the underlying biology of amyotrophic lateral sclerosis, *Ann Neurol*, 2009; 65(Suppl 1): S3–S9.

[7] Miller R.G., Mitchell J.D., Moore D.H., Riluzole for amyotrophic lateral sclerosis (ALS)/ motor neuron disease (MND), *Cochrane Database Syst Rev*, 2012; 3: CD001447.

[8] Suzuki M., Svendsen C.N., Combining growth factor and stem cell therapy for amyotrophic lateral sclerosis, *Trends Neurosci*, 2008; 31(4): 192–198.

[9] Tovar-Y-Romo L.B., Ramírez-Jarquín U.N., Lazo-Gómez R., Tapia R., Trophic factors as modulators of motor neuron physiology and survival: implications for ALS therapy, *Front Cell Neurosci*, 2014; 8: 61.

[10] Chen Y., Shao J.Z., Xiang L.X., Dong X.J., Zhang G.R., Mesenchymal stem cells: a promising candidate in regenerative medicine,. *Int J Biochem Cell Biol*, 2008; 40(5): 815–820.

[11] Mariano E.D., Batista C.M., Barbosa B.J., Marie S.K., Teixeira M.J., Morgalla M., et al., Current perspectives in stem cell therapy for spinal cord repair in humans: a review of work from the past 10 years, *Arq Neuropsiquiatr*, 2014; 72: 451–456.

[12] Salem H.K., Thiemermann C., Mesenchymal stromal cells: current understanding and clinical status, *Stem Cells*, 2010; 28: 585–596.

[13] Ferrero I., Mazzini L., Rustichelli D., Gunetti M., Mareschi K., Testa L., et al., Mesenchymal stem cells from healthy donors and sporadic amyotrophic lateral sclerosis patients, *Cell Transplant*, 2008; 17: 255–266.

[14] Kim C., Lee H.C., Sung J.J., Amyotrophic lateral sclerosis cell based therapy and novel therapeutic development, *Exp Neurobiol*, 2014; 23(3): 207–214.

[15] Traub R., Mitsumoto H., Rowland L.P., Research advances in amyotrophic lateral sclerosis, 2009 to 2010, *Curr Neurol Neurosci Rep*, 2011; 11(1): 67–77.

[16] Tabakow P., Jarmundowicz W., Czapiga B., Fortuna W., Miedzybrodzki R., Czyz M., Huber J., Szarek D., Okurowski S., Szewczyk P., Gorski A., Raisman G., Transplantation of autologous olfactory ensheathing cells in complete human spinal cord injury, *Cell Transplant*, 2013; 22(9): 1591–612.

[17] Pearse D., Bunge M., Designing cell- and gene-based regeneration strategies to repair the injured spinal cord, *J Neurotrauma*, 2006; 23: 438–452.

[18] Machalinski B., Lazewski-Banaszak P., Dąbkowska E., Paczkowska E., Gołąb-Janowska M., Nowacki P., The role of neurotrophic factors in regeneration of the nervous system, *Neurol Neurochir Pol*, 2012; 46(6): 579–590.

[19] Ciesler J., Sari Y., Neurotrophic peptides: potential drugs for treatment of amyotrophic lateral sclerosis and Alzheimer's disease, *Open J Neurosci*, 2013; 3: 1–13.

[20] Lindholm P., Saarma M., Novel CDNF/MANF family of neurotrophic factors, *Dev Neurobiol*, 2010; 70: 360–371.

[21] Nicaise C., Mitrecic D., Pochet R., Brain and spinal cord affected by amyotrophic lateral sclerosis induce differential growth factors expression in rat mesenchymal and neural stem cells, *Neuropathol Appl Neurobiol*, 2011; 37(2): 179–188.

[22] Goulda T.W., Oppenheim R., Motor neuron trophic factors: therapeutic use in ALS?, *Brain Res Rev*, 2011; 67(1–2): 1–39.

[23] Park S., Kim H. T., Yun S., Kim I. S., Lee J., Lee I. S., Park K.I., Growth factor-expressing human neural progenitor cell grafts protect motor neurons but do not ameliorate motor performance and survival in ALS mice, *Exp Mol Med*, 2009; 41: 487–500.

[24] Paczkowska E., Kaczyńska K., Pius-Sadowska E., Rogińska D., Kawa M., Ustianowski P et al., Humoral activity of cord blood-derived stem/progenitor cells: implications for stem cell-based adjuvant therapy of neurodegenerative disorders, *PLoS One*, 2013; 8(12): e83833.

[25] Barde Y.A., Edgar D., Thoenen H., Purification of a new neurotrophic factor from mammalian brain, *EMBO J*, 1982; 1(5): 549–553.

[26] Chao M.V., Neurotrophins and their receptors: a convergence point for many signalling pathways, *Nat Rev Neurosci*, 2003; 4: 299–309.

[27] Huang E.J., Reichardt L.F., Trk receptors: roles in neuronal signal transduction, *Annu Rev Biochem*, 2003; 72: 609–642.

[28] Conner J.M., Lauterborn J.C., Yan Q., Gall C.M., Varon S., Distribution of brain-derived neurotrophic factor (BDNF) protein and mRNA in the normal adult rat CNS: evidence for anterograde axonal transport, *J Neurosci*, 1997; 17: 2295–2313.

[29] Cheng P.L., Song A.H., Wong Y.H., Wang S., Zhang X., Poo M.M., *Proc Natl Acad Sci U S A*, 2011; 108(45): 18430–18435.

[30] Ji Y., Lu Y., Yang F., Shen W., Tang T.T., Feng L., Duan S., Lu B., Acute and gradual increases in BDNF concentration elicit distinct signaling and functions in neurons, *Nat Neurosci*, 2010; 13: 302–309.

[31] Vicario-Abejón C., Owens D., McKay R., Segal M., *Nat Rev Neurosci*, 2002; 3(12): 965–974.

[32] Park H., Poo M.M., *Nat Rev Neurosci*, 2013; 14(1): 7–23.

[33] Ikeda K., Klinkosz B., Greene T., Cedarbaum J.M., Wong V., Effects of brain-derived neurotrophic factor on motor dysfunction in wobbler mouse motor neuron disease., *Ann Neurol*, 1995; 37(4): 505–511.

[34] The BDNF Study Group, A controlled trial of recombinant methionyl human BDNF in ALS: The BDNF Study, *Neurology*, 1999; 52: 1427–1433.

[35] Ochs G., Penn R.D., York M., Giess R., Beck M., Tonn J. et al., A phase I/II trial of recombinant methionyl human brain derived neurotrophic factor administered by intrathecal infusion to patients with amyotrophic lateral sclerosis, *Amyotroph Lateral Scler Other Motor Neuron Disord*, 2000; 1(3): 201–206.

[36] Kalra S., Genge A., Arnold D.L., A prospective, randomized, placebo-controlled evaluation of corticoneuronal response to intrathecal BDNF therapy in ALS using magnetic resonance spectroscopy: feasibility and results, *Amyotroph Lateral Scler Other Motor Neuron Disord*, 2003; 4(1): 22–26.

[37] Beck M., Flachenecker P., Magnus T., Giess R., Reiners K., Toyka K.V., Naumann M., Autonomic dysfunction in ALS: a preliminary study on the effects of intrathecal BDNF, *Amyotroph Lateral Scler Other Motor Neuron Disord*, 2005; 6(2): 100–103.

[38] Dadon-Nachum M., Ben-Yaacov K., Ben-Zur T., Barhum Y., Yaffe D., Perlson E., Offen D., Transplanted modified muscle progenitor cells expressing a mixture of neurotrophic factors delay disease onset and enhance survival in the SOD1 mouse model of ALS, *J Mol Neurosci*, 2015; 55(3): 788–797.

[39] Krakora D., Mulcrone P., Meyer M., Lewis C., Bernau K., Gowing G. et al., Synergistic effects of GDNF and VEGF on lifespan and disease progression in a familial ALS rat model, *Mol Ther*, 2013; 21(8): 1602–1610.

[40] Lin L.-F.H., Doherty D., Lile J., Bektesh S., Collins F., GDNF: a glial cell line-derived neurotrophic factor for midbrain dopaminergic neruons, *Science*, 1993; 260: 1130–1132.

[41] Wang L.J., Lu Y.Y., Muramatsu S., Ikeguchi K., Fujimoto K., Okada T. et al., Neuroprotective effects of glial cell line-derived neurotrophic factor mediated by an adeno-associated virus vector in a transgenic animal model of amyotrophic lateral sclerosis, *J Neurosci*, 2002; 22: 6920–6928.

[42] Clarkson E.D., Zawada W.M., Freed C.R., GDNF reduces apoptosis in dopaminergic neurons in vitro, *Neuroreport*, 1995; 7(1): 145–149.

[43] Kitagawa H., Hayashi T., Mitsumoto Y., Koga N., Itoyama Y., Abe K., Reduction of ischemic brain injury by topical application of glial cell line-derived neurotrophic factor after permanent middle cerebral artery occlusion in rats, *Stroke*, 1998; 29: 1417–1422.

[44] Grundström E., Askmark H., Lindeberg J., Nygren I., Ebendal T., Aquilonius S.M., Increased expression of glial cell line-derived neurotrophic factor mRNA in muscle biopsies from patients with amyotrophic lateral sclerosis, *J Neurol Sci*, 1999; 162(2): 169–173.

[45] Grundström E., Lindholm D., Johansson A., Blennow K., Askmark H., GDNF but not BDNF is increased in cerebrospinal fluid in amyotrophic lateral sclerosis, *Neuroreport*, 2000; 11: 1781–1783.

[46] Saarma M., Sariola H., Other neurotrophic factors: glial cell line-derived neurotrophic factor (GDNF), *Microsc Res Tech*, 1999; 45: 292–302.

[47] Suzuki M., McHugh J., Tork C., Shelley B., Hayes A., Bellantuono I., Aebischer P., Svendsen C.N., Direct muscle delivery of GDNF with human mesenchymal stem cells improves motor neuron survival and function in a rat model of familial ALS, *Mol Ther*, 2008; 16: 2002–2010.

[48] Acsadi G., Anguelov R.A., Yang H., Toth G., Thomas R., Jani A., et al., Increased survival and function of SOD1 mice after glial cell-derived neurotrophic factor gene therapy, *Hum Gene Ther*, 2002; 13(9): 1047–1059.

[49] Manabe Y., Nagano I., Gazi M.S.A., Murakami T., Shiote M., Shoji M., Kitagawa H., Setoguchi Y., Abe K., Adenovirus-mediated gene transfer of glial cell line-derived neurotrophic factor prevents motor neuron loss of transgenic model mice for amyotrophic lateral sclerosis, *Apoptosis*, 2002; 7(4).

[50] Manabe Y., Nagano I., Gazi M.S.A., Murakami T., Shiote M., Shoji M., et al., Glial cell line-derived neurotrophic factor protein prevents motor neuron loss of transgenic model mice for amyotrophic lateral sclerosis, *Neurol Res*, 2003; 25(2): 195–200.

[51] Kastin A.J., Akerstrom V., Pan W., Glial cell line-derived neurotrophic factor does not enter normal mouse brain, *Neurosci Lett*, 2003; 340: 239–241.

[52] Senger D.R., Galli S.J., Dvorak A.M., Perruzzi C.A., Harvey V.S., Dvorak H.F., Tumor cells secrete a vascular permeability factor that promotes accumulation of ascites fluid, *Science*, 1983; 219, 983–985.

[53] Carmeliet P., Ferreira V., Breier G., Pollefeyt S., Kieckens L., Gertsenstein M., et al., Abnormal blood vessel development and lethality in embryos lacking a single VEGF allele, *Nature* 1996; 380(6573): 435–439.

[54] Coultas L., Chawengsaksophak K., Rossant J., Endothelial cells and VEGF in vascular development, *Nature*, 2005; 438(7070): 937–945.

[55] Schwartz C.M., Tavakoli T., Jamias C., Park S., Maudsley S., Martin B., Stromal factors SDF1α, sFRP1, and VEGFD induce dopaminergic neuron differentiation of human pluripotent stem cells, *J Neurosci Res*, 2012; 90: 1367–1381.

[56] Erskine L., Reijntjes S., Pratt T., Denti L., Schwarz Q., Vieira J.M., VEGF signaling through neuropilin 1 guides commissural axon crossing at the optic chiasm, *Neuron*, 2011; 70: 951–965.

[57] Jin K.L., Mao X.O., Greenberg D.A., Vascular endothelial growth factor: direct neuroprotective effect in in vitro ischemia, *Proc Natl Acad Sci U S A*, 2000; 97: 10242–10247.

[58] Matsuzaki H., Tamatani M., Yamaguchi A., Namikawa K., Kiyama H., Vitek M.P., Vascular endothelial growth factor rescues hippocampal neurons from glutamate-induced toxicity: signal transduction cascades, *FASEB J*, 2001; 15: 1218–1220.

[59] Ma Y., Liu W.,Wang Y., Chao X., Qu Y.,Wang K., VEGF protects rat cortical neurons from mechanical trauma injury induced apoptosis via the MEK/ERK pathway, *Brain Res Bull*, 2011; 86: 441–446.

[60] Oosthuyse, B., Moons, L., Storkebaum, E., Beck, H., Nuyens, D., Brusselmans, K., et al., Deletion of the hypoxia-response element in the vascular endothelial growth factor promoter causes motor neuron degeneration, *Nat Genet*, 2001; 28: 131–138.

[61] Azzouz M., Ralph G.S., Storkebaum E., Walmsley L.E., Mitrophanous K.A., Kingsman S.M.,Carmeliet P.,Mazarakis N.D., VEGF delivery with retrogradely transported lentivector prolongs survival in a mouse ALS model, *Nature*, 2004; 429: 413–417.

[62] Sakowski S.A., Heavener S.B., Lunn J.S., Fung K., Oh S.S., Spratt S.K., et al., Neuroprotection using gene therapy to induce vascular endothelial growth factor-A expression, *Gene Ther*, 2009; 16: 1292–1299.

[63] Kliem M.A., Heeke B.L., Franz C.K., Radovitskiy I., Raore B., Barrow E., et al., Intramuscular administration of a VEGF zinc finger transcription factor activator (VEGF-

ZFP-TF) improves functional outcomes in SOD1 rats, *Amyotroph Lateral Scler*, 2011; 12: 331–339.

[64] Hwang D.H., Lee H.J., Park I.H., Seok J.I., Kim B.G., Joo I.S., et al., Intrathecal transplantation of human neural stem cells overexpressing VEGF provide behavioral improvement, disease onset delay and survival extension in transgenic ALS mice, *Gene Ther*, 2009; 16: 1234–1244.

[65] Storkebaum E., Lambrechts D., Dewerchin M., Moreno-Murciano M.P., Appelmans S., Oh H., et al., Treatment of motoneurondegeneration by intracerebroventricular delivery of VEGF in a rat model of ALS, *Nat Neurosci*, 2005; 8: 85–92.

[66] Zheng C., Skold M.K., Li J., Nennesmo I., Fadeel B., Henter J.I., VEGF reduces astrogliosis and preserves neuromuscular junctions in ALS transgenic mice, *Biochem Biophys Res Commun*, 2007; 363: 989–993.

[67] Salmon W.D., Daughaday W., A hormonally controlled serum factor which stimulates sulfate incorporation by cartilage in vitro, *J Lab Clin Med*, 1957; 49: 825–836.

[68] Froesch E.R., Burgi H., Ramseier E.B.,et al., Antibody-suppressible and nonsuppressible insulin-like activities in human serum and their physiologic significance. An insulin assay with adipose tissue of increased precision and specificity, *J Clin Invest*, 1963; 42: 1816–1834.

[69] Laron Z., Insulin-like growth factor 1 (IGF-1): a growth hormone, *J Clin Pathol Mol Pathol*, 2001; 54: 311–316.

[70] Caroni P., Activity-sensitive signaling by muscle-derived insulin-like growth factors in the developing and regenerating neuromuscular system, *Ann N Y Acad Sci*, 1993; 692: 209–222.

[71] Bilak M.M., Corse A.M., Kuncl R.W., Additivity and potentiation of IGF-I and GDNF in the complete rescue of postnatal motor neurons, *Amyotroph Lateral Scler Other Motor Neuron Disord*, 2001; 2: 83–91.

[72] Lepore A.C., Haenggeli C., Gasmi M., Bishop K.M., Bartus R.T., Maragakis N.J., Rothstein J.D., Intraparenchymal spinal cord delivery of adeno-associated virus IGF-1 is protective in the SOD1G93A model of ALS, *Brain Res*, 2007; 1185: 256–265.

[73] Franz C.K., Federici T., Yang J., Backus C., Oh S.S., Teng Q., et al., Intraspinal cord delivery of IGF-I mediated by adeno-associated virus 2 is neuroprotective in a rat model of familial ALS, *Neurobiol Dis*, 2009; 33: 473–481.

[74] Sorenson E.J., Windbank A.J., Mandrekar J.N., Bamlet W.R., Appel S.H., Armon C., et al., Subcutaneous IGF-1 is not beneficial in 2-year ALS trial, *Neurology*, 2008; 71: 1770–1775.

[75] Nagano I., Shiote M., Murakami T., Kamada H., Hamakawa Y., Matsubara E., et al., Beneficial effects of intrathecal IGF-1 administration in patients with amyotrophic lateral sclerosis, *Neurol Res*, 2005; 27: 768–772.

[76] Kim Y.K., Park J.H., Park S.H., Lim B., Baek W.K., Suh S.I., et al., Protective role of glucagon-like peptide-1 against glucosamine-induced cytotoxicity in pancreatic beta cells, *Cell Physiol Biochem*, 2010; 25(2–3): 211–220.

[77] Hamilton A., Holscher C., Receptors for the incretin glucagonlike peptide-1 are expressed on neurons in the central nervous system, *Neuroreport*, 2009; 20(13): 1161–1166.

[78] Perry T., Haughey N.J., Mattson M.P., Egan J.M., Greig N.H.,Protection and reversal of excitotoxic neuronal damage byglucagon-like peptide-1 and exendin-4, *J Pharmacol Exp Ther*, 2002; 302(3): 881–888.

[79] During M.J., Cao L., Zuzga D.S., Francis J.S., Fitzsimons H.L., Jiao X., et al., Glucagon-like peptide-1 receptor is involved in learning and neuroprotection, *Nat Med*, 2003; 9(9): 1173–1179.

[80] Sun H., Knippenberg S., Thau N., Ragancokova D., Körner S., Huang D., Dengler R., Döhler K., Petri S., Therapeutic potential of N-acetyl-glucagon-like peptide-1 in primary motor neuron cultures derived from non-transgenic and SOD1-G93A ALS mice, *Cell Mol Neurobiol*, 2013; 33(3): 347–57.

[81] Knippenberg S., Thau N., Dengler R., Brinker T., Petri S., Intracerebroventricular injection of encapsulated human mesenchymal cells producing glucagon-like peptide 1 prolongs survival in a mouse model of ALS, *PLoS One*, 2012; 7(6): e36857.

Chapter 12

Molecular Taxonomy: Use of Transcriptional Profiles to Identify Different ALS Subtypes

Giovanna Morello, Francesca Luisa Conforti,
Antonio Gianmaria Spampinato and
Sebastiano Cavallaro

Additional information is available at the end of the chapter

http://dx.doi.org/10.5772/62988

Abstract

Advances in diagnostic techniques and high-throughput biotechnologies provide a compelling opportunity to improve the diagnosis and treatment of diseases by developing a "New Taxonomy" that defines diseases on the basis of their underlying molecular and environmental factors rather than on traditional physical signs and symptoms. Oncology represents the first interesting example of how genomic medicine has changed the understanding of diseases and their therapy. However, much work remains to be completed on the molecular characterization and classification of complex and multifactorial diseases, including neurodegenerative disorders. Our research group has recently shown the genomic heterogeneity of sporadic amyotrophic lateral sclerosis (SALS), identifying two divergent subtypes associated with differentially expressed genes and pathways and providing several potential biomarkers and therapeutic targets. This chapter reviews the results emerged from our work, highlighting how molecular characterization of SALS patients may provide a framework for developing a more precise and accurate classification of diseases that could revolutionize the diagnosis, therapy, and clinical decisions of diseases, leading to more individualized treatments and improved outcomes for patients.

Keywords: ALS, expression profiling, genomics, molecular taxonomy, pathway analysis, system biology

INTECH
open science | open minds

© 2016 The Author(s). Licensee InTech. This chapter is distributed under the terms of the Creative Commons Attribution License (http://creativecommons.org/licenses/by/3.0), which permits unrestricted use, distribution, and reproduction in any medium, provided the original work is properly cited.

1. Introduction

The current diagnosis and classification of diseases are primarily based on physical signs and symptoms that, despite providing valuable information about clinical course, are often not sufficient to fully characterize the complex and heterogeneous nature of many disorders.

The completion of the human genome sequencing together with advances in high-throughput genomic, proteomic, imaging, and other diagnostic techniques in the past decades has provided a framework for developing a new, more accurate, and refined "molecular taxonomy" of human diseases which implies the use of molecular data (i.e., gene expression, copy number variants, single nucleotide polymorphisms, and haplotype analysis) to classify patients into distinct subgroups with differing diagnostic, prognostic, or therapeutic implications. This new disease classification has profound implications not only providing new insights into studying mechanisms and environmental causes underpinning diseases but also facilitating the development of a more precise diagnosis and individualized treatment for optimal therapeutic efficacy [1–3]. One seminal example of how molecular data may translate into clinical practice is represented by the "drug repositioning "approach. In fact, many drugs that were abandoned at clinical stages because of their low efficacy and/or toxicity in a specific subtype of patients may be re-evaluated for their potential therapeutic role with the consequent possibility to reduce both the time and costs associated with drug discovery and development [4].

Oncology offers multiple examples of how genomic medicine has changed disease understanding and drove targeted therapeutic interventions. Numerous studies, in fact, have demonstrated the power and ability of gene expression profiling, and other molecular approaches, to classify and substratify patients with various types of cancer (e.g., glioblastoma, breast, and colon carcinoma) into selective clinically relevant subtypes characterized by similar clinicopathological features but different biological properties, prognostic biomarkers, and treatment options [5]. Based on these promising results, over the past years, this new molecular reclassification has been extended to other polygenic and multifactorial human disorders, including cardiovascular and rheumatic diseases and multiple sclerosis [6]. However, a lack of progress remains in the understanding of detailed molecular mechanisms of several neurological and neurodegenerative diseases mainly because of the limited access to human brain tissues. Thus, the patient-specific molecular diagnosis of many neurological disorders and the consequent translation of this into tailored clinical trials and specific treatments remain challenging tasks [7].

Recently, by using an unsupervised hierarchical clustering analysis on motor cortex samples of patients with sporadic amyotrophic lateral sclerosis (SALS), our research group has identified two greatly divergent subtypes, each associated with differentially expressed genes and biological pathways [8]. These experiments highlight, for the first time, the genomic heterogeneity of SALS, revealing new clues for defining molecular signatures for this disease that were not put in evidence by considering SALS as a single entity. Moreover, the altered pathways of biological molecules in SALS also provided a number of potential biomarkers and therapeutic targets that could be used for developing personalized diagnosis and treatment of amyotrophic lateral sclerosis (ALS) [9, 10].

In this chapter, we will first briefly review the current state of the art in the ALS classification system, showing how the recent advances in technology and genetic discoveries have revolutionized ALS research. Then, we will discuss our data, the experimental setup, and results, highlighting how the molecular characterization of SALS patients may provide a framework for developing a new taxonomy of the disease and establishing the foundation for personalized medicine in ALS.

2. Amyotrophic lateral sclerosis: an overview

ALS is a neurodegenerative disease characterized by the progressive muscular paralysis reflecting the degeneration of upper and lower motor neurons which leads to respiratory insufficiency and death after three to five years. ALS is the commonest of the motor unit diseases in Europe and North America and its incidence ranges from 1.7 to 2.3 cases per 100,000 population per year worldwide [11]. Currently, there is no cure or prevention for ALS and Riluzole is the only disease-modifying medication presently approved by the US Food and Drug Administration (FDA) for the treatment of ALS [12]. Riluzole is largely symptomatic and prolongs survival but only with a modest effect. Many clinical trials have been performed but have unfortunately had limited success [13]. Thus, the development of novel treatments and diagnostic research strategies is a goal of increasing urgency.

Accurately understanding the etiopathogenic mechanisms underlying ALS is a crucial step for developing effective diagnostic–therapeutic strategies. Approximately 95% of the cases are isolated or sporadic (SALS), while about 10% are familial (FALS), showing autosomal dominant, recessive, or X-linked inheritance. Although genetic studies in FALS are rendered difficult by the late onset of disease, its incomplete penetrance and the short survival of affected family members, several familial ALS loci, and genes have been identified [14–16], such as *SOD1*, *ALSIN*, *SETX*, *SPG11*, *FUS*, *VAPB*, *ANG*, *TARDBP*, *FIG4*, *OPTN*, *ATXN2*, and *C9ORF72*. The contribution of genetic risk factors also seems to be considerable into the sporadic form of the disease [16]. Despite the identification of several disease-linked mutations, the etiology and pathogenesis of ALS remain largely unknown, supporting the multifactorial and complex nature of this disease, in which multiple genetic variants, each of the small effects, combine with a variety of environmental triggers and risk factors [14, 16–18].

The diagnosis of ALS is primarily based on the clinical observation of symptoms, physical signs, progression, and electrodiagnostic testing, in accordance with the "El Escorial" criteria. These represent a catalog of clinical and diagnostic features, specified by the World Federation of Neurology (www.wfneurology.org), that aim to exclude "ALS-mimic" syndromes (i.e., cervical spondylotic myelopathy, multifocal motor neuropathy, and Kennedy's disease) and permit to classify ALS patients for research studies [19–21]. The broad clinical spectrum of ALS comprehends distinct phenotypes ranging from pure upper motor neuron disease to pure lower motor neuron disease, with several different intermediate forms (classic, flail arm, flail leg, pyramidal, respiratory, and bulbar), each characterized by different degrees of involvment of Upper Motor Neurons (UMN) and Lower Motor Neurons (LMN), body regions that are affected, degrees of involvement of other systems especially cognition and behavior, and progression rates [22].

Although clinical neurophysiology in ALS plays a fundamental role in both diagnosis and assessment of its severity and progression, the initial symptoms of ALS are often subtle (limb or shoulder weakness and difficulty in walking), leading to a delay in the diagnosis as well as misdiagnosis and, consequently, restricting the possibilities for effective preventive and therapeutic strategies [23]. Thus, the adequate integration of neurophysiological techniques and advanced biological methods is essential in order to obtain a better understanding of disease pathogenesis, support earlier diagnosis, inform about prognosis, and monitor ALS progression in clinical trials.

The advent of high-throughput techniques—microarrays and next-generation sequencing—has shed light on the pathophysiology of complex diseases, including ALS and oriented researchers from a single-molecule analysis toward a "system biology" approach, offering a better understanding of the molecular mechanisms that, interacting with each other, may contribute to ALS pathogenesis [4].

3. Transcriptional analysis in ALS

In the last decade, the quantification of the transcriptome has represented one of the most informative research strategies for both discovering and defining mechanisms of pathogenesis in ALS as well as facilitating the discovery of biomarkers or new therapeutic approaches [24, 25]. In this regard, high-throughput genomic technologies, such as DNA microarrays, have been developed to simultaneously screen, on a genome-wide scale, the expression of thousands of genes in parallel in the same experiment, providing a more detailed picture of the ALS-related profile of molecular changes occurring during the disease progression [24, 26–28]. Both ALS post-mortem tissues (e.g., brain, spinal cord, cerebrospinal fluid, and blood) and those taken from animal models have been investigated with this purpose, revealing the involvement of several cellular events into ALS pathobiology, including mitochondrial dysfunction, enhanced apoptosis, glutamate-mediated excitotoxicity, oxidative stress, protein misfolding/aggregation, abnormal calcium metabolism, and altered axonal transport and neuroinflammatory cascades [29, 30]. However, because of the inherent complexity of nervous tissue and the need for post-mortem material, the existing genomic studies of ALS were restricted to a limited number of post-mortem ALS samples (≤11 motor cortex and 14 spinal cord), which did not permit the inclusion of genome changes within a framework of pathways or networks [24, 26–28].

http://dx.doi.org/10.5772/62988

4. Toward a molecular classification of SALS patients: our experience

Recently, our research group has analyzed whole-genome expression profiles of motor cortex samples from control and SALS patients [8]. In particular, using an unsupervised hierarchical clustering, we were able to separate control from SALS patients and subdivide the latter into two different subgroups (SALS1 and SALS2), based on differentially expressed genes and pathways. This molecular stratification of SALS patients has permitted us to reveal a novel etiopathogenic mechanism that was not emerged by considering SALS as a single entity, providing new interesting opportunities for defining molecular signatures for the disease. Moreover, our analysis has revealed a good number of potential therapeutic targets for the treatment of ALS patients [9, 10]. In the following sections, we will review our results, highlighting their potentiality for developing a new molecular taxonomy of ALS disease moving increasingly toward the idea of a personalized medicine for patients.

4.1. Data and results

To uncover the entire spectrum of genes and pathways involved in ALS pathology, we have analyzed whole-genome expression profiles of motor cortex samples from control and SALS patients [8]. In particular, we monitored whole genome mRNA expression profiles of genes in motor cortex of control (10) and SALS (31) patients. Unsupervised hierarchical clustering was used to cluster control and SALS patients on the basis of their similarities measured over the most informative genes (9646). Transcriptomic profiles obtained in cortex samples produced a good separation of controls and SALS patients, segregating these latter into two greatly divergent groups: SALS1 and SALS2 (**Figure 1a**). Interestingly, this patient stratification was not related to technical variations (arrays hybridization) or patient demographics (gender, age at onset, age at death, survival time from the date of onset, post-mortem intervals (PMIs)) (**Figure 1a**). By comparing gene expression profiles in SALS patients to controls, we identified a good number of significantly differentially expressed genes: 4485 in SALS1 and 16144 in SALS2. Although some of these genes (1268) were differentially expressed in both pairwise comparisons, the majority of differentially expressed genes were cluster specific (**Figure 1b**). A larger number of genes (21,930) were differentially expressed between SALS1 and SALS2, indicating these clusters were greatly divergent at the genomic level. Moreover, in order to depict genome changes within a framework of pathways, the most informative genes were subjected to pathway analysis by using functional ontologies represented in the MetaCore repository [31]. Statistically significant canonical pathways emerged from our analysis were involved in different cellular processes: apoptosis and survival, cell adhesion, cytoskeleton remodeling and axonal transport, cell cycle, immune response, energy metabolism, and signal transduction (**Figures 2–5**).

4.2. Pathway analysis and exploration of potential drug targets in ALS

In the following sections, we will review functional clusters of coregulated genes and pathways emerged in our previous work in light of the main pharmacological targets present, potentially useful for the development of more effective and personalized treatments for

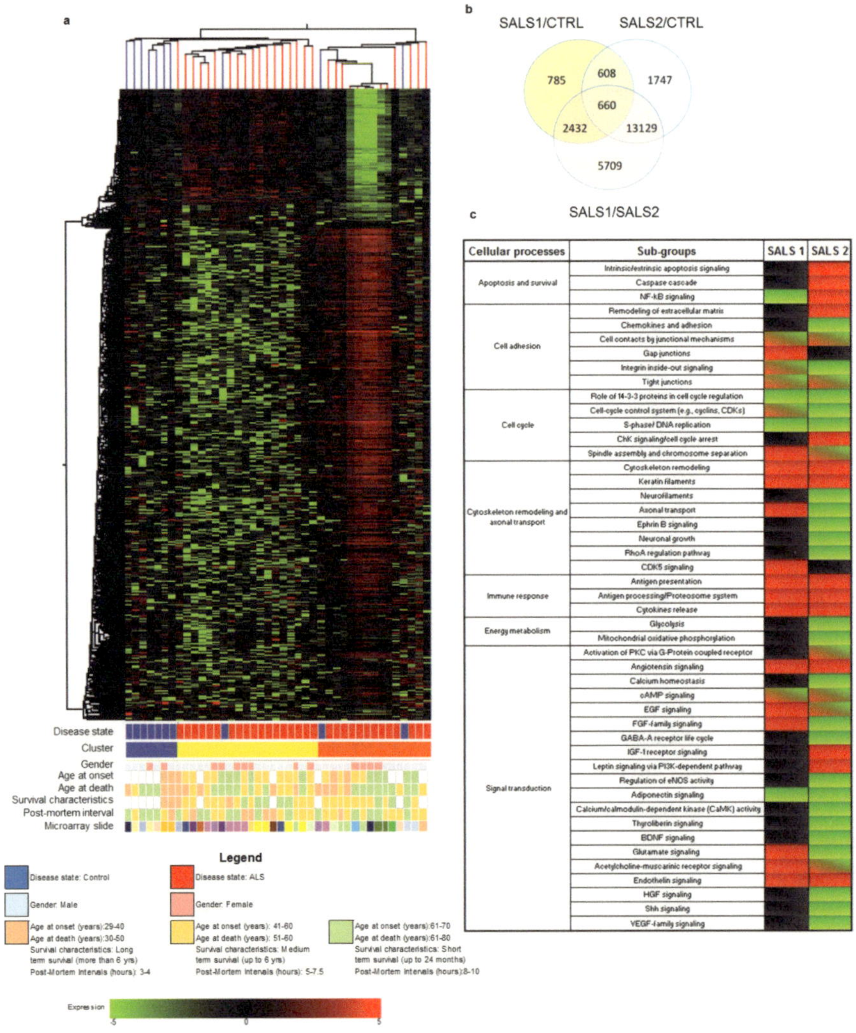

Figure 1. Panel a: Unsupervised hierarchical clustering of control and SALS patients and correlation between patient stratification and technical variation (array hybridization) or patient demographic (gender, age at onset, age at death, survival time from date of onset, and PMIs). Unsupervised hierarchical clustering (similarity measure: Pearson centered; linkage rule: average) was used to cluster control and SALS patients on the basis of their similarities measured over the most informative genes expressed in motor cortex (9646 genes with a standard deviation >1.5). Similarly, the same genes were clustered on the basis of their similarities measured over the motor cortex of control and SALS patients. In this two-dimensional presentation, each row represents a single gene and each column a motor cortex from control or SALS patients. In the "microarray slide" bar, samples hybridized on the same array are shown with the same color. As shown in the color bar, red indicates upregulation, green downregulation, and black no change. White squares indicate the n/a values. In the dendrograms shown (left and top), the length and the subdivision of the branches display the relatedness of the expression of the genes (left) and the motor cortex (top). Although SALS patients could be clearly distinguished on the basis of their motor cortex gene expression patterns, no significant association was found between their clinical characteristics and cluster assignment. **Panel b:** Venn diagrams of differentially expressed genes in the motor cortex of control and SALS (clusters 1 and 2) patients. **Panel c:** Pathways differentially deregulated in cluster SALS patients. Red boxes represent cellular processes mainly upregulated, green bars downregulated, red/green bars indicate signal pathways both up- and downregulated, and gray bars indicate no significant change when compared to controls.

ALS patients [8–10]. In particular, we focused our attention on primary targets of drugs actually undergoing to preclinical or clinical studies for several clinical diseases, including neurodegenerative [8, 9]. As described below and represented in **Figure 1c**, deregulation of identified genes and pathways in SALS patients was cluster specific.

4.2.1. Apoptosis and survival

A shift in the delicate balance between apoptosis- and survival-inducing genes plays a role in most neurodegenerative diseases, including ALS. We identified a number of genes, some encoding for potential drug targets, previously associated with apoptosis and survival that resulted deregulated in the cortex of SALS patients (**Figure 2a**) [8].

SALS2 patients showed increased expression of some genes involved in the triggering of the neuroinflammation and extrinsic apoptotic signaling cascade (Fas-L, FADD, RIPK1, and p38

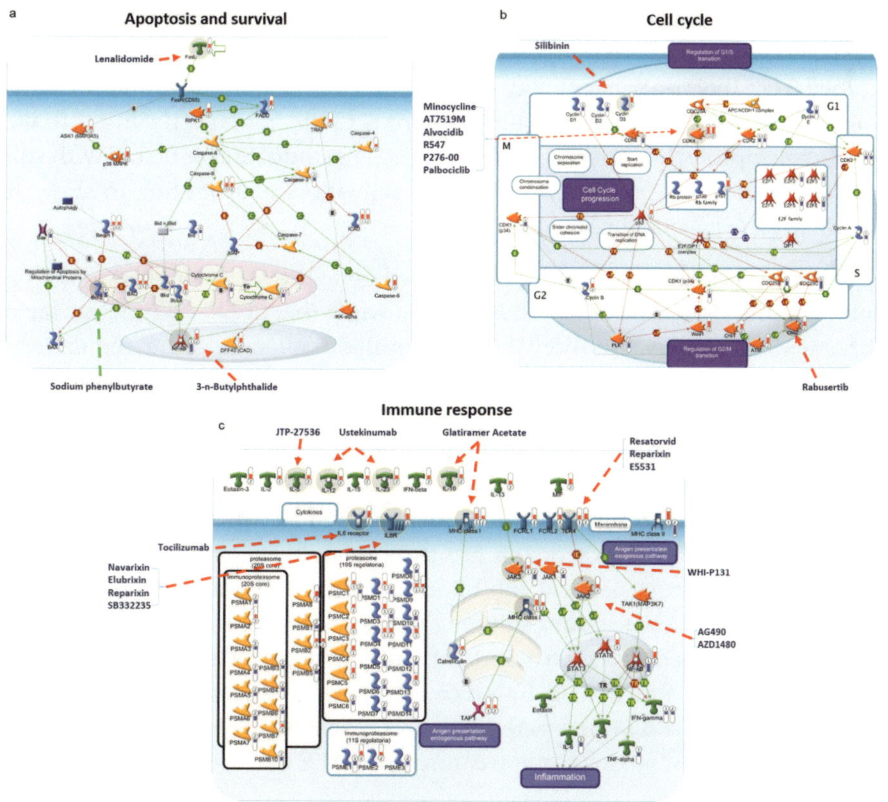

Figure 2. MetaCore analysis of altered signaling pathways in the motor cortex of SALS patients. Panel a: Apoptosis and survival. Panel b: Cell cycle. Panel c: Immune response. All maps are drawn from scratch by GeneGo annotators and manually curated and edited. Experimental data are visualized on the maps as blue (for downregulation) and red (upregulation) thermometers indicating expression ratio in the following conditions: 1 (SALS1/control) and 2 (SALS2/control). Some of the differentially expressed genes (highlighted with a yellow circle) are direct or indirect targets of experimental or therapeutic drugs. For each known drug target-pharmacological compound, we connect (dashed line) the drug to the target on which it acts. The line color indicates drug effect on target: red for inhibition and green for activation. Pathway objects and links are described separately in Supplementary Figure 1.

MAPK), accordingly with previous data found in degenerating spinal cord and cerebral cortex motor neurons of ALS mouse models [8]. Among these genes, Fas ligand (FasL or CD95L) may represent a possible target to block or slow the progressive degeneration of the motor neurons in ALS. In fact, preclinical studies have shown that Lenalidomide, a potent immunomodulatory agent that inactivates downstream effector caspases also by reducing the Fas-L expression, extends survival in transgenic mouse models of ALS [9]. Expression of genes encoding proteins (caspase-4, 6, 9, ICAD, and CAD) involved in one of the major processes responsible for the execution phase of cell apoptosis, the caspases signaling, resulted deregulated in SALS2 patients (**Figure 2a**), in accordance with previous findings showing their involvement in motoneuron degeneration in ALS [8].

Deregulated expression of pro- and antiapoptotic regulators (BAD, BID, BCL-2, BAX, and cytochrome c) involved in the mitochondrial intrinsic signaling pathway was also observed in SALS patients, supporting the evidence that the altered functionality of this system contributes to trigger motor neurons degeneration in both ALS patients and animal models [8]. Although the role of these factors in ALS pathogenesis should be further investigated, promising results were obtained from their pharmacological modulation. An example is represented by sodium phenylbutyrate, a programmed cell death inhibitor actually in phase II clinical trials for ALS that exerts its neuroprotective effects by pharmacological induction of BCL-2 with subsequent block both of cytochrome c release and caspase activation, contributing to slow the motor neuron death in ALS mice and patients [9].

The expression of Beclin1, a key autophagy-related gene previously linked to ALS neurodegeneration, was found increased in SALS patients, while that of NF-κB (nuclear factor kappa light chain enhancer of activated B cells) was identified with an opposite regulation in SALS patients (decreased in cluster 1 and increased in cluster 2) [8]. This apparent discrepancy may be explained by the controversial role of NF-κB on neurons. It is, in fact, a protein complex involved in various cellular mechanisms, including immune response and transcription regulation, cytokine production, and cellular responses to oxidative stress as well as processes of synaptic plasticity and memory. Although low levels of NF-κB have been related to loss of neuroprotection, its increased expression has been related to neuroinflammatory processes [32]. Several NF-κB pharmacological inhibitors, including dl-3-*n*-butylphthalide (dl-NBP), have been tested in preclinical studies showing to exert a neuroprotective role in ALS mainly by inhibiting programmed cell death and inflammation, reducing oxidative damage and improving mitochondrial function [9]. Based on these promising results, further studies aimed at defining the role of NF-κB in ALS pathogenesis are needed to elucidate its potentiality as a pharmacological target for personalized treatments of ALS patients.

4.2.2. Cell cycle

Progress in cell cycle is driven by oscillations in the activities of cyclin-dependent kinases (CDKs), which are controlled by periodic synthesis and degradation of cyclins as well as by other regulators. Alterations in gene expression and cellular distribution of these and other cell-cycle regulating proteins characterize several human neurodegenerative diseases, including ALS [33–35]. In accordance with this hypothesis, we observed deregulated expression of genes encoding key regulators of G1, S, M, and G2 phases (**Figure 2b**), some of them may represent an interesting candidate therapeutic target for ALS [9].

Increased expression of CDK4 and its regulatory subunit G1/S-specific cyclin-D3 were observed in SALS patients (**Figure 2b**), supporting the theory that dysregulation of the cyclin system may contribute to ALS neurodegeneration and that cell death may be the result of an unsuccessfully attempt by terminally differentiated neurons to re-entry into the cell cycle [8]. If so, drug inhibitors of the cell cycle might counteract neuronal degeneration in ALS, as suggested by *in vitro* studies on motor neurons. In fact, it has been observed that the pharmacological treatment with the CDK4 inhibitors (AT7519M, Alvocidib, R547, P276-00, Palbociclib, and Minocycline) currently studied for cancer treatment attenuates microgliosis and slows down the neuronal degeneration in a series of CNS disease models, including ALS [9]. Additionally, drugs inhibiting cyclin D3 signaling, including the natural flavonoid silibinin, also decrease CDK4 activity indirectly, with a consequent reduction of oxidative stress and inflammation. Given this, inhibitors of the cyclin–CDK complexes may represent a new promising avenue for ALS therapy and future clinical trials should be truly undertaken to measure their efficacy in ALS patients.

In accordance with previous observations in both SOD1 transgenic mice and ALS patients, in SALS2 patients we found the upregulation of Ataxia-telangiectasia-mutated (ATM), cell-cycle checkpoint kinases (CHK1/CHK2), and the tumor suppressor gene P53, whose increased levels have been associated with the arrest of the cell-cycle progression (**Figure 2b**) [8]. Although the role of CHK2 in ALS pathology remains unclear, our data suggest that an increased activity of this kinase may be the result of a DNA damage induced, for example, by diverse stress conditions, resulting in the alteration of neuronal apoptotic mechanisms. Therefore, pharmacological inhibitors of CHK2 (e.g., Rabusertib) may represent a promising therapeutic approach for delaying the progressive motor neurons degeneration in ALS.

4.2.3. Immune response

The immune response has been implicated in ALS and may contribute to the pathogenesis of disease or represent a response to damage. Reactive microglia and inflammatory processes have been observed to coincide with ALS onset and disease progression in SOD1 transgenic mice as well as post-mortem examinations of neural tissues in ALS patients show both innate and adaptive immunity activation [36, 37]. Similarly, we found differential expression of an extensive number of immune-related genes in the cortex of SALS patients (**Figure 2c**). While further explorations are needed to clarify the positive and negative effects of this system in ALS pathogenesis, its potential as a drug target is being explored [38].

Toll-like receptor 4 (TLR4) is among the immune-cell-specific genes upregulated in SALS patients, which is a marker of innate immunity response and monocyte/macrophage activation previously observed in reactive glial cells of spinal cords of ALS patients [8]. Several studies have shown that TLR4-signaling inhibition could reduce neuroinflammatory processes associated with ALS, supporting the potential therapeutic role of TLR4 inhibitors (Resatorvid, Reparixin, and E5531) in improving the neurological functionality recovery after brain injury and neuroinflammation [9].

SALS patients sowed differential expression of genes encoding Janus kinase (JAK-1, KAK-2, JAK-3, and Tyk-2) (**Figure 2c**), a family of tyrosine kinases mainly involved in the regulation of gene expression whose dysregulation has been already associated with inflammation and neurodegenerative diseases, including ALS [8]. The pharmacological blockade of JAK-STAT pathway with JAKs inhibitors (AG490, AZD1480, and WHI-P131) has shown neuroprotective effects also for slowing disease progression and increasing survival in an animal model of ALS [9].

In SALS patients, we also observed deregulated expression of several gene encoding proteins involved in antigen processing and presentation. Most of these genes were increased in SALS1 and reduced in SALS2 patients. Proteins involved in antigen presentation include major histocompatibility complex (MHC) class I and class II molecules (HLA-A, HLA-B, and HLA-C), TAP1, and calreticulin. MHC class I antigens were yet observed in the ALS affected tissues and their pharmacological inhibition with the immunomodulatory drug glatiramer acetate (GA) has shown neuroprotective effects in several neurological conditions [9]. This drug, clinically used for the treatment of multiple sclerosis, is currently object of phase II clinical trials for ALS. Proteins involved in antigen processing mainly belong to the proteasome/immunoproteasome system (**Figure 2c**), one of the major intracellular proteolytic mechanisms controlling the degradation of misfolded/abnormal proteins whose accumulation into damaged neurons represents a common hallmark in ALS. The deregulation of the constitutive and inducible proteasome subunits may not only influence the ubiquitin-mediated protein degradation but also lead to the generation of peptides that can be used by MHC I molecules for antigen presentation to the immune system, providing an interesting connection between the immune responses and proteasome function [39]. In this regard, SALS1 patients also showed the increased expression of serpin peptidase inhibitor, clade A, member 3 (SERPINA3), an acute phase reactant protein considered an important link between the immune/inflammatory response and proteasomal turnover [8]. Our findings are consistent with the previous results showing the upregulation of SERPINA3 in several ALS mouse models and human studies.

The upregulation of several cytokines and IFNβ was also observed in SALS2 patients (**Figure 2c**). Enhanced expression of IFNβ was already demonstrated in the spinal cord of SOD1 mice which seems to represent an early response to pathological changes in ALS. The downregulation of the potent anti-inflammatory cytokine interleukin-10 (IL-10) was observed in SALS2 patients (**Figure 2c**), sustaining the neuroprotective role of this factor against motor neuron injury in ALS [8]. It is of interest to note that glatiramer acetate, in addition to its activity as MHC regulator (as discussed above), also increases IL-10 levels suggesting that the multitarget action of this drug may provide an avenue for the treatment of ALS [9]. Although the pathogenic role of cytokines in ALS is still unknown, previous studies have associated their abnormal expression with the clinical status and some of these (IL8R, IL-5, IL-6R, IL-12, and IL-23) have been suggested as potential targets for the pharmacological treatment of ALS patients [9]. In this regard, different interleukin inhibitors, including those targeting the chemokine receptor interleukin 8 receptor (IL8R, also known as CXCR2) (Reparixin, Navarixin, Elubrixin, and SB332235) and IL-6 receptor (IL6R) (i.e., tocilizumab), showed excellent activity

http://dx.doi.org/10.5772/62988

in vitro against inflammatory cascade activation in SALS patients. In addition, the anti-IL-12/IL-23 monoclonal antibody ustekinumab has also shown neuroprotective properties, reversing cognitive decline related to Alzheimer's disease. Based on these evidences, further studies will be needed to elucidate the potential clinical benefits of these and other inflammatory cytokine inhibitors (such as JTP-27536) in the clinical treatment of ALS.

4.2.4. Cell adhesion

Dysfunction of the cell adhesion system may lead to alterations in cell–cell communication and the formation of multicellular structure, promoting the development of neurodegenerative diseases, such as ALS [40]. Consistently, our analysis has revealed differential expression of numerous genes involved in cell adhesion, mainly in SALS2 patients (**Figure 3a**). These genes encode for 12 integrin receptors (ITGA1, ITGA2, ITGA3, ITGA5, ITGA6, ITGA7, ITGA8, ITGA10, ITGA11, ITGAV, ITGB1, and ITGB4), three extracellular matrix molecules (Collagen IV, Laminin 1, and Fibronectin), seven components of tight junctions (Claudin-1, Claudin-3, Caludin-5, Jam1, Jam2, ZO-1, and ZO-2), and one component of Gap junctions (Connexin 43) [8]. A significant decrease in both protein and mRNA levels of tight junction components has been previously described in ALS patients and animal models. Although such a vast deregulation of integrins has not yet been described, changes in plasma Fibronectin levels were already found in ALS patients and were significantly correlated with the clinical progression of this disorder. A progressive decrease of Collagen IV has also been demonstrated in serum and vascular structures of ALS spinal cord while high levels of Laminin 1, previously observed in ALS spinal anterior horn, may represent a protective measure to aid neuronal survival. Integrins also play a role in the activation of focal adhesion kinase 1 (FAK-1) whose expression was upregulated in SALS patients (**Figure 3a**) as well as in other neurological diseases, such as Alzheimer's [8]. Interestingly, the pharmacological inhibition of FAK-1 signaling cascade by the administration of FAK-1 inhibitors (such as PF562271 and Sulindac) was observed to extend the survival of G93A SOD1 mice [9].

SALS2 patients also show the differential expression of four extracellular matrix metalloproteinases (MMP-1, 2, 9, and 13) together with the metallopeptidase inhibitor TIMP1. MMPs are a family of zinc-dependent endoproteinases that regulate the extracellular matrix structure and play an important role in synaptic remodeling, neuronal regeneration, and remyelination, modulation of blood–brain and blood–cerebrospinal fluid barrier permeability and leukocyte invasion in neuroinflammatory diseases [8]. Although the role of MMPs in ALS pathogenesis is currently unknown, their altered levels may reflect degenerative processes of motor neurons and tissues remodeling. Moreover, deletion of MMP-9 gene has shown to accelerate motor neuron disease and shorten survival in mutant SOD-1 mice. Several studies have sustained the potential role of MMP inhibitors as attractive candidates for ALS therapy and demonstrated the beneficial effects of compounds inhibiting MMP expression, synthesis, and activity in various neurodegenerative conditions [9]. Among these drugs, a particular attention should be addressed to thalidomide, a potent anti-inflammatory drug, which is able to reduce MMP-2 and increase the lifespan of ALS animal models. Although this drug has shown promising results in ALS patients, its clinical use is limited by a variety of side effects. Even so, other

MMPI inhibitors (Marimastat, Tanomastat, Batimastat, ONO4817, Doxycycline, Rebimastat, Pravastatin, S3304, Halofuginone, and Melphalan) in addition to their antineoplastic properties have also gained interest for their therapeutic effects in several neurodegenerative conditions, including Alzheimer's disease [9].

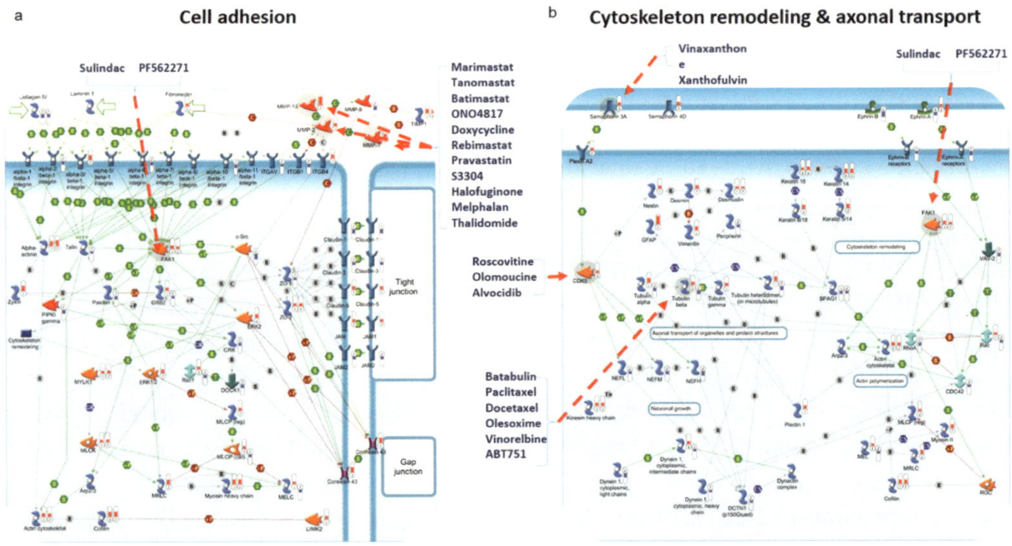

Figure 3. MetaCore analysis of altered signaling pathways in the motor cortex of SALS patients. Panel a: Cell adhesion. Panel b: Cytoskeleton remodeling and axonal transport. All maps are drawn from scratch by GeneGo annotators and manually curated and edited. Experimental data are visualized on the maps as blue (for downregulation) and red (upregulation) thermometers indicating expression ratio in the following conditions: 1 (SALS1/control) and 2 (SALS2/control). Some of the differentially expressed genes (highlighted with a yellow circle) are direct or indirect targets of experimental or therapeutic drugs. For each known drug target-pharmacological compound, we connect (dashed line) the drug to the target on which it acts. The line color indicates drug effect on target: red for inhibition and green for activation. Pathway objects and links are described separately in Supplementary Figure 1.

4.2.5. Cytoskeleton remodeling and axonal transport

The cytoskeleton is critical for neuronal maintenance and plasticity, neurite outgrowth, axonal caliber, and transport. Our analysis uncovered differential expression of genes encoding major components of the cytoskeleton in SALS patients, including intermediate filaments proteins (Nestin, GFAP, Desmin, Desmuslin, Vimentin, Peripherin, Keratins 5, 8, 14, and 18), Actin, Tubulin (alpha, beta, and gamma), Myosin, and all three neurofilament subunits (NEFL, NEFM, and NEFH) (**Figure 3b**).

Tubulin beta proteins (TUBBs) belong to the tubulin family of proteins that, together with alpha-tubulin, form and organize structures called microtubules. TUBBs are expressed in neurons which are involved in several processes, including neurogenesis and axon guidance and maintenance/remodeling. Differential expression of genes encoding TUBB1/TUBB3 was observed in SALS patients (**Figure 3b**), supporting previous data that propose tubulin system recovery as a possible mechanism for restoring the altered nerve signal in ALS [8]. In this regard, several studies support the ability of taxanes (Paclitaxel and Docetaxel) and other microtubule-targeting drugs (Batabulin, Vinorelbine, and ABT751) to restore lost nerve signals in neurodegenerative conditions, such as Alzheimer's [9]. Although the potential neurotoxicity of these drugs has limited their clinical use, the development of novel compounds may prevent this side effect. Among these novel compounds, olesoxime, a potent trophic factor able to promote neuronal survival and axonal sprouting, has shown prominent neuroprotective properties for motor neurons in both *in vitro* and *in vivo* models.

Despite the controversial role of neurofilaments (NFs) in ALS, their aberrant accumulation in the cell body and proximal axons of motor neurons is a hallmark of ALS [8]. A deletion of NEFL subunits in an ALS mouse model, in fact, is accompanied by an increase of the NEFH and NEFM subunits in the motor neuron cell bodies and their reduction in the axons, slowing the onset and progression of the disease. Increased expression of the NEFH subunit has similar effects, suggesting that NFs may act as buffer for processes that would otherwise be deleterious, for example, offering phosphorylation sites for dysregulated intracellular tyrosine kinases or reducing the axonal burden. Decreasing the axonal burden of NFs may thus protect motor neurons, at least in part, by enhancing axonal transport, a hypothesis supported by the observation of defects in slow axonal transport in presymptomatic ALS animal models.

Consistent with the view that impaired axonal transport may be involved in the degeneration of motor neurons, we observed in SALS2 patients the downregulation of cytoplasmic Dynein intermediate, light, and heavy chains, together with the p150Glued subunit of Dynactin (DCTN1), implicated in retrograde transport of cargoes, such as endosomes (**Figure 3b**). Mutations in the cytoplasmic Dynein heavy-chain gene have previously been found in two mouse models, Legs at odd angles (Loa) and Cramping 1 (Cra1), with late-onset motor neuron degeneration, while mutations of DCTN1 gene are responsible for a lower motor neuron disorder with vocal cord paresis. In addition to this, decreased expression of DCTN1 has been reported in motor neurons of patients with SALS suggesting that abnormalities in Dynactin may play a role in the pathogenesis of ALS [8].

Aberration in axon guidance may also result from differential expression of Semaphorins, Plexins, and Ephrins as well as of their receptors in SALS patients, together with their downstream signaling factors (Cdc42, Rac, and RhoA) (**Figure 3b**). Increased expression of Semaphorin 3A (SEMA3A), a protein involved in the regulation of axon and dendrite growth guidance and neural system development, has previously been associated with deadhesion or repulsion of motor axons away from the neuromuscular junction in terminal Schwann cell of SOD1G93A transgenic mice, probably resulting in axonal denervation and motor neuron degeneration [8]. An altered expression of SEMA3A, in fact, might lead to aberrant outgrowth of corticospinal tract fibers from the cortex, the inappropriate guidance of cranial motor axons and hyperfasciculation or defasciculation of both cranial nerves and MMC and LMC motor axons. Although these changes in SEMA3A expression might be small and may not cause obvious defects during early life, minor changes in motor neuron circuitry due to altered SEMA3A expression may result in motor connections, which are more vulnerable to additional genetic or environmental changes. Although the precise role of SEMA3A in the pathogenesis of ALS is unclear, vinaxanthone and xanthofulvin, two selective SEMA3A inhibitors, have shown to promote neuronal regeneration, suggesting a potential role of this and other SEMA3A modulatory drugs as protective agents against neurodegenerative conditions, including ALS [9]. Promising results have also been obtained by the pharmacological inhibition of downstream mediators of SEMA3A signaling cascade, such as cell division protein kinase 5 (CDK5), whose expression resulted augmented in SALS1 patients (**Figure 3b**), in accordance with previously published studies [8]. It has been, in fact, demonstrated that the treatment with CDK5 inhibitors, including olomoucine and roscovitine, is able to reduce neuronal death and microglial neurotoxicity as well as reverse axonal transport defects, contributing to reduce ALS neurodegeneration [9]. The promising effects shown by these and other CDK5 inhibitors (e.g., Alvocidib) encourage further studies aimed to evaluate the clinical utility of this drug class in ALS therapy.

Similarly to Semaphorins, Ephrins have a variety of important functions including axonal outgrowth and cytoskeletal structure development, neuronal connectivity, neuronal apoptosis, synaptic maturation, and plasticity. It is, therefore, plausible that variability in such molecules could contribute to the initiation and progression of neurodegenerative diseases. A marked increase of Ephrin A1 has previously been found in motor neurons of SALS patients and SNPs in several Ephrin and Eph receptor genes, including Ephrin B1, have been used to predict susceptibility, survival free, and age at onset of ALS [8]. Our findings in ALS motor cortex support the hypothesis that aberrant expression or function of Ephrins may induce pathological changes in motor neuron circuitry and contribute to ALS pathogenesis.

4.2.6. Energy metabolism

Energy metabolism is an extremely complicated series of chemical reactions that breakdown organic matter to harvest energy and involved two main processes: glycolysis and mitochondrial oxidative phosphorylation (**Figure 4**). Among the proteins implicated in the glycolysis process are 6-phosphofructokinase (PFKM and PFKP) and pyruvate kinase (KPYR and PKM2), and MDH1, some enzymes of the rate-limiting step that were previously linked to ALS [8]. These genes were mainly downregulated in SALS2 patients. In the same patients, we observed the coordinated decrease of several gene encoding proteins involved in the oxidative phosphorylation pathway, including those encoding proteins of respiratory complex I (36/46 subunits), II (SDHB and SDHD), III (7/11 subunits), IV (6/13 subunits), and V (10/14 subunits of the catalytic and membrane proton channel of ATP synthase), while a limited but significant number of these genes were increased in SALS1 (**Figure 4**). Our findings are in agreement with previous studies conducted on post-mortem ALS tissues in which an increase of complex I and a deficiency of complex IV are reported. This apparent discrepancy may be explained by the opposite behavior of SALS patients found in the present study (increase of complex I in SALS1 and decrease of complex IV in both clusters). Oxidative phosphorylation represents one of the major cellular energy supply systems and its deregulation has been widely reported to play an important role in ALS pathology [8]. Dysfunctional mitochondria, in fact, exhibit a reduction in bioenergetics efficiency, putting neurons at risk of death when energy demands exceed cellular energy production. Based on these findings, it appears evident that treatments designed to improve respiratory chain function may ameliorate the progression of this disorder. In this regard, some drugs that can reverse mitochondrial dysfunction (Acetyl-L-carnitine, Creatine, Minocycline, Olesoxime, Dexpramipexole, and Cyclosporine A) are currently in clinical trials for ALS, showing to be effective and well tolerated [9]. Promising preclinical results for ALS were also reported by other members of this drug class (Uridine, Pyruvate, and Dichloroacetate), supporting the idea that mitochondria-targeted therapies may restore bioenergetics defects observed in SALS2 patients.

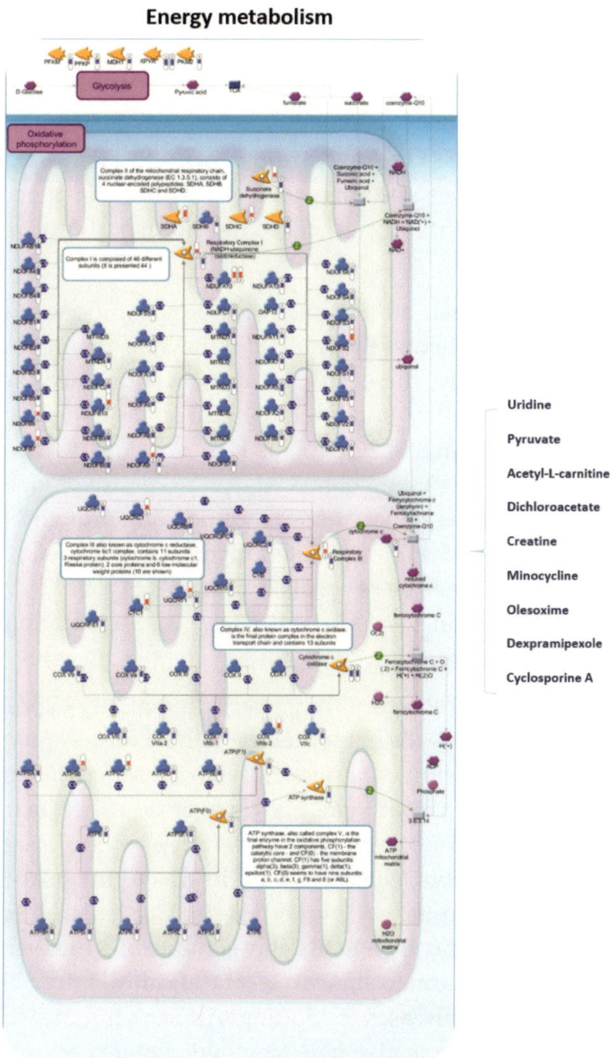

Figure 4. MetaCore analysis of altered energy metabolism pathways in the motor cortex of SALS patients. The map is drawn from scratch by GeneGo annotators and manually curated and edited. Experimental data are visualized on the maps as blue (for downregulation) and red (upregulation) thermometers indicating expression ratio in the following conditions: 1 (SALS1/control) and 2 (SALS2/control). Drugs potentially useful for reversing mitochondrial dysfunction are shown on the right side of the map. Pathway objects and links are described separately in Supplementary Figure 1.

4.2.7. Signal transduction

Neurosignaling involves the largest class of proteins and receptors that transmit chemical signals from the cell surface to their intracellular targets. This section, for the multitude of signaling cascades resulted altered in SALS patients, will be divided into two subsections (neuropeptides and receptors, and neuromodulation and ion homeostasis).

4.2.7.1. Neuropeptides and receptors

Neurotrophins is a protein family that, among other things, is able to influence the survival and death as well as the development, proliferation, and differentiation of neuronal and non-neuronal cells. The loss of neurotrophins and their receptors and the consequent deleterious effect on neuron health and stability is one of the major pathologic hallmarks of neurodegenerative disorders, including ALS [41]. In accordance with this concept, our results showed the differential expression of genes encoding several neuropeptides and relative receptors, many of them represented potential drug targets, in the motor cortex of SALS patients (**Figure 5a**).

Deregulated expression of diverse adipokines, including Adiponectin, Leptin, and their receptors, was found in SALS patients (**Figure 5a**) [8]. Beyond their peripheral effects on fat metabolism and insulin sensitivity, these proteins and receptors are expressed in the brain which regulate neuronal excitability and exert neurotrophic and neuroprotective effects. Decreased expression of PTCH1 in SALS2 patients is in agreement with the neuroprotective effects of Sonic hedgehog (Shh) signaling observed in ALS mouse models. The same patients also showed downregulated expression of three gene encoding proteins implicated in neurite outgrowth and ALS pathology: Myelin-associated glycoprotein (MAG), Reticulon-4, and its receptor. Anti-MAG antibodies have been yet observed in ALS patients, whereas a number of studies have implicated Reticulon-4 in ALS pathology, demonstrating a protective effect against ALS-like neurodegeneration.

Several trophic factors and their receptors were also differentially expressed in SALS cortex (**Figure 5a**) [8]. Among these, all are the epidermal growth factor receptors (EGFRs) and some of their ligands, according to previous findings in liquor of ALS patients. Evidence suggests that the activation of this signaling pathway may trigger quiescent astrocytes into reactive astrocytes and, consequently, activate the neurodegenerative process. Pharmacological studies showed that EGFR/ErbB2 inhibitors, clinically used in cancer treatment, have recently also gained interest for their neuroprotective properties [9]. Particularly, some of these drugs (Erlotinib, Genistein, and Masoprocol) seem to delay significantly disease onset in ALS animal models. Belonging to the same pharmacological class is Suramin, a drug actually in preclinical phase for several neurological diseases, including Alzheimer's and Parkinson's. Besides inhibiting EGF signaling, Suramin is also able to inhibit the activity of histone deacetylase (HDAC), nitric oxide synthase (NOS), and P2Y2, three proteins already widely associated with ALS pathogenesis [42, 43]. The promising preclinical results obtained with above-mentioned and other EGFR/ErbB2 inhibitors (PKI166, BMS690514, Canertinib, Gefitinib, and PD153035) stimulate their future developments and clinical validations in the hope of translating them into clinical practice.

http://dx.doi.org/10.5772/62988

Decreased levels of Neuregulin were observed in SALS patients, coherently with previous findings observed in cerebral spinal fluid of ALS patients, as well as aberrant Neuregulin signaling was detected in both ALS patients and SOD1 mice [8]. Moreover, altered expression of genes encoding three fibroblast growth factor receptors and seven of their ligands was detected in SALS patients (**Figure 5a**). Reduced expression of FGF9 may be consistent with its role as an autocrine or paracrine survival factor for motoneurons [8]. On the other hand, the release of FGF-1 from motor neurons is expected to happen in response to oxidative stress stimuli, leading to the accumulation of FGFR1 and activation of astrocytes that, in turn, could initiate or promote apoptotic processes in ALS. In support of this theory, studies conducted on FGFR inhibitors (e.g., PD166866) have shown promising effects, by preventing motor neuron apoptosis in ALS mouse models, sustaining the need for additional studies to further investigate the role of this and other inhibitors of FGF signal transduction (Orantinib, Brivanib, Dovitinib, Suramin, and Pentosan polysulfate) in ALS therapy [9].

SALS patients also showed altered expression of genes encoding brain-derived neurotrophic factor (BDNF), one member of the neurotrophin family of growth factors, and their receptors (TrkA, TrkB, TrkC, and NGFR) (**Figure 5a**), according to an extensive amount of data supporting their implication in ALS humans and animal models [8]. In particular, a prolonged TrkB activation may render motor neurons vulnerable to excitotoxic insult, contributing to developing ALS. Therefore, therapeutic strategies aimed to inhibit TrkB signaling may result promising for treating ALS. Although the development of TrkB inhibitors has been difficult, mainly because of the central role of BDNF in cognitive functions, some selective compounds (Cyclotraxin-B and Ana-12) have shown to decrease neurotoxicity without affecting neuronal survival [9].

The expression of vascular endothelial growth factors (VEGF-A, VEGF-B, VEGF-C, and VEGF-D) and their receptors (VEGF-R1, VEGF-R2, Neuropilin 1, and Neuropilin 2) was mainly downregulated in SALS2 patients (**Figure 5a**). There are extensive evidence linking this family of ligands and receptors to ALS pathology [44, 45] and treatment with VEGF was found to strongly protect motor neurons from excitotoxicity and prevent neuronal death in different models of ALS [8]. In addition, some drugs activating VEGF (SB-509 and Celecoxib) have been tested in phase II clinical trials for ALS, showing encouraging results [9].

The downregulation of hepatocyte growth factor (HGF) was observed in SALS2 patients, which is one of the most potent survival-promoting factors for motor neurons with potential therapeutic effects on ALS (**Figure 5a**) [8]. Likewise, decreased expression of thyrotropin-releasing hormone (TRH) receptor in SALS2 patients supports previous studies showing a reduction of this receptor in the spinal cord of ALS patients and may explain the conflicting results obtained by TRH therapy. Masoprocol is among TRHR agonist, which, besides its EGFR inhibitor activity, is also able to exert neuroprotective effects through anti-inflammatory and antioxidant properties as well as by reducing the glutamate neurotoxicity. In addition, Taltirelin, another TRH analog, also exerts neuroprotective effects in several neurodegenerative conditions, contributing to make these attractive candidates for restore damaged or maladaptive neural systems in ALS patients [9].

The expression of several gene encoding G-protein coupled receptors and/or their ligands is resulted altered in SALS patients (**Figure 5a**). Some of these, such as the Muscarinic acetylcholine receptors, the endothelin-1, and its receptor EDNR-B, have been previously associated with ALS pathology and pharmacological approaches, aimed to repair these defective neuromodulatory signaling, are thought to slow motor neuron degeneration in ALS [8]. Several preclinical and clinical studies have corroborated this hypothesis, suggesting that muscarinic agonists (such as Cevimeline, Xanomeline, Bethanechol, and Clozapine) may be able to restore neuronal loss associated with diverse CNS disorders, including ALS. In the same way, evidence has demonstrated that EDNR-B antagonists (such as BQ-788, Bosentan, and IRL-2500) exert neuroprotective and neuroinflammatory properties [9].

Differential expression of leukemia inhibitory factor (LIF) and its receptor emerged from our analysis is consistent with a study proposing LIF as a modifier gene in ALS, while that of Angiotensin II and its type-1 receptor (AGTR1) is in agreement with previous studies showing altered levels of Angiotensin II in liquor of ALS patients [8]. Moreover, angiotensin signaling pathway has been recently proposed as a new potential target in ALS therapy [9]. In fact, agents able to block AGTR1 (ARBs), such as Telmisartan, Olmesartan, and Candesartan, in addition to their clinical usefulness as antihypertensive agents have also shown neuroprotective effects in Alzheimer's and other neuronal diseases. Among these drugs, olmesartan has manifested neurotrophic properties on spinal motor neurons *in vitro* and *in vivo*. This drug class also exerts its neuroprotective actions by significantly enhancing GLT-1 expression, whose loss of function has been widely implicated in the pathogenesis of ALS.

The upregulation of purinergic receptor P2Y2 found in SALS patients (**Figure 5a**) is in agreement with previous studies as well as that of insulin-like growth factor 1 receptor (IGFR-1) that supports the critical role of this signaling cascade in ALS pathogenesis [8]. In this regard, the inhibition of the IGF signaling pathway has been seen to increase lifespan and prevent neurodegeneration in a variety of model organisms [9]. Simvastatin is among IGF receptor inhibitors, which has shown to reduce the excitotoxicity and neuronal death occurring in neurodegenerative diseases, such as Alzheimer's and Parkinson's, suggesting that treatment with this and other IGF receptor inhibitors (such as Masoprocol, BMS-754807, and Linsitinib) may represent a potential strategy for the treatment of ALS.

4.2.7.2. Ion homeostasis

A number of genes encoding proteins and/or their receptors involved in the regulation of ion homeostasis were deregulated in the motor cortex of SALS patients and some of them (CACNA1C, GRIAs, and GABRs) may be taken into account as targets in ALS therapy (**Figure 5a**).

Decreased expression of L-type voltage-gated calcium channels (CACNA1C) (**Figure 5a**) is consistent with the presence of immunoglobulins against this L-type voltage-gated calcium channels in ALS patients, which correlate with disease progression and exert neurotoxicity [8]. The downregulation of three subunits of the *N*-methyl-d-aspartate (NMDA) receptor (GRIN1, GRIN2A, and GRIN2D) observed in SALS2 patients (**Figure 5a**) is in agreement with previous studies in animal models and with a large literature indicating that a dysfunction of these ligand-gated cation channels may be an underlying molecular mechanism in ALS [8]. Three subunits of the alpha-amino-3-hydroxy-5-methyl-4-isoxazole propionate (AMPA) glutamate receptor were differentially expressed in SALS patients: GRIA1 increased in SALS1 patients, whereas GRIA2 and GRIA3 were reduced in SALS2 (**Figure 5a**). Similar changes in expression of GRIA1 and GRIA2 have been reported in SOD1 mice, whereas in human a defect in the editing of the messenger RNA encoding GRIA2 has been previously reported. AMPA receptors lacking the GRIA2 subunit are permeable to Ca2+ and the entrance of this cation might be responsible for the selective vulnerability of spinal motoneurons in ALS. These results are in accordance with the theory that the receptor-mediated glutamate toxicity, together with alteration in neuronal calcium homeostasis, may induce pathological changes associated with motor neurons in ALS. Therefore, pharmacological strategies aimed to minimize glutamate-mediated neurotoxicity and restore impaired calcium homeostasis could result useful for the treatment of the ALS condition. In this regard, preclinical studies conducted on FPL 64176 and Bay K 8644, two CACNA1C agonists, have highlighted neuroprotective effects exerted by these compounds in ALS [9]. Moreover, the administration of AMPA receptor antagonists has

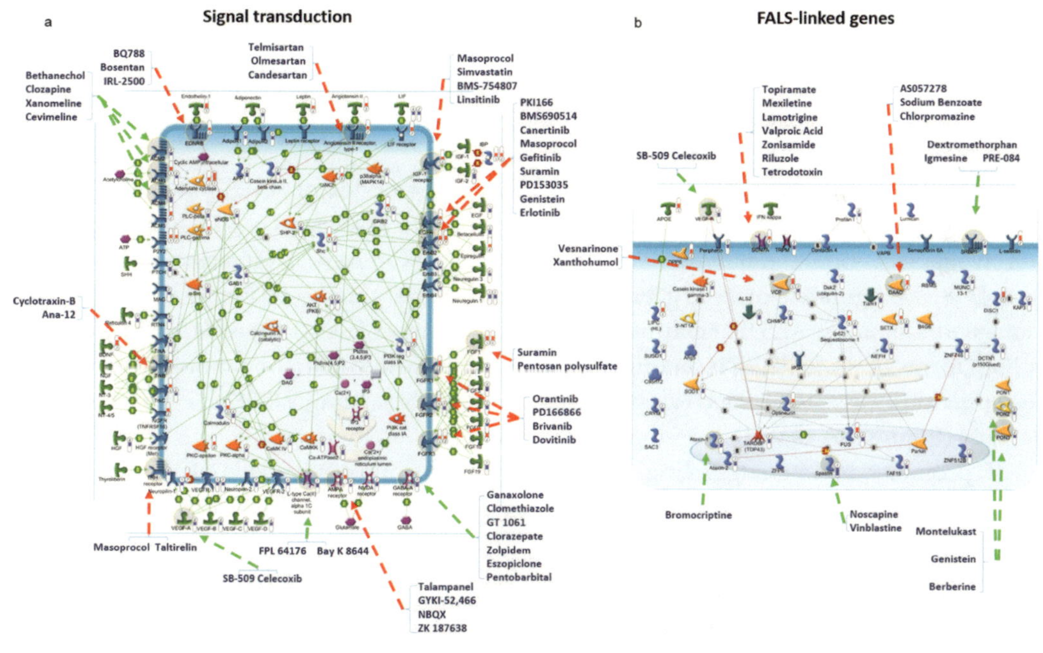

Figure 5. MetaCore analysis of altered signaling pathways in the motor cortex of SALS patients. Panel a: Signal transduction. Panel b: FALS-linked genes. All maps are drawn from scratch by GeneGo annotators and manually curated and edited. Experimental data are visualized on the maps as blue (for downregulation) and red (upregulation) thermometers indicating expression ratio in the following conditions: 1 (SALS1/control) and 2 (SALS2/control). Some of the differentially expressed genes (highlighted with a yellow circle) are direct or indirect targets of experimental or therapeutic drugs. For each known drug target-pharmacological compound, we connect (dashed line) the drug to the target on which it acts. The line color indicates drug effect on target: red for inhibition and green for activation. Pathway objects and links are described separately in Supplementary Figure 1.

shown promising effects by re-establishing Ca2+ homeostasis and reducing glutamate excitotoxicity. Among these, ZK 187638, NBQX, and GYKI-52,466 have shown protective effects on motor neurons in ALS animal models, by improving motor functions and prolonging survival. Moreover, also talampanel, another exponent of this drug class, has shown promising results in preclinical stages for ALS, but only a limited efficacy has been observed when tested in ALS patients. This clinical failure may be at least partly explained by the differential expression of GRIA1 and GRIA2 observed in SALS patients (**Figure 5a**). In the light of this, further studies are needed to re-evaluate the potential therapeutic benefits of talampanel for the personalized treatment of ALS patients.

Downregulated expression of six subunits of the gamma-aminobutyric acid type A receptor (GABA-A) was also found in SALS2 patients (**Figure 5a**) [8]. Although impaired GABAergic signaling has been previously observed in the motor cortex of ALS patients, little is known about its receptor composition. The few studies present in the literature confirm the reduced expression of the alpha1 subunit in ALS patients. This may suggest GABA-A signaling agonists as potential therapeutic agents able to reduce or prevent the progressive degeneration of motor neurons occurring in ALS. In accordance with this theory, some GABA-A agonists (Ganaxolone, Clomethiazole, GT 1061, Clorazepate, Zolpidem, Eszopiclone, Pentobarbital, and GT 1061) have shown neuroprotective properties in several neurological conditions by preventing excitotoxicity and neuronal loss [9].

4.2.8. Genes previously linked to FALS

Our analysis has revealed differential expression in the cortex of SALS patients of a large number of genes whose mutations have been previously associated with FALS (**Figure 5b**) and available in online databases, such as OMIM, ALSGene, ALS mutation database, and ALSoD [8]. Deregulation of these genes provides a potential common pathogenic link between familiar and sporadic ALS that may lead to the development of new strategies for the treatment of both forms of ALS. VEGF is among these whose protective effects on motor neurons have been previously discussed. Decreased expression of gene encoding VEGF was found in SALS2 patients (**Figure 5b**) as well as in individuals homozygous for a variety of mutations in the VEGF promoter region, suggesting the loss of the neuroprotective role of this factor may contribute to both forms of ALS [8].

Reduced expression of the sigma-1 receptor (SRBP1) and Spastin, an ATPase microtubules-binding protein necessary for normal neurite outgrowth, was also found in SALS2 patients (**Figure 5b**). Mutations in SRBP1 and SPAST (also known as SPG4) genes were proposed as potential genetic risk factors in ALS [46, 47]. These observations support the neuroprotective role of these proteins in maintaining physiological motor neurons functions, including proliferation, survival, and death, and highlight their potential role as a new therapeutic target in both forms of ALS. In this regard, some microtubule-targeting drugs (Noscapine and Vinblastine) and SRBP1 pharmacological ligands (Igmesine, Dextromethorphan, and PRE-084) have shown to exert neuroprotective effects in a variety of neurodegenerative diseases, including ALS [9].

http://dx.doi.org/10.5772/62988

In SALS2 patients, we also observed the increased expression of voltage-gated sodium channel (SCN7) (**Figure 5b**), according to previous literature data reporting an abnormal increase in the persistent Na+ currents in animal models of ALS [48]. Therefore, pharmacological agents that can restore sodium current, reducing consequently the neuronal hyperexcitability, may represent innovative strategies to treat both familial and sporadic ALS. In this regard, the only approved treatment for ALS, Riluzole, is able to block sodium currents, reducing the motor neuronal hyperexcitability and the firing rate observed in ALS [49]. Other sodium channel blockers (Topiramate, Mexiletine, Lamotrigine, Valproic Acid, Zonisamide, Riluzole, and Tetrodotoxin) have also shown promising results in human and animal models of several neurodegenerative diseases, including ALS [9].

Decreased expression of Ataxin-1 (ATXN1), a protein mainly implicated in mRNA processing by forming an RNA-dependent complex with PolyQ binding protein-1 (PQBP-1), was found in SALS2 patients (**Figure 5b**). ATXN1 normally contains a polyglutamine (polyQ) tract with 22–23 repeats while an augmented number of polyQ repeats (23–34) may increase genetic risk for ALS [50]. Thus, alterations of ATXN-1 functions may be involved in the development of both sporadic and familial ALS and its pharmacological modulation may represent a potential therapeutic strategy against ALS. Bromocriptine is among the agents that prevent mutant ATXN-1 aggregation and the consequent neurotoxicity, which is an FDA-approved drug for the treatment of Parkinson's disease that has also shown promising results in preclinical stages for ALS [9].

SALS patients showed deregulated expression of genes involved in the regulation of the oxidative stress response. Among these, the upregulation of D-amino acid oxidase (DAAO), a flavoenzyme localized in motor neurons that metabolizes D-serine, was found in SALS2 patients (**Figure 5b**), coherently with the observation that altered DAAO activity which leads to an increased accumulation of D-serine in ALS mouse models and patients [51]. Moreover, a mutation in DAAO gene (R199W) has been associated with classical adult onset familial ALS [52]. Drugs inhibiting or controlling the activity of D-serine and DAAO enzymes may thus represent therapeutic strategies for treating both forms of ALS. Recent studies have, in fact, demonstrated that DAO inhibitors (AS057278, Sodium Benzoate, and Chlorpromazine) show promising beneficial effects in several neuronal conditions, including Alzheimer's [9].

Decreased expression of genes encoding for PON2 and PON3, two enzymes involved in the prevention of oxidative damage [53], was also observed in SALS2 patients (**Figure 5b**) and mutations in these two genes have been associated with both familial and sporadic ALS [54]. Decreased expression of PON2 and PON3 was also observed in SALS2 patients (**Figure 5b**), supporting the neuroprotective role exerted by these factors and their modulators into preventing or reducing neurodegeneration in ALS. Among drugs that are able to improve PON-2/PON-3 activity, genistein (previously mentioned for its activity as EGFR/ErbB2 inhibitor) has shown promising results in preclinical studies for ALS and other PON-activating drugs (Montelukast and Berberine) have manifested neuroprotective effects in several animal models of neuronal diseases [9].

Another potential genetic risk factor in FALS patients is gene encoding Valosin-containing protein (VCP), a protein belonging to the ATP-binding cassette superfamily, involved in a multitude of cellular processes, such as vesicle transport and protein degradation. In accordance with literature studies, *VCP* mutations represent one of the major genetic causes of frontotemporal dementia but, recently, a specific mutation in this gene (p.R191Q) has been detected in some cases of FALS [55]. In our analysis, we observed the differential expression of *VCP* in SALS patients (**Figure 5b**). Moreover, several studies have highlighted the existence of a link between alterations in VCP functionality and the toxic gain of function of full-length TDP-43 [56]. The latter is a DNA/RNA binding protein, involved in several processes, including transcription, pre-mRNA splicing, mRNA stability, and mRNA transport [57]. Because of various types of insults, such as dysregulation in calcium homeostasis and oxidative damage, TDP-43 can migrate from the nucleus to the cytoplasm which can cause sequestration of RNA stress granule as well as a loss or gain of splicing functions. Although several studies have focused their attention on the role of TDP-43 in ALS etiopathogenesis, additional investigations are needed. Recent literature data showed the presence of aberrant nuclear or cytoplasmic TDP-43 inclusions in the nervous tissue of ALS patients [58]. It is thus evident that the pharmacological modulation of VCP may represent a promising strategy for ALS treatment, also through the reduction of TDP-43-mediated motor neuron toxicity. Some VCP inhibitors (Vesnarinone and Xanthohumol) have, in fact, demonstrated how to prevent neuronal death and inflammatory processes occurring in diverse neurological conditions [9].

5. Conclusion

ALS is a fatal neurodegenerative disease characterized by the influence of diverse mechanisms that interacting among each other promote the development and progression of the disease. Despite intensive research, ALS is still incurable and the only approved drug, Riluzole, conveys only modest benefits to patients. This clinical failure may be mainly due to the actual classification of ALS diseases, which is mainly based on clinical observation of symptoms and physical signs and does not take into account the complexity and heterogeneity of molecular pathogenic mechanisms underlying ALS.

The advent of high-throughput techniques in the biomedical sciences has provided a framework for developing a new, more accurate, and refined "molecular taxonomy" of human diseases that implies the use of molecular data to classify patients into distinct subgroups with differing diagnostic, prognostic, or therapeutic implications. In our previous work, we used unsupervised hierarchical clustering to identify two subgroups of SALS patients, characterized by their gene expression pattern, and revealed new clues to pathogenesis and potential therapeutic targets.

We argue that, as it is already happening in the genomic cancer field, our genomic analysis in combination with other "omics" data will complement and augment existing phenotypic information, providing a much deeper understanding of etiopathogenic mechanisms, which may have been masked by considering SALS as a single entity, and facilitating the development of a more precise diagnosis and individualized treatments for ALS patients.

Author details

Giovanna Morello, Francesca Luisa Conforti, Antonio Gianmaria Spampinato and Sebastiano Cavallaro*

*Address all correspondence to: sebastiano.cavallaro@cnr.it

Institute of Neurological Sciences, Italian National Research Council, Catania and Mangone (CS), Italy

References

[1] Perou CM, Sorlie T, Eisen MB, van de Rijn M, Jeffrey SS, Rees CA, et al. Molecular portraits of human breast tumours. Nature. 2000;406(6797):747. DOI: 52.10.1038/35021093.

[2] Sorlie T, Perou CM, Tibshirani R, Aas T, Geisler S, Johnsen H, et al. Gene expression patterns of breast carcinomas distinguish tumor subclasses with clinical implications. Proc Natl Acad Sci USA. 2001;98(19):10869. DOI: 74.10.1073/pnas.191367098.

[3] Hu Z, Fan C, Oh DS, Marron JS, He X, Qaqish BF, et al. The molecular portraits of breast tumors are conserved across microarray platforms. BMC Genom. 2006;7:96. DOI: 96.10.1186/1471-2164-7-96.

[4] Iorio F, Rittman T, Ge H, Menden M, Saez-Rodriguez J. Transcriptional data: a new gateway to drug repositioning? Drug Discov Today. 2013;18(7–8):350. DOI: 7.10.1016/j.drudis.2012.07.014.

[5] Bertucci F, Houlgatte R, Benziane A, Granjeaud S, Adelaide J, Tagett R, et al. Gene expression profiling of primary breast carcinomas using arrays of candidate genes. Human Molecul Genet. 2000;9(20):2981–2991.

[6] Chan IS, Ginsburg GS. Personalized medicine: progress and promise. Annu Rev Genom Human Genet. 2011;12:217. DOI: 44.10.1146/annurev-genom-082410-101446.

[7] Neuroscience Biomarkers and Biosignatures: Converging Technologies, Emerging Partnerships, Workshop Summary. The National Academies Collection: Reports funded by National Institutes of Health, Washington, DC. DOI: 2008.10.17226/11947.

[8] Aronica E, Baas F, Iyer A, ten Asbroek AL, Morello G, Cavallaro S. Molecular classification of amyotrophic lateral sclerosis by unsupervised clustering of gene expression in motor cortex. Neurobiol Dis. 2015;74:359. DOI: 76.10.1016/j.nbd.2014.12.002.

[9] Morello G, Cavallaro S. Transcriptional analysis reveals distinct subtypes in amyotrophic lateral sclerosis: implications for personalized therapy. Future Medicinal Chem. 2015;7(10):1335. DOI: 59.10.4155/fmc.15.60.

[10] Morello G, Conforti FL, Parenti R, D'Agata V, Cavallaro S. Selection of potential pharmacological targets in ALS based on whole-genome expression profiling. Curr Medicinal Chem. 2015;22(17):2004–2021.

[11] Beghi E, Logroscino G, Chio A, Hardiman O, Mitchell D, Swingler R, et al. The epidemiology of ALS and the role of population-based registries. Biochim Biophys Acta. 2006;1762(11–12):1150. DOI: 7.10.1016/j.bbadis.2006.09.008.

[12] Jenkins TM, Hollinger H, McDermott CJ. The evidence for symptomatic treatments in amyotrophic lateral sclerosis. Curr Opin Neurol. 2014;27(5):524. DOI: 31.10.1097/WCO.0000000000000135.

[13] Venkova-Hristova K, Christov A, Kamaluddin Z, Kobalka P, Hensley K. Progress in therapy development for amyotrophic lateral sclerosis. Neurol Res Int. 2012;2012:187234. DOI: 187234.10.1155/2012/187234.

[14] Simpson CL, Al Chalabi A. Amyotrophic lateral sclerosis as a complex genetic disease. Biochim Biophys Acta. 2006;1762(11–12):973–985.

[15] Valdmanis PN, Rouleau GA. Genetics of familial amyotrophic lateral sclerosis. Neurology. 2008;70(2):144–152.

[16] Andersen PM, Al-Chalabi A. Clinical genetics of amyotrophic lateral sclerosis: what do we really know? Nat Rev Neurol. 2011;7(11):603. doi: 10.1038/nrneurol.2011.150.

[17] Armon C. Environmental risk factors for amyotrophic lateral sclerosis. Neuroepidemiology. 2001;20(1):2. DOI: 6.54751.

[18] Majoor-Krakauer D, Willems PJ, Hofman A. Genetic epidemiology of amyotrophic lateral sclerosis. Clin Genet. 2003;63(2):83–101.

[19] Morris J. Amyotrophic lateral sclerosis (ALS) and related motor neuron diseases: an overview. Neurodiagn J. 2015;55(3):180–194.

[20] Brooks BR, Miller RG, Swash M, Munsat TL, World Federation of Neurology Research Group on Motor Neuron Diseases. El Escorial revisited: revised criteria for the diagnosis of amyotrophic lateral sclerosis. Amyotrophic lateral sclerosis and other motor neuron disorders. World Fed Neurol Res Group Motor Neuron Dis. 2000;1(5):293–299.

[21] Beghi E, Balzarini C, Bogliun G, Logroscino G, Manfredi L, Mazzini L, et al. Reliability of the El Escorial diagnostic criteria for amyotrophic lateral sclerosis. Neuroepidemiology. 2002;21(6):265. DOI:10.1159/000065524.

[22] Ravits J, Appel S, Baloh RH, Barohn R, Brooks BR, Elman L, et al. Deciphering amyotrophic lateral sclerosis: what phenotype, neuropathology and genetics are telling us about pathogenesis. Amyotrophic Lateral Sclerosis Frontotemporal Degen. 2013;14 (Suppl. 1):5. DOI: 18.10.3109/21678421.2013.778548.

[23] Nzwalo H, de Abreu D, Swash M, Pinto S, de Carvalho M. Delayed diagnosis in ALS: the problem continues. J Neurological Sci. 2014;343(1–2):173. DOI: 5.10.1016/j.jns. 2014.06.003.

[24] Cox LE, Ferraiuolo L, Goodall EF, Heath PR, Higginbottom A, Mortiboys H, et al. Mutations in CHMP2B in lower motor neuron predominant amyotrophic lateral sclerosis (ALS). PloS One. 2010;5(3):e9872. DOI: e9872.10.1371/journal.pone.0009872.

[25] Ferraiuolo L, Heath PR, Holden H, Kasher P, Kirby J, Shaw PJ. Microarray analysis of the cellular pathways involved in the adaptation to and progression of motor neuron injury in the SOD1 G93A mouse model of familial ALS. J Neurosci. 2007;27(34):9201. DOI: 19.10.1523/JNEUROSCI.1470-07.2007.

[26] Offen D, Barhum Y, Melamed E, Embacher N, Schindler C, Ransmayr G. Spinal cord mRNA profile in patients with ALS: comparison with transgenic mice expressing the human SOD-1 mutant. J Mol Neurosci. 2009;38(2):85–93.

[27] Wang XS, Simmons Z, Liu W, Boyer PJ, Connor JR. Differential expression of genes in amyotrophic lateral sclerosis revealed by profiling the post mortem cortex. Amyotroph Lateral Scler. 2006;7(4):201–210.

[28] Lederer CW, Torrisi A, Pantelidou M, Santama N, Cavallaro S. Pathways and genes differentially expressed in the motor cortex of patients with sporadic amyotrophic lateral sclerosis. BMC Genom. 2007;8(1):26.

[29] Ferraiuolo L, Kirby J, Grierson AJ, Sendtner M, Shaw PJ. Molecular pathways of motor neuron injury in amyotrophic lateral sclerosis. Nat Rev Neurol. 2011;7(11):616. DOI: 30.10.1038/nrneurol.2011.152.

[30] Peviani M, Caron I, Pizzasegola C, Gensano F, Tortarolo M, Bendotti C. Unraveling the complexity of amyotrophic lateral sclerosis: recent advances from the transgenic mutant SOD1 mice. CNS Neurol Disorders Drug Targets. 2010;9(4):491–503.

[31] Nikolsky Y, Kirillov E, Zuev R, Rakhmatulin E, Nikolskaya T. Functional analysis of OMICs data and small molecule compounds in an integrated "knowledge-based" platform. Methods Mol Biol. 2009;563:177. DOI: 96.10.1007/978-1-60761-175-2_10.

[32] Camandola S, Mattson MP. NF-kappa B as a therapeutic target in neurodegenerative diseases. Expert Opin Therapeutic Targets. 2007;11(2):123. DOI: 32.10.1517/14728222.11.2.123.

[33] Currais A, Hortobagyi T, Soriano S. The neuronal cell cycle as a mechanism of pathogenesis in Alzheimer's disease. Aging (Albany, NY). 2009;1(4):363–371.

[34] Vincent I, Pae CI, Hallows JL. The cell cycle and human neurodegenerative disease. Prog Cell Cycle Res. 2003;5:31–41.

[35] Yang Y, Herrup K. Cell division in the CNS: protective response or lethal event in post-mitotic neurons? Biochim Biophys Acta. 2007;1772(4):457. DOI: 66.S0925-4439(06)00199-2[pii]10.1016/j.bbadis.2006.10.002.

[36] Sta M, Sylva-Steenland RM, Casula M, de Jong JM, Troost D, Aronica E, et al. Innate and adaptive immunity in amyotrophic lateral sclerosis: evidence of complement activation. Neurobiol Dis. 2011;42(3):211. DOI: 20.S0969-9961(11)00003-9 [pii]10.1016/j.nbd.2011.01.002.

[37] Barbeito AG, Mesci P, Boillee S. Motor neuron-immune interactions: the vicious circle of ALS. J Neural Transm. 2010;117(8):981. DOI: 1000.10.1007/s00702-010-0429-0.

[38] Calvo A, Moglia C, Balma M, Chio A. Involvement of immune response in the pathogenesis of amyotrophic lateral sclerosis: a therapeutic opportunity? CNS Neurological Disorders Drug Targets. 2010;9(3):325–330.

[39] Bendotti C, Marino M, Cheroni C, Fontana E, Crippa V, Poletti A, et al. Dysfunction of constitutive and inducible ubiquitin–proteasome system in amyotrophic lateral sclerosis: implication for protein aggregation and immune response. Prog Neurobiol. 2012;97(2):101. DOI: 26.S0301-0082(11)00179-1 [pii]10.1016/j.pneurobio.2011.10.001.

[40] Boutahar N, Wierinckx A, Camdessanche JP, Antoine JC, Reynaud E, Lassabliere F, et al. Differential effect of oxidative or excitotoxic stress on the transcriptional profile of amyotrophic lateral sclerosis-linked mutant SOD1 cultured neurons. J Neurosci Res. 2011;89(9):1439. DOI: 50.10.1002/jnr.22672.

[41] Chao MV, Rajagopal R, Lee FS. Neurotrophin signalling in health and disease. Clin Sci. 2006;110(2):167. DOI: 73.10.1042/CS20050163.

[42] Janssen C, Schmalbach S, Boeselt S, Sarlette A, Dengler R, Petri S. Differential histone deacetylase mRNA expression patterns in amyotrophic lateral sclerosis. J Neuropathol Exp Neurol. 2010;69(6):573. DOI: 81.10.1097/NEN.0b013e3181ddd404.

[43] Carlesi C, Pasquali L, Piazza S, Lo Gerfo A, Caldarazzo Ienco E, Alessi R, et al. Strategies for clinical approach to neurodegeneration in Amyotrophic lateral sclerosis. Arch Ital Biol. 2011;149(1):151. DOI: 67.10.4449/aib.v149i1.1267.

[44] Lunn JS, Sakowski SA, Kim B, Rosenberg AA, Feldman EL. Vascular endothelial growth factor prevents G93A-SOD1-induced motor neuron degeneration. Dev Neurobiol. 2009;69(13):871. DOI: 84.10.1002/dneu.20747.

[45] Brockington A, Wharton SB, Fernando M, Gelsthorpe CH, Baxter L, Ince PG, et al. Expression of vascular endothelial growth factor and its receptors in the central nervous system in amyotrophic lateral sclerosis. J Neuropathol Exp Neurol. 2006;65(1):26. DOI: 36.00005072-200601000-00004 [pii].

[46] Al-Saif A, Al-Mohanna F, Bohlega S. A mutation in sigma-1 receptor causes juvenile amyotrophic lateral sclerosis. Ann Neurol. 2011;70(6):913. DOI: 9.10.1002/ana.22534.

[47] Meyer T, Schwan A, Dullinger JS, Brocke J, Hoffmann KT, Nolte CH, et al. Early-onset ALS with long-term survival associated with spastin gene mutation. Neurology. 2005;65(1):141. DOI: 3.10.1212/01.wnl.0000167130.31618.0a.

[48] Nutini M, Spalloni A, Florenzano F, Westenbroek RE, Marini C, Catterall WA, et al. Increased expression of the beta3 subunit of voltage-gated Na+ channels in the spinal cord of the SOD1G93A mouse. Mol Cell Neurosci. 2011;47(2):108. DOI: 18.10.1016/j.mcn.2011.03.005.

[49] Bellingham MC. Pre- and postsynaptic mechanisms underlying inhibition of hypoglossal motor neuron excitability by riluzole. J Neurophysiol. 2013;110(5):1047. DOI: 61.10.1152/jn.00587.2012.

[50] Conforti FL, Spataro R, Sproviero W, Mazzei R, Cavalcanti F, Condino F, et al. Ataxin-1 and ataxin-2 intermediate-length PolyQ expansions in amyotrophic lateral sclerosis. Neurology. 2012;79(24):2315. DOI: 20.10.1212/WNL.0b013e318278b618.

[51] Sasabe J, Miyoshi Y, Suzuki M, Mita M, Konno R, Matsuoka M, et al. D-amino acid oxidase controls motoneuron degeneration through D-serine. Proc Natl Acad Sci USA. 2012;109(2):627. DOI: 32.10.1073/pnas.1114639109.

[52] Mitchell J, Paul P, Chen HJ, Morris A, Payling M, Falchi M, et al. Familial amyotrophic lateral sclerosis is associated with a mutation in D-amino acid oxidase. Proc Natl Acad Sci USA. 2010;107(16):7556. DOI: 61.10.1073/pnas.0914128107.

[53] Giordano G, Cole TB, Furlong CE, Costa LG. Paraoxonase 2 (PON2) in the mouse central nervous system: a neuroprotective role? Toxicol Appl Pharmacol. 2011;256(3):369. DOI: 78.10.1016/j.taap.2011.02.014.

[54] Saeed M, Siddique N, Hung WY, Usacheva E, Liu E, Sufit RL, et al. Paraoxonase cluster polymorphisms are associated with sporadic ALS. Neurology. 2006;67(5):771. DOI: 6.10.1212/01.wnl.0000227187.52002.88.

[55] Gonzalez-Perez P, Cirulli ET, Drory VE, Dabby R, Nisipeanu P, Carasso RL, et al. Novel mutation in VCP gene causes atypical amyotrophic lateral sclerosis. Neurology. 2012;79(22):2201. DOI: 8.10.1212/WNL.0b013e318275963b.

[56] Rodriguez-Ortiz CJ, Hoshino H, Cheng D, Liu-Yescevitz L, Blurton-Jones M, Wolozin B, et al. Neuronal-specific overexpression of a mutant valosin-containing protein associated with IBMPFD promotes aberrant ubiquitin and TDP-43 accumulation and cognitive dysfunction in transgenic mice. Am J Pathol. 2013;183(2):504. DOI: 15.10.1016/j.ajpath.2013.04.014.

[57] Budini M, Baralle FE, Buratti E. Regulation of gene expression by TDP-43 and FUS/TLS in frontotemporal lobar degeneration. Curr Alzheimer Res. 2011;8(3):237–245.

[58] Lagier-Tourenne C, Cleveland DW. Rethinking ALS: the FUS about TDP-43. Cell. 2009;136(6):1001. DOI: 4.10.1016/j.cell.2009.03.006.

Chapter 13

Amyotrophic Lateral Sclerosis: Role of the Canonical Wnt/Beta-Catenin Pathway and PPAR Gamma

Yves Lecarpentier and Alexandre Vallée

Additional information is available at the end of the chapter

http://dx.doi.org/10.5772/63152

Abstract

Amyotrophic lateral sclerosis (ALS) is one of the most common adult-onset debilitating neurodegenerative diseases (NDs) which is characterized by a chronic progressive degeneration of upper and lower motor neurons, resulting in muscular atrophy, paralysis and ultimately death. It has been established that in ALS, the canonical Wnt/beta-catenin pathway is upregulated. Peroxisome proliferator-activated receptor gamma (PPAR gamma) generally varies in opposite way compared with the Wnt/beta-catenin signaling. Several studies carried out on ALS transgenic mice have shown the beneficial effects induced after treatment by PPAR agonists partly due to anti-inflammatory effects induced by PPAR gamma. The coupling between the Wnt/beta-catenin signaling and PPAR gamma has led to divide NDs into two classes: NDs in which the Wnt/beta-catenin pathway is upregulated whereas PPAR gamma is downregulated (ALS, Parkinson's disease, Huntington's disease and Friedreich's ataxia); and NDs in which the Wnt-beta-catenin pathway is downregulated while PPAR gamma is upregulated (Alzheimer's disease, bipolar disorder and schizophrenia).

Keywords: Wnt/beta-catenin, PPAR gamma, amyotrophic lateral sclerosis, riluzole, ALS

1. Introduction

Neurodegenerative diseases (NDs) are frequent and often present a pejorative prognosis. Two major systems play a key role in the pathophysiology of NDs, i.e., the canonical Wnt/beta-catenin pathway and PPAR gamma. Several studies have demonstrated the opposite interaction between the canonical Wnt/beta-catenin pathway and the PPAR gamma [1–7]. It has recently been shown that certain NDs can be divided into two classes [8]: on one hand, NDs

INTECH
open science | open minds

© 2016 The Author(s). Licensee InTech. This chapter is distributed under the terms of the Creative Commons Attribution License (http://creativecommons.org/licenses/by/3.0), which permits unrestricted use, distribution, and reproduction in any medium, provided the original work is properly cited.

in which the Wnt/beta-catenin pathway is upregulated whereas PPAR gamma is downregulated. Among these NDs, we find amyotrophic lateral sclerosis (ALS), Parkinson's disease, Huntington's disease and Friedreich's ataxia. PPAR agonists exert protective effects in ALS neurons of transgenic mice and may represent therapeutic targets in human ALS. On the other hand, NDs in which the Wnt-beta-catenin pathway is downregulated while PPAR gamma is upregulated. Among these NDs, we find Alzheimer's disease, bipolar disorder and schizophrenia. This list is not exhaustive.

2. Amyotrophic lateral sclerosis (ALS)

ALS is one of the most common adult-onset debilitating NDs with the prevalence of about 5 per 100,000 individuals. The pathophysiology of ALS in humans is particularly complex, due to the numerous interconnected pathological processes and, today, has not been fully elucidated. However, it remains to determine those really responsible for the disease from those simply involved in its development. ALS has been first described by J.M. Charcot in 1869. ALS is a fatal neurodegenerative disorder and is characterized by chronic progressive degeneration of upper and lower motor neurons, resulting in muscular atrophy, paralysis and ultimately death. And, 82% of ALS are sporadic. The most frequent mutations in inherited or familial ALS (FALS) are found in the gene for Cu, Zn superoxide dismutase (SOD1). Among numerous abnormalities, this FALS presents glutamate toxicity, axonal transport defects, aberrant neurotrophic factors, mitochondrial dysfunction [9]. Numerous in vivo studies have used transgenic mice expressing FALS mutants of human SOD1 [10]. This transgenic model develops a progressive motor neuron pathology which is reminiscent of the human ALS phenotype [11]. The human sporadic ALS differs little clinically from SOD1-related FALS. Both forms of ALS induce degeneration of motor neurons which leads to paralysis and death within 3–5 years from the appearance of the first symptoms. Today, no pharmacological therapeutic can really stop the progression of the disease. Although riluzole is approved for ALS patients, the benefits of this drug are marginal [12–15].

3. Canonical Wnt/beta-catenin pathway

Wnt signaling plays a key role in carcinogenesis, embryonic development, cell fate, cell migration and NDs [16, 17]. A hallmark of the canonical Wnt pathway activation by Wnt ligands is the increase in the cytoplasmic beta-catenin protein level, the subsequent nuclear translocation and further activation of beta-catenin specific gene transcription [4, 18–20]. In the absence of Wnt ligands, beta-catenin is recruited into a destruction complex that contains adenomatous polyposis coli (APC) and Axin, which facilitate the phosphorylation of beta-catenin by glycogen synthase kinase-3beta (GSK-3beta). GSK-3beta phosphorylates the N-terminal domain of beta-catenin, thereby targeting it for ubiquitination and proteasomal degradation. In the presence of a Wnt ligand, the binding of Wnt to Frizzled (Fzd) leads to activation of the phosphoprotein Dishevelled (Dsh). Dsh recruits Axin and the destruction

http://dx.doi.org/10.5772/63152

complex to the plasma membrane, where Axin directly binds to the cytoplasmic tail of the low-density lipoprotein-receptor-related proteins (LRP5-6). The activation of Dsh also leads to the inhibition of GSK-3beta by phosphorylation, which further reduces the phosphorylation and degradation of beta-catenin. The beta-catenin degradation complex is inactivated with recruitment of Axin to the plasma membrane, thus stabilizing the non-phosphorylated beta-catenin which translocates to the nucleus. Beta-catenin binds to T cell/lymphoid-enhancing binding (Tcf/Lef) transcription factors. The resulting complex becomes active by displacing Grouchos, leading to activation of numerous target genes including c-myc, cyclin D1, TIFF-1, Axin-2, CD44, Cox2, MMP-7, PPAR beta/delta, [21–23]. Upregulation of the canonical Wnt/beta-catenin pathway is observed in metabolic diseases such as type 2 diabetes, hypertension, in cancers (colon, lung, breast, leukemias) and certain NDs. Downregulation is observed in osteoporosis, cardiac hypoxia, cardiac hypertrophy, arrhythmogenic right ventricular dysplasia/cardiomyopathy (ARVC) and certain NDs [8].

4. PPAR gamma

Peroxisome proliferator-activated receptor gamma (PPAR gamma) is a ligand-activated transcriptional factor that belongs to the nuclear hormone receptor superfamily. PPAR gamma regulates the expression or activity of a large number of genes in a variety of signaling pathways, including regulation of insulin sensitivity, glucose homeostasis, lipid metabolism, immune responses, inflammation, redox balance, cardiovascular integrity and cell fate [24, 25]. PPAR gamma is expressed in various cell types, such as adipose tissues, immune cells and brain cells including microglia and astrocytes which contribute to anti-inflammatory response in the central nervous system. During the past decade, the role of PPAR gamma in neurodegeneration has been established. The administration of PPAR gamma ligands has been shown to be beneficial in many NDs such as ALS, Alzheimer's disease, Parkinson's disease, multiple sclerosis, Huntington's disease and stroke [26]. PPAR gamma has been shown to have anti-inflammatory and neuroprotective effects [27, 28]. Astrocytic GLT1/EAAT2 gene is a target of PPAR gamma, leading to neuroprotection by increasing the glutamate uptake [29]. PPAR gamma is a direct transcriptional modulator of the pyruvate carboxylase gene [30]. Given the fact that ALS patients suffer from massive weight loss, this provides a possible explanation for the potential protective effects of pioglitazone through increased lipogenesis.

5. PPAR gamma activation induces repression of the beta-catenin pathway

The thiazolidinedione PPAR gamma agonists (TZDs), troglitazone, rosiglitazone and pioglitazone, and a non-thiazolidinedione PPAR gamma activator, GW1929, inhibit the beta-catenin-induced transcription in a PPAR gamma-dependent fashion [1–3, 5]. Troglitazone-mediated activation of PPAR gamma is associated with an inhibition of beta-catenin at a post-transcriptional level. The functional interaction between beta-catenin and PPAR gamma involves the Tcf/Lef factor-binding domain of beta-catenin and a catenin-binding domain within PPAR gamma [5]. Treatment with PPAR gamma agonists decreases mRNA and protein levels of beta-catenin in 3T3L1 adipocytes [1]. TZDs induce a reduction in the levels of cytoplasmic beta-catenin in hepatocytes [3]. PPAR gamma suppresses Wnt/beta-catenin pathway during adipogenesis [2].

6. Deactivation of the Wnt/beta-catenin pathway induces activation of PPAR gamma

Inhibition of Wnt/beta-catenin pathway leads to an increase in transcription of PPAR gamma. Activation of the Wnt/beta-catenin signaling leads to osteogenesis, but not to adipogenesis. The canonical Wnt/beta-catenin-PPAR gamma system regulates the molecular switching of osteablastogenesis versus adipogenesis [6]. Wnt signaling maintains preadipocytes in an undifferentiated state through inhibition of both adipogenic transcription factors C/EBP alpha and PPAR gamma. Deactivation of Wnt/beta catenin pathway and activation of PPAR gamma are observed in ARVD [4, 31]. Taken together, these studies suggest that the canonical Wnt/beta-catenin signaling downregulates PPAR gamma expression, inhibition of Wnt/beta-catenin signaling upregulates PPAR gamma expression and PPAR gamma agonists inhibit the canonical Wnt/beta-catenin pathway.

7. ALS and Wnt/beta-catenin pathway

The canonical Wnt/beta-catenin signaling is involved in numerous NDs, particularly in ALS. Several studies have shown that this pathway is upregulated in motor neurons of ASL model mice [32–35]. In the spinal cord of SOD1(G93A) ALS transgenic mice, expression of Wnt2, Wnt7a and GSK-3beta has been determined [32]. Both Wnt2, Wnt7a mRNA and protein in the spinal cord of ALS mice have been found to be upregulated when compared with wild type. The immune-reactivity of Wnt2 and Wnt7a is strong in ALS adult transgenic mice, whereas it is weak in wild-type mice. Neurodegeneration upregulates the expression of Wnt2 and Wnt7a in the spinal cord of ALS mice, which in turn activates Wnt signaling and inhibits GSK-3beta activity in ALS adult transgenic mice. Expression of Wnt3a, beta-catenin and Cyclin D1, three key molecules of the Wnt/beta-catenin signaling, have been determined in the adult spinal cord of SOD1(G93A) ALS transgenic mice at different stages [33]. It has been found that mRNA and protein of Wnt3a and Cyclin D1 in the spinal cord of the ALS mice are upregulated compared with wild-type mice. Moreover, beta-catenin translocates from the cell membrane to the nucleus and subsequently activated transcription of the target gene Cyclin D1. Wnt3a, beta-catenin and Cyclin D1 are also expressed in both neurons and astrocytes. For the authors, these findings suggest that neurodegeneration activates the Wnt/beta-catenin pathway, in the spinal cord of adult ALS transgenic mice. Changes in Wnt5a and Fzd2 expression in the spinal cord of SOD1(G93A) transgenic mice (ALS), SOD1(G93A) transfected NSC-34 cells and primary cultures of astrocytes from SOD1(G93A) transgenic mice have been observed [35]. Expression of Wnt1 and Fzd1 has been found to be increased in the spinal cords of SOD1G93A

http://dx.doi.org/10.5772/63152

ALS transgenic mice [34]. In the in vitro model of ALS (G93A mutated forms of human Cu/Zn superoxide dismutase-1; SOD1), a cytosolic aggregation of beta-catenin has been observed. This suggests that Wnt/beta-catenin pathway could play critical role in the neurodegeneration of motor neurons in ALS [36]. Beta-catenin is activated in a subset of myofibers in extraocular muscles and limb muscles in ALS subjects [37].

8. ALS and riluzole

Today, no really efficient treatment exists for ALS [38, 39]. However, riluzole has been approved for the treatment of ALS in most countries and is tested in people based on results supporting a role of glutamate toxicity in ALS. Riluzole has numerous pharmacodynamics properties, i.e., presynaptic inhibition of the glutamate release, inhibition of G-protein-dependent processes, modulation of N-methyl-D-aspartate ionotropic receptor and blockade of the voltage-gated sodium channel, etc. [39]. Two trials [12, 13] have demonstrated the weak efficacy of riluzole in ALS with prolongation of median survival by 2 to 3 months and safety of riluzole. Thus, riluzole appears to slow the progression of ALS, and may improve survival in patients with disease of bulbar onset [12]. Riluzole is well tolerated and lengthens survival of patients with ALS [13]. Two other studies have led to almost the same conclusions [14, 15]. The FDA-approved drug, riluzole, 100 mg daily is reasonably safe and probably prolongs median survival by about 2 to 3 months in patients with ALS.

Importantly, riluzole has been found to be an enhancer of the Wnt/beta-catenin signaling in melanoma [40]. For the authors, treating melanoma cells with riluzole in vitro enhances the ability of WNT3A to regulate gene expression, promote pigmentation and decrease cell proliferation. Like WNT3A, riluzole decreases metastases in a mouse melanoma model. Moreover, riluzole enhances Wnt/beta-catenin signaling in the primary screen both in HT22 neuronal cells and in adult hippocampal progenitor cells [40]. As the Wnt/beta-catenin pathway is upregulated, at least in genetic ALS mice [32–35], this can partly explain poor results in trials testing riluzole in ALS as shown previously [12–15]. Lithium, an activator of the Wnt/beta catenin signaling, has also been evaluated as a treatment for ALS [41]. Surprisingly, in ALS patients treated with lithium, the disease progression has been shown to be markedly attenuated. In the genetic ALS G93A mouse model, there is a marked neuroprotection induced by lithium, which delayed disease onset and duration and augmented the life span. The use of the enhancer Wnt/beta-catenin lithium can be discussed in ALS in which the Wnt/beta-catenin pathway has been shown to be upregulated in several animal studies [32–35]. GSK-3beta-inhibitor lithium chloride enhances activation of the canonical Wnt signaling [42–44]. Lithium activates downstream components of the Wnt signaling pathway in vivo, leading to an increase of the beta-catenin protein. This pathway is implicated in the pathophysiology and treatment of bipolar disorder [45, 46]. Riluzole reduces symptoms of obsessive-compulsive disorder, unipolar and bipolar depression and generalized anxiety disorder [47]. This is not surprising due to the fact that the Wnt/beta-catenin pathway is downregulated in bipolar syndrome [8] and that like lithium, riluzole is an enhancer of Wnt/beta-catenin signaling.

9. ALS and PPAR gamma

In ALS, expression of PPAR gamma (mARN and protein) has not been precisely investigated in neurons. However, the upregulation of Wnt/beta-catenin signaling observed in ALS suggests that PPAR gamma might be downregulated due to the fact that these two systems generally operate in the opposite way [1–3, 5]. Neuroinflammation is a common pathological feature in NDs, particularly in ALS. PPAR gamma may be a key regulator of neuroinflammation. PPAR gamma inhibits NF-kappaB-mediated inflammatory signaling at multiple sites [48]. PPAR gamma might be a relevant regulator of neuroinflammation and possibly a new target for the development of therapeutic strategies for ALS. A potentially therapeutic pathway in ALS may be the activation by PPAR gamma agonists due to their ability to block neuropathological damages caused by inflammation [49]. The neuroprotective effect of pioglitazone has been demonstrated in G93A SOD1 transgenic mouse model of ALS and shows a significant increase in their survival. Pioglitazone protects motor neurons against p38-mediated neuronal death and NF-kappaB-mediated glial inflammation via a PPAR gamma-independent mechanism [50]. In ALS, PPAR gamma controls natural protective mechanisms against lipid peroxidation [51]. PPAR gamma-driven transcription selectively increases in the spinal cord of hSOD1G93A mice. This is correlated with the upregulation of lipid detoxification enzymes such as the lipoprotein lipase and glutathione S-transferase alpha-2, implied in scavenging lipid peroxidation by-products. Anticipation of protective reactions by pharmacological PPAR gamma modulation of the transcriptional activity attenuates neurodegeneration induced by lipid peroxidation. PPAR gamma activation is neuroprotective in a Drosophila model of ALS [52]. This Drosophila model of ALS based on TDP-43 recapitulates several aspects of ALS pathophysiology. Pioglitazone rescues TDP-43-dependent locomotor dysfunction in motor neurons and glia. PPAR gamma activation in neurons and glia is partially neuroprotective and restores metabolic alterations in ALS. Superoxide dismutase (SOD1)-G93A transgenic mice benefit from oral treatment with the PPAR gamma agonist pioglitazone [53]. Pioglitazone-treated transgenic mice reveal improved muscle strength and body weight, exhibit a delayed disease onset and survive significantly longer than non-treated SOD1-G93A mice. Pioglitazone-induced neuroprotection of motor neurons of the spinal cord is complete at day 90. There is also preservation of the median fiber diameter of the quadriceps muscle, indicating a morphological and functional protection of motor neurons induced by pioglitazone. However, in a phase II double-blind controlled clinical trial, the PPAR gamma agonist pioglitazone in combination with riluzole does not increase survival in ALS patients [54].

PPAR gamma coactivator-1alpha (PGC-1alpha) is a transcriptional coactivator that works together with the transcription factor PPAR gamma in the regulation of mitochondrial biogenesis. PGC-1alpha plays a role in several neurodegenerative pathologies [26]. PGC-1alpha protects neurons and alters disease progression in a PGC-1alpha transgenic mice crossed with SOD1 mutant G93A DL mice [55]. In these mice, the progression of the disease has been shown to be significantly slower. There is also a markedly improved performance on the rotarod test associated with an improved motor activity with a decreased loss of motor neurons and less degeneration of neuromuscular junctions. By using a double transgenic mouse model where PGC-1alpha is over-expressed in a SOD1 transgenic mouse (TgSOD1-G93A/

PGC-1alpha), it has been found that motor function and survival are improved [56]. This is accompanied by a reduction of motor neuron loss, a restoration of mitochondrial electron transport chain activities and an inhibition of stress signaling in the spinal cord. Thus, in the double-transgenic mice, there are improved motor performance, slowed ALS progression, decreased weight loss, and reduced motor neuronal death. Survival and disease improvement are greater in higher-expressing PGC-1alpha mice. Therefore, PPAR gamma is a possible target for ALS as it functions as a transcription factor that interacts with PGC-1alpha. Elevated PGC-1alpha activity sustains mitochondrial biogenesis and muscle function without extending survival in a mouse model of inherited ALS [57]. Increasing PGC-1alpha activity in muscles represents an attractive therapy for maintaining muscle function during the progression of ALS.

10. Conclusions

PPAR agonists represent promising therapeutics for NDs such as multiple sclerosis, ALS and Alzheimer's disease (AD). Their activation affects many pathological mechanisms. PPAR activation can weaken or reprogram the immune response, stimulate metabolism, improve mitochondrial function, promote axon growth and induce progenitor cells to differentiate into myelinating oligodendrocytes [58]. The mechanisms of action of PPAR agonists are various and may be useful at many stages of diseases. Type, timing and dose of PPAR agonists may vary depending on injury severity, progression of disease or cellular targets such as neurons, microglia, oligodendrocytes, and may explain a number of conflicting results in several studies. PPAR gamma may be useful due to its anti-inflammatory properties. Moreover, PPAR gamma agonists induce beta-catenin inhibition [3, 5], which represents a rationale to use it when the Wnt/beta-catenin pathway is upregulated such as in Parkinson's disease, multiple sclerosis, ALS, Huntington's disease and Friedreich's ataxia [8]. However, in AD, PPAR gamma levels (mRNA and protein) have been found to be elevated in brain tissues [59, 60]. Although PPAR gamma expression is high in AD, PPAR gamma agonists have been used in AD humans and various AD animal models and have been shown to induce beneficial effects, partly due to their anti-inflammatory effects [61–67]. Even if the PPAR gamma agonist pioglitazone, in combination with riluzole, does not increase survival in ALS patients [54], PPAR gamma represents a useful therapeutic target in several animal models. Inhibition of the Wnt/beta-catenin pathway might also represent a therapeutic approach in ALS animal model.

Acknowledgements

We thank Dr Michel Grivaux, Director of the Clinical Research Center, Meaux Hospital, and Mr Vincent Gobert, Administrative Manager of the Clinical Research Center, Meaux hospital, France.

Author details

Yves Lecarpentier[1*] and Alexandre Vallée[2]

*Address all correspondence to: yves.c.lecarpentier@gmail.com

1 Clinical Research Center, Meaux Hôpital, Meaux, France

2 Jules Verne University of Picardie, Amiens, France and Experimental and Clinical Neurosciences Laboratory, University of Poitiers, France

References

[1] Gerhold DL, Liu F, Jiang G, Li Z, Xu J, Lu M, Sachs JR, Bagchi A, Fridman A, Holder DJ et al.: Gene expression profile of adipocyte differentiation and its regulation by peroxisome proliferator-activated receptor-gamma agonists. Endocrinology 2002, 143(6):2106–2118. DOI: 10.1210/endo.143.6.8842

[2] Moldes M, Zuo Y, Morrison RF, Silva D, Park BH, Liu J, Farmer SR: Peroxisome-proliferator-activated receptor gamma suppresses Wnt/beta-catenin signalling during adipogenesis. Biochemistry journal 2003, 376(Pt 3):607–613.

[3] Sharma C, Pradeep A, Wong L, Rana A, Rana B: Peroxisome proliferator-activated receptor gamma activation can regulate beta-catenin levels via a proteasome-mediated and adenomatous polyposis coli-independent pathway. The journal of biological chemistry 2004, 279(34):35583–35594. DOI: 10.1074/jbc.M403143200

[4] Garcia-Gras E, Lombardi R, Giocondo MJ, Willerson JT, Schneider MD, Khoury DS, Marian AJ: Suppression of canonical Wnt/beta-catenin signaling by nuclear plakoglobin recapitulates phenotype of arrhythmogenic right ventricular cardiomyopathy. The journal of clinical investigation 2006, 116(7):2012–2021.

[5] Liu J, Wang H, Zuo Y, Farmer SR: Functional interaction between peroxisome proliferator-activated receptor gamma and beta-catenin. Molecular and cellular biology 2006, 26(15):5827–5837. DOI: 26/15/5827 [pii]10.1128/MCB.00441-06

[6] Takada I, Kouzmenko AP, Kato S: Wnt and PPARgamma signaling in osteoblastogenesis and adipogenesis. Nat Rev Rheumatol 2009, 5(8):442–447.

[7] Lu D, Carson DA: Repression of beta-catenin signaling by PPAR gamma ligands. European journal of pharmacology 2010, 636(1–3):198–202. DOI: 10.1016/j.ejphar.2010.03.010

[8] Lecarpentier Y, Claes V, Duthoit G, Hebert JL: Circadian rhythms, Wnt/beta-catenin pathway and PPAR alpha/gamma profiles in diseases with primary or secondary cardiac dysfunction. Front physiology 2014, 5:429. DOI: 10.3389/fphys.2014.00429

[9] Redler RL, Dokholyan NV: The complex molecular biology of amyotrophic lateral sclerosis (ALS). Progress in molecular biologyand translational science 2012, 107:215–262. DOI: 10.1016/B978-0-12-385883-2.00002-3

[10] Rosen DR: Mutations in Cu/Zn superoxide dismutase gene are associated with familial amyotrophic lateral sclerosis. Nature 1993, 364(6435):362. DOI: 10.1038/364362c0

[11] Turner BJ, Talbot K: Transgenics, toxicity and therapeutics in rodent models of mutant SOD1-mediated familial ALS. Progress in neurobiology 2008, 85(1):94–134. DOI: 10.1016/j.pneurobio.2008.01.001

[12] Bensimon G, Lacomblez L, Meininger V: A controlled trial of riluzole in amyotrophic lateral sclerosis. ALS/Riluzole Study Group. The New England journal of medicine 1994, 330(9):585–591. DOI: 10.1056/NEJM199403033300901

[13] Lacomblez L, Bensimon G, Leigh PN, Guillet P, Meininger V: Dose-ranging study of riluzole in amyotrophic lateral sclerosis. Amyotrophic Lateral Sclerosis/Riluzole Study Group II. Lancet 1996, 347(9013):1425–1431.

[14] Miller RG, Mitchell JD, Lyon M, Moore DH: Riluzole for amyotrophic lateral sclerosis (ALS)/motor neuron disease (MND). Amyotrophic lateral sclerosis and other motor neuron disorders: official publication of the world federation of neurology, research group on motor neuron diseases 2003, 4(3):191–206.

[15] Miller RG, Mitchell JD, Moore DH: Riluzole for amyotrophic lateral sclerosis (ALS)/ motor neuron disease (MND). The Cochrane database of systematic reviews 2012, 3:CD001447. DOI: 10.1002/14651858.CD001447.pub3

[16] Moon RT, Kohn AD, De Ferrari GV, Kaykas A: WNT and beta-catenin signalling: diseases and therapies. Nature review genetics 2004, 5(9):691–701. DOI: 10.1038/nrg1427

[17] Clevers H, Nusse R: Wnt/beta-catenin signaling and disease. Cell 2012, 149(6):1192–1205. DOI: 10.1016/j.cell.2012.05.012

[18] Barker N, Clevers H: Mining the Wnt pathway for cancer therapeutics. Nature review drug discovery 2006, 5(12):997–1014. DOI: 10.1038/nrd2154

[19] Ben-Ze'ev A, Geiger B: Differential molecular interactions of beta-catenin and plakoglobin in adhesion, signaling and cancer. Current opinions in cellular biology 1998, 10(5):629–639. DOI: S0955-0674(98)80039-2 [pii]

[20] Sen-Chowdhry S, Syrris P, McKenna WJ: Genetics of right ventricular cardiomyopathy. Journal of cardiovascular electrophysiology 2005, 16(8):927–935. DOI: JCE40842 [pii]

[21] He TC, Sparks AB, Rago C, Hermeking H, Zawel L, da Costa LT, Morin PJ, Vogelstein B, Kinzler KW: Identification of c-MYC as a target of the APC pathway. Science 1998, 281(5382):1509–1512.

[22] Shtutman M, Zhurinsky J, Simcha I, Albanese C, D'Amico M, Pestell R, Ben-Ze'ev A: The cyclin D1 gene is a target of the beta-catenin/LEF-1 pathway. Proceedings of the national academy of sciences of the United States of America 1999, 96(10):5522–5527.

[23] Angers S, Moon RT: Proximal events in Wnt signal transduction. Nature reviews molecular cell biology 2009, 10(7):468–477. DOI: 10.1038/nrm2717

[24] Elbrecht A, Chen Y, Cullinan CA, Hayes N, Leibowitz M, Moller DE, Berger J: Molecular cloning, expression and characterization of human peroxisome proliferator activated receptors gamma 1 and gamma 2. Biochemical and biophysical research communications 1996, 224(2):431–437.

[25] Fajas L, Auboeuf D, Raspe E, Schoonjans K, Lefebvre AM, Saladin R, Najib J, Laville M, Fruchart JC, Deeb S et al.: The organization, promoter analysis, and expression of the human PPARgamma gene. The journal of biological chemistry 1997, 272(30):18779–18789.

[26] Katsouri L, Blondrath K, Sastre M: Peroxisome proliferator-activated receptor-gamma cofactors in neurodegeneration. IUBMB life 2012, 64(12):958–964. DOI: 10.1002/iub.1097

[27] Kapadia R, Yi JH, Vemuganti R: Mechanisms of anti-inflammatory and neuroprotective actions of PPAR-gamma agonists. Frontiers in bioscience: a journal and virtual library 2008, 13:1813–1826.

[28] Gray E, Ginty M, Kemp K, Scolding N, Wilkins A: The PPAR-gamma agonist pioglitazone protects cortical neurons from inflammatory mediators via improvement in peroxisomal function. Journal of neuroinflammation 2012, 9:63. DOI: 10.1186/1742-2094-9-63

[29] Romera C, Hurtado O, Mallolas J, Pereira MP, Morales JR, Romera A, Serena J, Vivancos J, Nombela F, Lorenzo P et al.: Ischemic preconditioning reveals that GLT1/EAAT2 glutamate transporter is a novel PPARgamma target gene involved in neuroprotection. Journal of cerebral blood flow and metabolism: official journal of the international society of cerebral blood flow and metabolism 2007, 27(7):1327–1338. DOI: 10.1038/sj.jcbfm.9600438

[30] Jitrapakdee S, Slawik M, Medina-Gomez G, Campbell M, Wallace JC, Sethi JK, O'Rahilly S, Vidal-Puig AJ: The peroxisome proliferator-activated receptor-gamma regulates murine pyruvate carboxylase gene expression in vivo and in vitro. The journal of biological chemistry 2005, 280(29):27466–27476. DOI: 10.1074/jbc.M503836200

[31] Djouadi F, Lecarpentier Y, Hebert JL, Charron P, Bastin J, Coirault C: A potential link between PPAR signaling and the pathogenesis of arrhythmogenic right ventricular cardiomyopathy (ARVC). Cardiovascular research 2009,84:83–90.

[32] Chen Y, Guan Y, Zhang Z, Liu H, Wang S, Yu L, Wu X, Wang X: Wnt signaling pathway is involved in the pathogenesis of amyotrophic lateral sclerosis in adult transgenic mice. Neurological research 2012, 34(4):390–399. DOI: 10.1179/1743132812Y.0000000027

[33] Chen Y, Guan Y, Liu H, Wu X, Yu L, Wang S, Zhao C, Du H, Wang X: Activation of the Wnt/beta-catenin signaling pathway is associated with glial proliferation in the adult spinal cord of ALS transgenic mice. Biochemical and biophysical research communications 2012, 420(2):397–403. DOI: 10.1016/j.bbrc.2012.03.006

[34] Wang S, Guan Y, Chen Y, Li X, Zhang C, Yu L, Zhou F, Wang X: Role of Wnt1 and Fzd1 in the spinal cord pathogenesis of amyotrophic lateral sclerosis-transgenic mice. Biotechnology Letters 2013, 35(8):1199–1207. DOI: 10.1007/s10529-013-1199-1

[35] Li X, Guan Y, Chen Y, Zhang C, Shi C, Zhou F, Yu L, Juan J, Wang X: Expression of Wnt5a and its receptor Fzd2 is changed in the spinal cord of adult amyotrophic lateral sclerosis transgenic mice. International journal of clinical and. experimental pathology 2013, 6(7):1245–1260.

[36] Pinto C, Cardenas P, Osses N, Henriquez JP: Characterization of Wnt/beta-catenin and BMP/Smad signaling pathways in an in vitro model of amyotrophic lateral sclerosis. Frontiers in cellular neuroscience 2013, 7:239. DOI: 10.3389/fncel.2013.00239

[37] McLoon LK, Harandi VM, Brannstrom T, Andersen PM, Liu JX: Wnt and extraocular muscle sparing in amyotrophic lateral sclerosis. Investigative ophthalmology & visual science 2014, 55(9):5482–5496. DOI: 10.1167/iovs.14-14886

[38] Carter GT, Krivickas LS, Weydt P, Weiss MD, Miller RG: Drug therapy for amyotrophic lateral sclerosis: where are we now? IDrugs: the investigational drugs journal 2003, 6(2): 147–153.

[39] Aggarwal S, Cudkowicz M: ALS drug development: reflections from the past and a way forward. Neurotherapeutics: the journal of the American society for experimental neurotherapeutics 2008, 5(4):516–527. DOI: 10.1016/j.nurt.2008.08.002

[40] Biechele TL, Camp ND, Fass DM, Kulikauskas RM, Robin NC, White BD, Taraska CM, Moore EC, Muster J, Karmacharya R et al.: Chemical-genetic screen identifies riluzole as an enhancer of Wnt/beta-catenin signaling in melanoma. Chemistry & biology 2010, 17(11):1177–1182. DOI: 10.1016/j.chembiol.2010.08.012

[41] Fornai F, Longone P, Cafaro L, Kastsiuchenka O, Ferrucci M, Manca ML, Lazzeri G, Spalloni A, Bellio N, Lenzi P et al.: Lithium delays progression of amyotrophic lateral sclerosis. Proceedings of the national academy of sciences of the United States of America 2008, 105(6):2052–2057. DOI: 10.1073/pnas.0708022105

[42] Hedgepeth CM, Conrad LJ, Zhang J, Huang HC, Lee VM, Klein PS: Activation of the Wnt signaling pathway: a molecular mechanism for lithium action. Developmental biology 1997, 185(1):82–91. DOI: 10.1006/dbio.1997.8552

[43] Sinha D, Wang Z, Ruchalski KL, Levine JS, Krishnan S, Lieberthal W, Schwartz JH, Borkan SC: Lithium activates the Wnt and phosphatidylinositol 3-kinase Akt signaling

pathways to promote cell survival in the absence of soluble survival factors. American journal of physiology renal physiology 2005, 288(4):F703–713. DOI: 10.1152/ajprenal.00189.2004

[44] Galli C, Piemontese M, Lumetti S, Manfredi E, Macaluso GM, Passeri G: GSK3b-inhibitor lithium chloride enhances activation of Wnt canonical signaling and osteoblast differentiation on hydrophilic titanium surfaces. Clinical oral implants research 2013, 24(8):921–927. DOI: 10.1111/j.1600-0501.2012.02488.x

[45] Gould TD, Manji HK: The Wnt signaling pathway in bipolar disorder. Neuroscientist 2002, 8(5):497–511.

[46] Valvezan AJ, Klein PS: GSK-3 and Wnt signaling in neurogenesis and bipolar disorder. Front Mol Neurosci 2012, 5:1. DOI: 10.3389/fnmol.2012.00001

[47] Pittenger C, Coric V, Banasr M, Bloch M, Krystal JH, Sanacora G: Riluzole in the treatment of mood and anxiety disorders. CNS drugs 2008, 22(9):761–786.

[48] Chen YC, Wu JS, Tsai HD, Huang CY, Chen JJ, Sun GY, Lin TN: Peroxisome proliferator-activated receptor gamma (PPAR-gamma) and neurodegenerative disorders. Molecular neurobiology 2012, 46(1):114–124. DOI: 10.1007/s12035-012-8259-8

[49] Kiaei M: Peroxisome proliferator-activated receptor-gamma in amyotrophic lateral sclerosis and Huntington's disease. PPAR research 2008, 2008:418765.

[50] Shibata N, Kawaguchi-Niida M, Yamamoto T, Toi S, Hirano A, Kobayashi M: Effects of the PPARgamma activator pioglitazone on p38 MAP kinase and IkappaBalpha in the spinal cord of a transgenic mouse model of amyotrophic lateral sclerosis. Neuropathology: official journal of the Japanese society of neuropathology 2008, 28(4):387–398. DOI: 10.1111/j.1440-1789.2008.00890.x

[51] Benedusi V, Martorana F, Brambilla L, Maggi A, Rossi D: The peroxisome proliferator-activated receptor gamma (PPARgamma) controls natural protective mechanisms against lipid peroxidation in amyotrophic lateral sclerosis. The journal of biological chemistry 2012, 287(43):35899–35911. DOI: 10.1074/jbc.M112.366419

[52] Joardar A, Menzl J, Podolsky TC, Manzo E, Estes PS, Ashford S, Zarnescu DC: PPAR gamma activation is neuroprotective in a Drosophila model of ALS based on TDP-43. Human molecular genetics 2015, 24(6):1741–1754. DOI: 10.1093/hmg/ddu587

[53] Schutz B, Reimann J, Dumitrescu-Ozimek L, Kappes-Horn K, Landreth GE, Schurmann B, Zimmer A, Heneka MT: The oral antidiabetic pioglitazone protects from neurodegeneration and amyotrophic lateral sclerosis-like symptoms in superoxide dismutase-G93A transgenic mice. The journal of neuroscience: the official journal of the society for neuroscience 2005, 25(34):7805–7812. DOI: 10.1523/JNEUROSCI.2038-05.2005

[54] Dupuis L, Dengler R, Heneka MT, Meyer T, Zierz S, Kassubek J, Fischer W, Steiner F, Lindauer E, Otto M et al.: A randomized, double blind, placebo-controlled trial of

pioglitazone in combination with riluzole in amyotrophic lateral sclerosis. PloS one 2012, 7(6):e37885. DOI: 10.1371/journal.pone.0037885

[55] Liang H, Ward WF, Jang YC, Bhattacharya A, Bokov AF, Li Y, Jernigan A, Richardson A, Van Remmen H: PGC-1alpha protects neurons and alters disease progression in an amyotrophic lateral sclerosis mouse model. Muscle nerve 2011, 44(6):947–956. DOI: 10.1002/mus.22217

[56] Zhao W, Varghese M, Yemul S, Pan Y, Cheng A, Marano P, Hassan S, Vempati P, Chen F, Qian X et al.: Peroxisome proliferator activator receptor gamma coactivator-1alpha (PGC-1alpha) improves motor performance and survival in a mouse model of amyotrophic lateral sclerosis. Molecular neurodegeneration 2011, 6(1):51. DOI: 10.1186/1750-1326-6-51

[57] Da Cruz S, Parone PA, Lopes VS, Lillo C, McAlonis-Downes M, Lee SK, Vetto AP, Petrosyan S, Marsala M, Murphy AN et al.: Elevated PGC-1alpha activity sustains mitochondrial biogenesis and muscle function without extending survival in a mouse model of inherited ALS. Cell metabolism 2012, 15(5):778–786. DOI: 10.1016/j.cmet.2012.03.019

[58] Mandrekar-Colucci S, Sauerbeck A, Popovich PG, McTigue DM: PPAR agonists as therapeutics for CNS trauma and neurological diseases. ASN neuro 2013, 5(5):e00129. DOI: 10.1042/AN20130030

[59] Kitamura Y, Shimohama S, Koike H, Kakimura J, Matsuoka Y, Nomura Y, Gebicke-Haerter PJ, Taniguchi T: Increased expression of cyclooxygenases and peroxisome proliferator-activated receptor-gamma in Alzheimer's disease brains. Biochemical and biophysical research communications 1999, 254(3):582–586.

[60] de la Monte SM, Wands JR: Molecular indices of oxidative stress and mitochondrial dysfunction occur early and often progress with severity of Alzheimer's disease. Journal of Alzheimer's disease 2006, 9(2):167–181.

[61] Combs CK, Johnson DE, Karlo JC, Cannady SB, Landreth GE: Inflammatory mechanisms in Alzheimer's disease: inhibition of beta-amyloid-stimulated proinflammatory responses and neurotoxicity by PPARgamma agonists. The journal of neuroscience: the official journal of the society for neuroscience 2000, 20(2):558–567.

[62] Sastre M, Dewachter I, Landreth GE, Willson TM, Klockgether T, van Leuven F, Heneka MT: Nonsteroidal anti-inflammatory drugs and peroxisome proliferator-activated receptor-gamma agonists modulate immunostimulated processing of amyloid precursor protein through regulation of beta-secretase. The journal of neuroscience: the official journal of the society for neuroscience 2003, 23(30):9796–9804.

[63] Camacho IE, Serneels L, Spittaels K, Merchiers P, Dominguez D, De Strooper B: Peroxisome-proliferator-activated receptor gamma induces a clearance mechanism for the amyloid-beta peptide. The journal of neuroscience: the official journal of the society for neuroscience 2004, 24(48):10908–10917. DOI: 10.1523/JNEUROSCI.3987-04.2004

[64] d'Abramo C, Massone S, Zingg JM, Pizzuti A, Marambaud P, Dalla Piccola B, Azzi A, Marinari UM, Pronzato MA, Ricciarelli R: Role of peroxisome proliferator-activated receptor gamma in amyloid precursor protein processing and amyloid beta-mediated cell death. Biochemistry journal 2005, 391(Pt 3):693–698. DOI: 10.1042/BJ20050560

[65] Pedersen WA, McMillan PJ, Kulstad JJ, Leverenz JB, Craft S, Haynatzki GR: Rosiglitazone attenuates learning and memory deficits in Tg2576 Alzheimer mice. Experimental neurology 2006, 199(2):265–273. DOI: 10.1016/j.expneurol.2006.01.018

[66] Risner ME, Saunders AM, Altman JF, Ormandy GC, Craft S, Foley IM, Zvartau-Hind ME, Hosford DA, Roses AD: Efficacy of rosiglitazone in a genetically defined population with mild-to-moderate Alzheimer's disease. Pharmacogenomics journal 2006, 6(4): 246–254. DOI: 10.1038/sj.tpj.6500369

[67] Escribano L, Simon AM, Gimeno E, Cuadrado-Tejedor M, Lopez de Maturana R, Garcia-Osta A, Ricobaraza A, Perez-Mediavilla A, Del Rio J, Frechilla D: Rosiglitazone rescues memory impairment in Alzheimer's transgenic mice: mechanisms involving a reduced amyloid and tau pathology. Neuropsychopharmacology: official publication of the American college of neuropsychopharmacology 2010, 35(7):1593–1604. DOI: 10.1038/npp.2010.32